CBR Institute for
Biomedical Research
SUC & WST

Bone Graft Substitutes

Edited by
Cato T. Laurencin, M. D., Ph. D.

Chair, Department of Orthopaedic Surgery
University Professor and Lillian T. Pratt Distinguished Professor
of Orthopaedic Surgery
Professor of Biomedical Engineering and Chemical Engineering
University of Virginia

ASTM Stock Number: Mono6

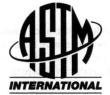

ASTM International
100 Barr Harbor Drive
PO Box C700
West Conshohocken, PA 19428-2959

Developed in conjunction with
American Academy of Orthopaedic Surgeons
6300 N. River Rd.
Rosemont, IL 60018

Printed in the U. S. A.

Library of Congress Cataloging-in-Publication Data

Bone graft substitutes / Cato T. Laurencin, editor.
    p. cm.
    Includes index.
    ISBN 0-8031-3356-1
      1. Bone substitutes.   2. Bone-grafting.   I. Laurencin, Cato T.

RD755.6.B66 2003
617.48710592—dc21

2002043799

Photocopy Rights

Publisher:

ASTM International
100 Barr Harbor Drive
PO Box C700
West Conshohocken, PA 19428-2959
Phone: (610) 832-9585   Fax: (610) 832-9555
ISBN: 0-8031-3356-1
ASTM Stock Number: Mono 6

Developed in conjunction with:
American Academy of Orthopaedic Surgeons
6300 N. River Road
Rosemont, IL 60018

Printed in Bridgeport, NJ
March 2003

Dedication

This book is dedicated to my wife Cynthia and our children, Tiberius, Michaela, and Victoria.

Contributors

C. Mauli Agrawal, Ph.D., P.E.
Professor of Orthopaedics and Engineering
Director, Center for Clinical Bioengineering
The University of Texas Health Science Center
Houston, TX

Mohamed Attawia, M.B.B. Ch.
Senior Product Development Engineer,
  Osteobiologics
DePuy AcroMed, a Johnson & Johnson Company
Raynham, MA

Mark D. Borden, Ph.D.
Senior Product Development Scientist
Interpore Cross International
Irvine, CA

Barbara D. Boyan, Ph.D.
Price Gilbert, Jr. Chair in Tissue Engineering
Wallace H. Coulter Department of Biomedical
  Engineering at Georgia Tech and Emory
  University
Institute of Bioengineering and Bioscience
Georgia Institute of Technology
Atlanta, GA

Scott P. Bruder, M.D., Ph.D.
Worldwide Vice President, Orthobiologics
DePuy Orthopaedics, DePuy AcroMed, and
  Mitek Worldwide, a Division of Ethicon Inc.,
Johnson & Johnson Companies
Raynham, MA

Robert W. Bucholz, M.D.
Professor and Chairman
Department of Orthopaedic Surgery
University of Texas Southwestern Medical School
Dallas, TX

Emilie V. Cheung, M.D.
Orthopaedic Surgical Resident
Department of Orthopedic Surgery
Drexel University School of Medicine
Philadelphia, PA

Kim Fitzgerald, B.S.
Senior Product Director
DePuy AcroMed, a Johnson & Johnson Company
Raynham, MA

Sergio J. Gadaleta, Ph.D.
Manager, Regulatory Affairs
Mitek Worldwide, a Division of Ethicon Inc.,
  a Johnson and Johnson Company
Norwood, MA

Warren O. Haggard, Ph.D.
Vice President of Research
Wright Medical Technology, Inc.
Arlington, TN

Scott Hofer, D.O.
Major, United States Army Medical Corps
Orthopaedic Surgery Service
William Beaumont Army Medical Center
El Paso, TX

Joshua J. Jacobs, M.D.
Crown Family Professor of Orthopaedic Surgery
Rush Medical College
St Luke's Medical Center
Chicago, IL

David M. Joyce, B.S.
Case Western Reserve University
Cleveland, OH

Michael J. Joyce, M.D.
Orthopaedic Surgeon: Cleveland Clinic Foundation
Past-President (1997-1999) American Association
  Tissue Banks
Associate Clinical Professor of Orthopaedic
  Surgery: Case Western Reserve University
Cleveland, OH

Sudha Kadiyala, Ph.D.
Director, Bone and Spinal Technologies
DePuy AcroMed, a Johnson & Johnson Company
Raynham, MA

Dhirendra S. Katti, Ph.D.
Assistant Professor of Orthopaedics and
  Biomedical Engineering
University of Virginia
Charlottesville, VA

Yusuf Khan, M.S.
Research Fellow
Center for Advanced Biomaterials and Tissue
  Engineering
Drexel University
Philadelphia, PA

John S. Kirkpatrick, M.D.
Associate Professor, Division of Orthopaedic
  Surgery
University of Alabama at Birmingham,
  Chief, Division of Orthopaedic Surgery,
Birmingham Veterans Administration Medical
  Center
Birmingham, AL

Karl H. Kraus, D.V.M.
Professor
Orthopedic Research Laboratory
Tufts University School of Veterinary Medicine
North Grafton, MA

Joseph M. Lane, M.D.
Professor of Orthopaedic Surgery
Assistant Dean, Medical Students
Weill Medical College of Cornell University
Chief, Metabolic Bone Diseases and Orthopaedic
  Surgery
Hospital for Special Surgery
New York, NY

Cato T. Laurencin, M.D., Ph.D.
Lillian T. Pratt Distinguished Professor and
  Chair, Department of Orthopaedic Surgery
University Professor
Professor of Biomedical Engineering and
  Chemical Engineering
University of Virginia
Charlottesville, VA

Jack Lemons, Ph.D.
Professor and Director of Laboratory Surgical
  Research
Division of Orthopaedic Surgery
University of Alabama at Birmingham
Birmingham, AL

Seth S. Leopold, M.D.
Associate Professor
Department of Orthopaedics and Sports Medicine
University of Washington Medical Center
Seattle, WA

Jay R. Lieberman, M.D.
Associate Professor
Department of Orthopaedic Surgery
David Geffen School of Medicine at UCLA
Los Angeles, CA

Treena Livingston Arinzeh, Ph.D.
Assistant Professor
Department of Biomedical Engineering
New Jersey Institute of Technology
University Heights
Newark, NJ

Christoph H. Lohmann, M.D
Department of Orthopaedics, University of Texas
  Health Science Center at San Antonio
San Antonio, TX
Department of Orthopaedics, University of
  Hamburg-Eppendorf
Hamburg, Germany

Marc Long, Ph.D.
Project Manager, Bone Graft Substitute Team,
  Research Projects
Smith & Nephew, Inc.
Memphis, TN

**Jacquelyn McMillan, M.B.B.Ch., F.R.C.S.Ed.,
  F.R.C.S. (Trauma & Orthopaedics)**
Research Fellow
Georgia Tech/Emory Center for the Engineering
  of Living Tissues
Institute of Bioengineering and Bioscience
Georgia Institute of Technology
Atlanta, GA

Jack E. Parr, Ph.D.
Chief Scientific Officer
Wright Medical Technology, Inc.
Arlington, TN

**Ashley R. Poynton M.D., F.R.C.S.I., F.R.C.S.
  (Trauma & Orthopaedics)**
Spine Fellow
Hospital for Special Surgery
Weill-Cornell University Medical College
New York, NY

Don M. Ranly, D.D.S., Ph.D.
Principal Research Scientist
Wallace H. Coulter Department of Biomedical
  Engineering at Georgia Tech and Emory
  University
Institute of Bioengineering and Bioscience
Georgia Institute of Technology
Atlanta, GA

A Hari Reddi, Ph.D.
Lawrence J. Ellison Professor of Orthopaedic
  Research
Center for Tissue Regeneration and Repair
Department of Orthopaedic Surgery
University of California at Davis
Sacramento, CA

Kelly C. Richelsoph, M.S.
Senior Project Engineer
Wright Medical Technology, Inc.
Arlington, TN

Randy N. Rosier, M.D., Ph.D.
Professor and Chairman
Department of Orthopaedic Surgery
The University of Rochester
Rochester, NY

T. Kuber Sampath, Ph.D.
Vice President
Orthopedic Research & Development
Cell and Protein Therapeutic Division
Genzyme Corporation
Framingham, MA

Zvi Schwartz, D.M.D, Ph.D.
Professor
Wallace H. Coulter Department of Biomedical
  Engineering at Georgia Tech and Emory
  University
Institute of Bioengineering and Bioscience
Georgia Institute of Technology
Atlanta, GA

Edwin C. Shors, Ph.D.
Vice President, Research and New Technology
Interpore Cross International
Irvine, CA

Robert Talac, M.D., Ph.D.
Research Fellow
Departments of Orthopedic Surgery and
  Bioengineering
Mayo Clinic
Rochester, MN

William W. Tomford, M.D.
Professor of Orthopedic Surgery
Harvard Medical School
Massachusetts General Hospital
Cambridge, MA

Peter G. Whang, M.D.
Resident Physician
Department of Orthopaedic Surgery
David Geffen School of Medicine at UCLA
Los Angeles, CA

Michael J. Yaszemski, M.D., Ph.D.
Associate Professor of Orthopedic Surgery and
  Biomedical Engineering
Director, Tissue Engineering and Polymeric
  Biomaterials Laboratory
Departments of Orthopedic Surgery and
  Biomedical Engineering
Mayo Clinic
Rochester, MN

Foreword

In 1997, the leadership of the American Society for Testing and Materials (ASTM International) Committee F04 on Medical and Surgical Materials and Devices created a broad-based standards development activity in Tissue Engineered Medical Products (TEMPs). This was a proactive initiative borne out of the realization that in the near future a large number of medical products will be introduced into the marketplace that are fundamentally different from the current generation of products fabricated from conventional engineering materials. These new products will be based on some combination of cells, growth factors, human tissue and biologic or non-biologic biodegradable scaffoldings. Unlike previous standards development activities, the TEMPs standards initiative is occurring prior to or concurrent with the commercial introduction of the vast majority of the products to be covered by the standards. This situation provides a unique opportunity for consensus standards to accelerate the product development phase and regulatory processes (by virtue of the establishment of a common nomenclature and standardized test methods) in order to bring these promising treatment modalities to the patient in an expeditious fashion.

To produce the most relevant and useful standards, it is critical that the best science and the latest scientific developments are brought to bear. Thus, ASTM Committee F04 regularly conducts workshops and scientific symposia in targeted areas where the science is rapidly evolving and the need for standards is pressing. This volume entitled "Bone Graft Substitutes," edited by Dr. Cato Laurencin represents, in large part, the proceedings of a workshop held in November 2000 in Orlando, FL during ASTM committee week activities. Dr. Laurencin organized this workshop with help from Dr. Mohamed Attawia and recruited an impressive array of speakers, most of whom are recognized as leaders in their respective scientific, clinical and regulatory fields. The symposium organization effort was a cooperative endeavor between ASTM Committee F04 and the American Academy of Orthopaedic Surgeons Biological Implants Committee, and Biomedical Engineering Committee.

Bone defects resulting from traumatic, neoplastic, degenerative, inflammatory and congenital diseases are commonly seen in the clinical arena. Autologous bone grafting remains as the "gold standard" in treating such defects. In addition, autologous bone grafting is widely used to promote bone healing in the absence of bone defects in arthrodesis (fusion) procedures and in the treatment of delayed fracture healing. Unfortunately, only limited quantities of bone autograft are available and the harvesting of the graft can be associated with substantial morbidity. Thus, there is a great need for autologous bone graft substitutes—a need that can be filled by allograft tissue, synthetic bone graft substitutes, tissue-engineered bone products or a combination of the three. In this volume, the state of the art and science of bone grafting is presented in the context of the role of standards in the development, manufacturing, processing, testing, and regulation of bone graft substitute materials.

This monograph is divided into three sections. The first section presents a summary of the clinical use of bone allografts and allograft-based bone graft substitutes. This section includes a chapter on allograft tissue banking and safety and a chapter on potential areas of standards development. The second section addresses the use of cells and growth factors as bone graft substitutes. Representatives from academia, industry, and the regulatory communities present their perspectives on the exciting opportunities and formidable challenges involved in bringing scientific advances in the field of bone tissue engineering to the patient care arena. The final section addresses the use of synthetic materials, including polymers and ceramics, for bone graft substitutes. As in the other two sections, there is a chapter addressing the regulatory and standards issues involved. All sections begin with an overview by some of the leading authorities in the field.

Overall, this is a unique monograph exploring not only the clinical and scientific aspects of bone grafting, but also the practical issues of bringing promising new bone graft substitutes to the marketplace in a fashion which insures their safety and efficacy. Dr. Laurencin, the editor of this book, is to be commended for his tireless efforts in bringing this project to fruition. He has assembled an accomplished multidisciplinary panel of authors who collectively have produced a comprehensive and authoritative summary of a complex field. This volume will serve as a foundation for future standards development activities in this area.

Joshua J. Jacobs, M.D.
Chairman, ASTM Committee F04

Jack Lemons, Ph.D.
Past Chairman, ASTM Committee F04

Contents

SECTION III: POLYMERS, CERAMICS, AND OTHER SYNTHETIC MATERIALS FOR BONE GRAFT SUBSTITUTES
Section Leaders: Mauli Agrawal, Ph.D., P.E. and Dhirendra S. Katti, Ph.D.

Preface

In November 2000 a workshop sponsored by the American Society for Testing and Materials (ASTM International) brought together individuals from academia, industry, and regulatory bodies to examine important issues surrounding the development of Bone Graft Substitutes for Clinical Use. The effort, co-sponsored by the American Academy of Orthopaedic Surgeons (AAOS) achieved unprecedented success, and with the backing of ASTM International and AAOS a monograph largely based on the proceedings of that workshop has been produced. As with the workshop, the monograph provides various perspectives on the variety of bone graft substitutes currently available, and proposed for use. There is a special emphasis on outlining the challenges in the development, evaluation and use of these materials, along with analyses of regulatory and standards development concepts.

There are a number of individuals whose efforts in producing this monograph must be acknowledged. Dr. Barbara Boyan was the first individual I called, and came at her own expense to the workshop to provide a lead lecture. Not surprisingly, she was the first to answer the call for manuscripts for the book. I am indebted to her. Dr. Joseph Lane and Dr. Kuber Sampath also gave lead lectures and provided outstanding manuscripts for the book, while Dr. Arnold Kaplan re-routed a trip around the world to participate in the workshop. Drs. Jack Lemons and Joshua Jacobs, the leadership of ASTM International, were the catalysts for the workshop, and encouraged the production of this monograph, while Dr. Mauli Agrawal provided significant support in his roles as ASTM International publications committee liaison and section leader for the book. In addition, the production staff at ASTM must be commended for their work. Led by Ms. Kathy Dernoga, their diligence and professionalism made this book a reality. On the Academy side, Dr. Randy Rosier, Chair of the Biological Implants Committee and Ms. Jeanne Kennedy must be thanked for their encouragement throughout the development of the workshop and monograph.

I must thank the inner circle of individuals who helped me on this project. This includes my good friends and colleagues Dr. Mohamed Attawia and Dr. Dhirendra Katti who were active in all phases of the work. Finally I must thank my clinical mentors, Dr. Henry Mankin, Dr. Charles Epps, and Dr. Augustus White and especially my research mentor Dr. Robert Langer who taught me science, and who has been the guiding light for my career.

To all who have helped in producing this monograph, I give thanks.

Cato T. Laurencin, M.D., Ph.D.

Bone Grafts and Bone Graft Substitutes: A Brief History

Bone Grafts and Bone Graft Substitutes: A Brief History

by Cato T. Laurencin, M.D., Ph.D. and Yusuf Khan, M.S.

INTRODUCTION

THE ORIGIN OF THE FIELD OF MEDICINE as a formal discipline has been traced to Africa by many historians. Imhotep's descriptions of ailments and treatments were found written on papyrus and translated in the mid-1800s by Edwin Smith [1]. Among the medical descriptions included in Imhotep's writings are cervical dislocations, skull fractures, and compound fractures [1]. Indeed, mummies found in Egyptian tombs have been found with crude braces constructed from wood planks and linen straps on their limbs representing some of the earliest accounts of orthopedics [2]. The use of autografts, allografts, and bone graft substitutes has interesting origins as well. The use of each graft type dates back several hundred years to apparently crude yet inspired methods and theories, which nonetheless set the stage for what we today consider state-of-the-art. Below is a brief history of each graft sub-group.

Autografts were first used as far back as the early 1800s. After a trephination, the practice of drilling holes in the skull to release pressure, Walther repaired the defect by refilling the hole with the original bone plug [3]. This repair resulted in good healing and informally began the practice of autografting. In the late 1800s, more reports of autografting emerged: Seydel used tibial periosteal flaps to close a cranial defect and Bergmann used a fibular graft to close a tibial defect [4]. By the early 1920s, more than 1600 autograft procedures had been documented [4]. Early structural limitations of cancellous autograft tissue delayed its full emergence, however, which did not occur until more modern tools of external and internal fixation were available [4]. One of the primary reasons for the success of autografts is its ability to be osteoinductive, which is due to the presence of blood, factors, and proteins within the graft that stimulate and facilitate healing. Although investigational attention to these factors has intensified during the past 30 years, the notion that the body's own fluids could provide stimulus for healing and bone growth dates back further than that. Early attempts at non-union treatments involved sawing both ends of the fracture to expose fresh bone, rubbing both ends of the bone together, and splinting the wound to allow some limited motion in hopes of stimulating inflammation, and thus healing [5]. Although early surgeons may not have realized it, this procedure may have stimulated the recruitment of growth factors as well as inflammatory elements. A similar approach to non-unions was described by Physick in 1802 when he repaired a fracture non-union by running a seton, or a small bundle of fibers, through and between both ends of the fracture, with the hopes of stimulating an exaggerated immune response, thus stimulating healing [6].

Allograft use has been reported as far back as the late 1800s when Macewen reported on the implantation of a tibial graft from one child to another [7,8]. In the early 1900s, cadaveric and fresh allografts were used as in the case of a transplant of cadaver cartilage to a patient and another of a fresh bone allograft from parent to child for the treatment of spina bifida [3,9]. The earliest collections of allograft tissue, or bone banks, were established in the beginning of the 20th century when Bauer refrigerated bone samples for three weeks and then implanted them in dogs. Allografts were prepared for storage at this point by either chilling or heating, but it was soon determined that boiling the bone samples rendered them inferior in healing to autografts as the endogenous proteins and factors were undoubtedly destroyed during heating [9]. The big leap forward in bone banking came during World War II when new methods of bone storage preparation were studied including freezing, freeze-drying, deproteinating, irradiating, autoclaving, demineralizing, and chemically treating the harvested bone. Although initially prompted by the US Navy to help combat war injuries, the expansion of bone banking continued with a new focus on civilian needs. Many of today's currently held beliefs and understandings about bone bank tissues came from the Naval projects [8]. It was about this time that the use of fresh allograft tissue declined sharply in orthopedic procedures, giving rise to the need for better allograft treatments and bone graft substitutes in general.

Some of the first evidence for the use of bone graft substitutes, crude as it may be, have been found in prehistoric skulls with gold and silver plates and even remnants of coconut shells found in place of cranial defects [3]. In more recent times, several synthetic materials have been utilized as either bone graft substitutes or internal fixation devices. Several metals, including platinum, vitallium, tantalum, stainless steel, and titanium, have been used for joint replacements or fracture fixations. Polymers, including polyethylene, silicon rubber, acrylic resins, polymethylmethacrylates, and others, have been used, as have ceramics, in place of bone grafts. In their infancy, they were more suited for replacement rather than regeneration of bone tissue.

The current generation of bone graft substitutes, however, has been designed with both replacement and regeneration in mind. Materials are either designed with living tissue structures in mind, or are combined with factors, proteins, and other tissues to encourage rapid and complete healing. Some of the more successful materials have been around for decades. Calcium sulfate, for instance, also known as Gypsum or Plaster of Paris, was used in the late 1800s by Dreesman to fill bone voids [10] and is still used today as a bone graft substitute with very good clinical results. The newest generation of bone grafts and bone graft substitutes, of which this book is the focus, continues a long tradition.

Between 1998 and 1999, the number of bone graft procedures in the United States climbed from 300,000 to 500,000 with the estimated cost of these procedures approaching $2.5 billion per year [11,12]. Also in 1998, nine of ten bone graft procedures utilized autograft or allograft tissue [11]. The autograft, tissue harvested from the patient (commonly the iliac crest but other regions as well) and implanted within the patient at another site, is the current gold standard of bone grafts because of its inherent osteoconductivity, osteogenicity, and osteoinductivity [13]. Osteoconductivity describes a graft that supports the attachment of new osteoblasts and osteoprogenitor cells onto a structure with an interconnected pore system that allows these cells and others, to migrate. Osteogenicity describes a graft that supplies and supports the growth of its native bone healing cells. Osteoinductivity describes a graft that can induce non-differentiated stem cells or osteoprogenitor cells to differentiate into osteoblasts.

Although autografts provide the best replacement tissue to a defect site, the harvesting procedure requires an additional surgery at the donor-site, which can result in its own complications, most commonly pain and risk of infection. This donor-site morbidity occurs in approximately 20% of all cases [13–15]. Supply limitations are a problem as well for the autograft, further limiting its desirability. There are several categories of bone graft substitutes encompassing varied materials, material sources, and origin (natural vs. synthetic). Accordingly, a bone graft classification system, described in Table 1, has been developed by us that describes these groups based on their material makeup.

TABLE 1—Description of classification system for bone graft substitutes. Many of the currently available bone graft substitutes fall within one or more of the following groups.

CLASS	DESCRIPTION
Allograft-based	Allograft bone used alone or in combination with other materials
Cell-based	Utilize cells to generate new tissue either alone or seeded onto a support matrix
Factor-based	Natural and recombinant growth factors used alone or in combination with other materials
Ceramic-based	Includes calcium phosphate, calcium sulfate, and bioactive glasses used alone or in combination
Polymer-based	Both degradable and non-degradable polymers used alone and in combination with other materials

Allograft-Based

Prior to the 1980s, allograft tissue was primarily used as a substitute for autografts in large defect sites, but since then allograft tissue use has expanded from approximately 5,000 to 10,000 cases in 1985 to almost 150,000 in 1996 [16]. The coordination of donor screening and tissue processing methodologies has reduced the risk of allograft tissue and thus it has become a more attractive alternative to autograft. With the increase in acceptance of allograft tissue, a number of products have emerged that are allograft-based but also used in combination with other materials.

Cell-Based

To differentiate mesenchymal stem cells in vitro to the osteogenic lineage, stem cells are cultured in the presence of certain additives. After culture in these additives, phenotypic assays and staining has confirmed the osteoblast-like cell phenotype of the stem cell [17]. The addition of TGF-β, BMP-2, -4, and -7, to culture media has also been used to guide the stem cells toward the osteogenic lineage. However, the interaction between stem cells and potential use in bone graft substitutes is still being explored.

Factor-Based

Many proteins in bone regulate cellular activity by binding to receptors on cell surfaces and therefore stimulate the intracellular environment. Generally this activity translates to a protein kinase that induces a series of events that result in the transcription of mRNA and ultimately into the formation of a protein to be used intra- or extra-cellularly. The simultaneous activity of many factors acting on a cell results in the controlled production and resorption of bone. These factors, residing in the extracellular matrix of bone, include transforming growth factor-β (TGF-β), insulin-like growth factor (I and II)(IGF), platelet-derived growth factor (PDGF), fibroblast growth factor (FGF) and the bone morphogenetic proteins (BMPs). These factors have been isolated and some have been synthesized, allowing for the examination of function of the factors both alone and in combination. The ability to isolate appropriate factors from bone, synthesize them in large quantities, and reapply them in concentrated amounts to accelerate bone healing has produced many possibilities for bone graft substitutes. Much work has been done and continues in the research setting, while some products have appeared on the market for clinical use.

Ceramic-Based

Many of the currently available bone graft substitutes contain ceramics, including calcium sulfate, bioactive glass, and calcium phosphates. The use of ceramics, especially calcium phosphates, is motivated by the fact that the primary inorganic component of bone is calcium hydroxyapatite (HA), a subset of the calcium phosphate group. Calcium phosphates are also osteoconductive, osteointegrative, and in some cases osteoinductive [18]. They often require exposure to high temperature for scaffold formation and have brittle properties. To combat the brittle nature, they are frequently combined with other materials to form a composite.

Polymer-Based

The final group of bone graft substitutes are polymer-based groups. Polymers present some options that the other groups do not. For instance, there are many polymers that are potential candidates for bone graft substitutes representing different physical, mechanical, and chemical properties. These polymers used today can be loosely divided into natural polymers and synthetic polymers, which can be divided further into degradable and non-degradable materials.

CONCLUSIONS

Bone graft substitutes are substances with varied forms and characteristics all utilized to affect the repair of musculoskeletal tissues. This book provides an in depth discussion of the various classes of substitutes with special attention to enormously important issues involving both the regulation of these materials and the development of standards for fabrication and characterization.

REFERENCES

[1]   Smith E., *The Edwin Smith Papyrus*, Bern, Stuttgart, 1966.

[2]   Wangensteen O. W. and Wangensteen S. D., *The Rise of Surgery*, Minneapolis, University of Minnesota Press, 1978.

[3]   Sanan A. and Haines S. J., "Repairing Holes in the Head: A History of Cranioplasty," *Neurosurgery*, Vol. 40, 1997, pp. 588–602.

[4]   Meeder P. J. and Eggers C., "The History of Autogenous Bone Grafting," *Injury*, Vol. 25, 1994, pp. A2–A4.

[5]   Friedenberg Z. B., "Musculoskeletal Surgery in Eighteenth Century America," *Clin Orthop Rel Res*, Vol. 374, 2000, pp. 10–16.

[6]   Cooper D. Y., "The Evolution of Orthopedic Surgeons from Bone and Joint Surgery at the University of Pennsylvania," *Clin Orthop Rel Res*, Vol. 2000, 374, pp. 17–35.

[7]   Czitrom A. A. and Gross A. E., *Allografts in Orthopedic Practice*, Williams & Wilkins, Baltimore, 1992.

[8]   Friedlaender G. E., Mankin H. J., and Sell K. W., *Osteochondral Allografts Biology, Banking, and Clinical Applications*, Little, Brown, and Co., Boston, 1983.

[9]   Urist M. R., O'Connor B. T., and Burwell R. G., *Bone Grafts, Derivatives and Substitutes*, Butterworth and Heinemann, Oxford, 1994.

[10] Tay B. K., Patel V. V., and Bradford D. S., "Calcium Sulfate- and Calcium Phosphate-based Bone Substitutes. Mimicry of the Mineral Phase of Bone," *Orthop Clin North Am*, Vol. 30, 1999, pp. 615–623.

[11] Editor, "Bone Grafts and Bone Graft Substitutes," *Orthopedic Network News*, Vol. 10, 1999, pp. 10–17.

[12] Bostrom M. P., Saleh K. J., and Einhorn T. A., "Osteoinductive Growth Factors in Preclinical Fracture and Long Bone Defects Models," *Orthop Clin North Am*, Vol. 30, 1999, pp. 647–58.

[13] Perry C. R., "Bone Repair Techniques, Bone Graft, and Bone Graft Substitutes," *Clin Orthop Rel Res*, Vol. 360, 1999, pp. 71–86.

[14] Fleming J. E., Cornell C. N., and Muschler G. F., "Bone Cells and Matrices in Orthopedic Tissue Engineering," *Orthop Clin North Am*, Vol. 31, 2000, pp. 357–374.

[15] Lane J. M. and Khan S. N., "Bone Grafts of the 20th Century: Multiple Purposes, Materials and Goals," *Orthopedics Today*, Available at: http://www.slackinc.com/bone/ortoday/200001/lane.asp (5/3/2000).

[16] Boyce T., Edwards J., and Scarborough N., "Allograft Bone: The Influence of Processing on Safety and Performance," *Orthop Clin North Am*, Vol. 30, 1999, pp. 571–581.

[17] Jaiswal N., Haynesworth S. E., Caplan A. I., and Bruder S. P., "Osteogenic Differentiation of Purified, Culture-expanded Human Mesenchymal Stem Cells In Vitro," *J Cell Biochem*, Vol. 64, 1997, pp. 295–312.

[18] Ripamonti U., "Osteoinduction in Porous Hydroxyapatite Implanted in Heterotopic Sites of Different Animal Models," *Biomaterials*, Vol. 17, 1995, pp. 31–35.

Section I: Allograft-Based Bone Graft Substitutes

OVERVIEW

Estimates of the number of surgical procedures performed annually in the United States that utilize some form of bone graft are now near 800,000. This number includes autograft procedures, which account for approximately 40–50%. The remaining number of over 400,000 indicates that there are a lot of allograft bone grafts being implanted. This section reviews the state-of-the-art in bone allografts and concentrates on allograft-based bone graft substitutes.

Bone allografts have been used since the late 19th century, but the types of grafts historically used were long bone grafts transplanted for skeletal reconstruction. The U.S. Navy Bone Bank in Bethesda, Maryland pioneered the preparation of freeze-dried cancellous bone during the 1960s. These allografts were mostly used as extenders for autograft bone by scoliosis surgeons. Cases employing these allografts numbered less than 10,000 annually. The current popularity of the use of allograft bone began in the mid 1980s due to applications in failed joint arthroplasties, instrumented spine surgery and arthroscopic sports medicine surgical techniques.

As the use of bone allografts has increased, investigation and research into how these grafts heal and are incorporated into the skeleton has also increased. Clearly the most significant advance in the science of bone grafting has been the discovery of bone morphogenetic proteins (BMP) as growth factors involved in bone formation. Originally described in 1965, these molecules first became available for use by surgeons in the form of demineralized cortical bone. This form was difficult to prepare, and the osteoinductive activity of the graft was not easily assessed. A more concentrated and useful form was produced as demineralized bone matrix, which still represents the most popular structure. Recently two BMPs have become available as pure proteins, but their cost is high and their application is somewhat restricted.

This section was written primarily to provide surgeons with knowledge of the currently available options in allograft bone grafts. Although the information provided is applicable to the use of large bone grafts such as osteochondral allografts, these chapters focus on smaller bone allografts because these types of bone grafts account for about 80% of the allografts used today. These grafts are "allograft-based" because by definition they contain human tissue, generally in the form of demineralized bone matrix that is derived from highly processed human cortical bone. The demineralized bone is attached to a non-bone, synthetic carrier, which allows the graft to be easily shaped or molded by the surgeon to fit a particular surgical application. These grafts are "substitutes" because strictly speaking they are not pure bone. These grafts contain a substrate such as glycerol, calcium sulfate or animal collagen, which, as noted, serves as the carrier of the demineralized bone. An "allograft-based bone graft substitute" should not be confused with a purely synthetic bone graft that contains only an inert substance such as calcium sulfate or hydroxyapatite.

This section contains five chapters. The first chapter reviews the differences between mineralized and demineralized bone to highlight the applicability of the latter. The authors analyze several issues concerning the use of demineralized bone such as its efficacy and safety, variations in demineralized bone products available to surgeons, and the value of adding autograft bone to this form of allograft. The second chapter provides a succinct overview of tissue banking with an in-depth discussion of safety and how processing can affect the safety of allografts. It also provides an analysis of recently reported infections in the use of soft tissue and bone allografts. The third chapter reviews the results of clinical applications of allograft-based bone grafts and notes which of these applications have been most successful and which have not met with expected results. Similar to the first chapter, this chapter provides an extensive reference list for those interested in original sources. The fourth chapter reviews products currently available commercially and their specific formulations of demineralized bone matrix. There are significant differences that should be considered in the use of these types of bone grafts.

The fifth chapter is an attempt to respond to a problem that is raised directly by the fourth chapter and indirectly by the three prior chapters. This concern is that "a method of assessing the osteoinductivity of the(se) ... product(s) needs to be established." This volume on Bone Graft Substitutes is sponsored by the American Academy of Orthopaedic Surgeons as well as by ASTM International. This latter organization is active in developing standards in the area of orthopedic devices and products, including the field of tissue-engineered products. One of the major concerns facing orthopedic surgeons who use these products is the comparative effectiveness and reliability of grafts. Unless standard methods and assays for testing these characteristics are available, surgeons will be unable to predict the end result of the use of these products. This final chapter proposes guidelines to accomplish the task of measuring the effectiveness of these grafts and setting standards for their future development.

Taken together, these five chapters attempt to diminish the confusion that is currently present in choosing when to use an allograft-based bone graft substitute and which product to use. They review the basic science involved in the advantages provided by this type of graft, the current clinical experience in its use, the safety concerns involved in its processing, the chemical differences among products, and an outline of the current regulatory and standardized testing of products available. Bone grafting is clearly a dynamic field of interest to tissue banks, medical device companies, orthopedic surgeons, basic scientists and governmental agencies. These chapters should provide answers to some of the questions raised about bone allografts by each of these groups. It should also provoke questions that will stimulate and guide them in future research.

William W. Tomford, M.D.

Section Leader

Review of the State of the Art: Allograft-Based Systems for Use as Bone Graft Substitutes

by Ashley R. Poynton,[1] M.D., F.R.C.S.I., F.R.C.S. (Tr & Orth) and Joseph M. Lane,[2] M.D.

INTRODUCTION

THE IDEAL BONE GRAFT SUBSTITUTE should contain all three prerequisites for new bone formation. These are osteoinductive factors that induce bone formation, osteoconductive matrix to provide both physical support and direction to the reparative process, and osteogenic stem cells that are capable of differentiating towards bone forming cells. No allograft system contains all three of these factors. Allograft osteogenic cells do not survive transplantation and the osteoinductive capacity of many allograft systems is variable. When one or more of these vital ingredients is absent the host environment must be relied upon to produce the missing factor. Fusion and union rates using autograft remains the gold standard in clinical practice and the results of any bone graft substitute must be compared to autograft. Autograft has major disadvantages that are well documented and include donor site morbidity, increased operative time and blood loss, and often, most importantly, limited quantity [1]. Allograft bone is a widely used alternative; however, its inherent properties are dependent on many factors that affect its efficacy. To make those who use allograft bone products aware of these factors is the purpose of this article. Two categories of allograft exist, mineralized and demineralized; each will be considered in turn.

MINERALIZED ALLOGRAFT

Mineralized allograft is available in several forms; namely, fresh, frozen, and freeze-dried. The processing, sterilization, and preservation techniques used to prepare these grafts may significantly affect their properties [2]. Thus, the osteoinductivity, osteoconductivity, immunogenicity, mechanical strength, and potential for disease transmission may differ between similar types of allografts, depending on techniques employed in their production [2]. Transmission of HIV, hepatitis B, and C remain a concern with all human-derived products; however, the risks of transmission of these viral agents are extremely low [2–5]. Donor screening and the use of processing techniques that have been validated to clear viruses means that the risk of transmission is

[1] Fellow Departments of Metabolic Bone Diseases and Orthopaedic Surgery, Weill-Cornell University Medical, College, Hospital for Special Surgery, 535 East 70th Street, New York, NY 10021.
[2] Chief, Departments of Metabolic Bone Diseases and Orthopaedic Surgery, Weill-Cornell University Medical, College, Hospital for Special Surgery, 535 East 70th Street, New York, NY 10021.

approximately 1 in 1.6 million for HIV [2,3]. There have been two reports (four patients) of HIV transmission from musculoskeletal allografts since 1980 [6,7]. In the first case donor screening was not undertaken and processing was limited [6]. In the second case 3 patients were infected by unprocessed musculoskeletal graft from a seronegative donor [7]. These cases highlight the importance of rigorous donor screening and raise concern regarding the use of unprocessed grafts. Concern regarding prion-related disease transmission by allograft bone might become an issue in the future.

Fresh allograft bone is rarely used; it is mainly osteochondral in nature and replaces joint surfaces. No processing or preservation is required. However, the speed with which the grafting transfers need to be performed leaves little time to test for disease or sterility. Obviously the donors are screened, but this screening may fail to detect carriers who have not seroconverted. Fresh allograft evokes an intense immune response [8–10], thus compromising its ability to incorporate and making it clearly inferior to autograft [10,11]. Most allografts are either frozen or freeze-dried. Frozen allografts are maintained at temperatures below −60°C to diminish degradation by enzymes, affording decreased immunogenicity [12]. Osteochondral allografts undergo a much more controlled slow freeze with use of a cryopreservative (glycerol or dimethylsulfoxide) for the cartilage. There is controversy regarding the viability of frozen cartilage. Recent studies looking at isolated in vitro chondrocyte viability following freezing at temperatures ranging from −80°C to −150°C suggest that 65–85% of cells remain viable [13,14]. Studies that have evaluated viability of cartilage slices following similar freezing have shown viability ranging from 19% to >50% [15,16]. Freezing does not seem to adversely affect the mechanical properties of allograft bone [17].

Freeze-drying (lyophilization) involves the removal of water from the frozen tissue, after which the tissues are vacuum-packed and stored at room temperature for up to 5 years [18]. Such methods decrease antigenicity even further and may reduce the limited osteoinductive properties [2,12]. These grafts become more brittle with freeze-drying and undergo biomechanical alteration with loss of compressive, bending and torsional strength [19,20]. These changes appear to be associated with damage in the bone matrix, specifically microcracks along the collagen fibers [21] a phenomenon that is exacerbated by gamma irradiation [22,23]. The material properties of freeze-dried allograft can be partially regained with rehydration prior to the grafting procedure [24,25]. In all freezing techniques, the osteoprogenitor cells are destroyed, the osteoconductive properties are largely retained in terms of their cancellous and cortical structure, and deeply bound, limited, osteoinductive material present in the graft may be only partially retained [2,12].

Sterility is an important consideration for allograft use as a number of sterilization techniques are associated with decreased biological performance [2]. In order to achieve sterility, the allograft may be aseptically processed or terminally sterilized. Aseptic sterilization is labor intensive and increases costs [2]. Terminal sterilization circumvents these problems but may alter graft viability. Gamma irradiation is a common modality of terminal sterilization; however, it may significantly weaken the graft particularly in the case of cortical bone [20]. This appears to be greatest for grafts subjected to torsional or bending loads [26,27]. The effects of gamma irradiation and freeze-drying are cumulative [2]. The mechanical properties of cancellous bone are less affected by gamma irradiation [2]. Ethylene oxide is another commonly used sterilization agent. Although it has little effect on graft mechanical properties it may have significant effects on the biological viability of the graft and has been associated with poor incorporation of mineralized allografts and sub-optimal clinical outcome [28].

Mineralized allografts have a large range of clinically proven uses, both structural and non-structural [12,29]; knowledge of factors influencing efficacy will ensure appropriate usage.

DEMINERALIZED ALLOGRAFT

Acid demineralization of allograft bone leaves behind a composite of noncollagenous proteins, bone growth factors, and collagen. The resultant product is known as demineralized bone matrix (DBM). A series of low molecular weight glycoproteins that include bone morphogenetic proteins (BMPs) are said to be the most important bone growth factors contained in DBM [29,30]; however other factors such as osteopontin, osteocalcin, and osteonectin may also be important. Nevertheless BMPs are credited with providing DBM with osteoinductive potential. However, controversy exists regarding the osteoinductive potential of some commercially available DBM products [31–34]. There have been few prospective randomized trials to determine clinical efficacy of DBM. The evidence that exists at present mainly stems from animal studies and non-randomized usually uncontrolled, clinical series. Despite this, an array of DBM products are commercially available and are in widespread clinical use. DBM is classified as processed tissue and; therefore, has not come under the same rigorous scrutiny of the Food and Drug Administration as a drug or medical device would. Consequently there are several important issues in relation to these products that must be highlighted and are as follows:

1. The effect of variation in processing and sterilization on DBM viability and efficacy.
2. The safety profile of DBM and how it may be affected by processing chemicals and various additives.
3. The effect of formulation and orientation of DBM on efficacy.
4. How efficacious/viable is a given DBM product and should manufacturers provide a measure of viability?
5. Can the efficacy of DBM be enhanced using autogenous bone marrow?
6. Specific applications for which DBM has shown efficacy.

The Effect of Variation in Processing and Sterilization on DBM Viability and Efficacy

The osteoinductive properties of DBM may be affected significantly by processing techniques [2,35] and potential users of these materials must be aware of this.

Standard demineralization occurs as follows: long bone segments are placed in 0.6 N hydrochloric acid for 24 hours at a mass per volume ratio of 1 g bone to 100 mL acid solution. The acid is removed by thoroughly washing in sterile water and the remaining material is lyophilized [36]. Modifications of the standard technique include pulverizing the bone before demineralization with 0.5 N HCl, 25 mEq/g for 3 hours followed by rinsing in sterile water, absolute alcohol and ethyl ether [37]. Manufacturers may vary the processing method including acid concentration [38–41] and duration of demineralization [39,42,43]. An array of solvents may be introduced during the process. These include ethanol, methanol, ether, chloroform, chloroform:methanol, and chloroform:ether [42,44]. Duration of post-demineralization washing also varies [40,41]. Following the demineralization process DBM must be stored either frozen or in a lyophilized form at room temperature [18,42].

It is vitally important that clinicians who use DBM understand that variations in processing may lead to significant differences in efficacy. The manufacturer may not necessarily give this information. Several forms of processing are known to affect the biological properties or bone-forming capacity of DBM; some may be deleterious while others are beneficial. Processing steps that are known to have a negative effect on osteoinduction include: preprocessing storage of >24 hours at temperatures of 25°C or higher, pulverization that yields particle sizes <75 μm, certain chelating agents such as EDTA, various acid-alcohol preparations, alternative decalcifying solutions, excessive heat during processing, multiple freeze-thaw cycles and tissue fixatives [2,35]. Methods that have a beneficial effect on osteoinduction include: decalcification with HCl (0.6 N), defatting with chloroform: ethanol, detergent rinsing, alcohol treatment, antibiotics such as oxytetracycline, erythromycin and merthiolate, and lyophilization [2,35].

Another important influence on DBM viability is the method of sterilization. Ethylene oxide is commonly used to sterilize DBM despite being shown to attenuate its osteoinductive potential [2,35,45–47]. Exposure of DBM to ethylene oxide for durations required to kill common bacterial pathogens results in marked reduction of its osteoinductivity most likely due to destruction of BMPs and other osteoinductive factors [46]. This effect of ethylene oxide has been shown to be dose-dependent [46]. Terminal sterilization using gamma radiation has the same deleterious effect on osteoinductivity [47–50]. Other methods of sterilization such as the use of ethanol may have less potential to reduce osteoinductive properties of DBM. Ethanol is effective in reducing bacterial load and does not affect the osteoinductive potential of DBM [51,52]. Grafton® DBM (Osteotech Inc., Eatontown, NJ) is processed by means of a patented technique that incorporates a permeation treatment that does not expose tissue to ethylene oxide or gamma radiation. This may protect more of the BMPs contained within the graft [12].

Despite some DBM products being terminally sterilized with ethylene oxide or irradiation their osteoconductive ability remains intact. This fact may explain the varying results with the use of DBM for different applications. In cases where osseous defects are small and the host environment receptive DBM used alone has been shown to result in bone formation [53–55]. In more challenging environments such as posterolateral spine fusion, certain formulations of DBM used alone may fail to form a solid fusion as osteoconduction combined with limited osteoinduction in this setting is not sufficient to induce bone formation [56,57].

Therefore, it is clear that both processing and sterilization techniques have significant effects on DBM viability. It is imperative that clinicians understand this and are aware how these factors influence the efficacy of a particular DBM product for a particular clinical situation.

The Safety Profile of DBM and How It May Be Affected by Processing Chemicals and Additives

A major issue with regard to the safety profile of any allogeneic product is the risk of disease transmission. In the case of DBM these risks are very small indeed. Meticulous donor screening, processing techniques, and sterilization serve to minimize the chances of transmission of viral-related disease such as HIV and hepatitis [3]. The demineralization process had been shown to reduce the infectivity risk of hepatitis A, B, and C, HIV to $<10^6$, and poliovirus to $<10^{12}$ [3]. Processing technique may have an influence on the bio-burden of DBM; therefore, the onus should be on the manufacturer to disclose any significant variations in processing that may influence this.

With the occurrence of prion-related diseases, particularly in Europe, concerns of prion transmission have arisen. Little is known about the effect of demineralization and further processing on prion viability. This may become a significant issue in the future; however, at present the risks are low due to the very low prevalence of prion-related disease in the general community.

The safety profile of DBM may potentially be influenced by chemical processing and by post-processing addition of factors or chemicals. Chemicals used and factors added vary between manufacturers. It must be noted; however, that no adverse effects have been reported in humans secondary to the use of processed DBM since its introduction in 1992. Nevertheless there is still potential for toxicity. This has been highlighted by two recent articles concerning DBM and glycerol toxicity [58,59]. Both of these studies evaluated Grafton putty-DBM, which is DBM combined with glycerol using a process that results in a product with a putty-like consistency that contains 79–85% glycerol. Glycerol has been shown to have toxic effects on muscles leading to myonecrosis [60,61]. Muscle breakdown products may result in renal failure and death [62,63]. This effect of glycerol had been used to create a reproducible animal model of renal failure [63]. Bostrum et al. [58] in a study initially intended to investigate osteoinductive efficacy of different DBM materials, found that 8 of 9 rats implanted with Grafton putty died 1–4 days post-operatively. Pathological analysis indicated that the cause of death was hemorrhagic necrosis of the kidneys, most likely caused by a toxic effect on the glomeruli and tubules. The authors suggested that the causative agent was the glycerol contained in the graft material [58]. It must be noted that the dose of Grafton and, hence, glycerol used in this study was more than 8 times the maximum dose recommended in humans. The rat model used in this investigation was athymic, which may increase susceptibility to toxicity [58].

Wang et al. [59] investigated the dose-dependent toxicity of Grafton putty in athymic rats. Three different doses of Grafton were used. All rats died in the high dose group, 50% died in the intermediate dose group, and all survived in the low dose group. The LD_{50} for Grafton was calculated as 0.00469 mL/g [59]. This is comparable to the previously known LD_{50} for glycerol (0.00442 mL/g) [64]. The results of this study suggest that high doses of Grafton in humans have the potential to cause renal failure. The authors' recommendations are that the clinical usage of Grafton putty in humans should be limited to no more than 2 mL/kg body weight, and it should be used with caution in those with low body weight and those with pre-existing renal compromise [59].

It must be pointed out that Grafton has a track record of 10 years of widespread clinical usage in more than 400,000 grafting procedures without any documented reports of adverse effects [65,66]. The doses examined by Wang et al. [59] are equivalent to a total volume, in the human, of 140 to more than 500 mL of Grafton. Such doses are unlikely to be used in the human clinical setting. These studies serve to show the potential hazards of a common additive to DBM. It is vital that the safety profile of all additives are known and clearly given by the manufacturers of each DBM product.

The Effect of Formulation and Orientation of DBM on Efficacy

Commercially available DBM exists in flowable forms (gel), pliable forms that maintain dimensional integrity (flex), and moldable forms that maintain cohesiveness (putty) [67]. The latter two formulations are fiber based, whereas the former is particle based. Grafton DBM exists in all three formulations. The fiber containing forms have shown improved handling characteristics compared with the gel [67]. The effect of DBM formulation on bone forming potential has been investigated [68,69].

The athymic heterotopic implant rat model developed by Edwards et al. [69] in which DBM is implanted intramuscularly is well accepted as a valid model to assess osteoinductive potential. Using this model Grafton gel-DBM, flex-DBM, and putty-DBM have been shown to have equivalent osteoinductive capacities [68]. However, despite having similar osteoinductive properties, it has been shown that the different formulations may act differently in vivo, particularly in the situation of posterolateral intertransverse spinal fusion. This has been shown in a series of studies using the Boden animal model [70] of posterolateral intertransverse process spinal fusion. In these studies using a rabbit model it has been shown that certain formulations of DBM, when used alone, are insufficient to promote fusion in the intertransverse process region when compared to autograft [71,72]. This was also noted in a primate model [72]. Similarly, Grafton gel-DBM did not increase fusion rate when added to a standard amount of iliac crest autograft in a rabbit model [73]. The addition of gel-DBM to a less than standard amount of autograft did result in fusion rates that were comparable to autograft alone. Gel-DBM was most effective in producing autograft fusion rates when used with autograft in a 3:1 ratio. The conclusions from these studies were that Grafton gel-DBM showed properties of a viable graft extender. When added to autologous bone, it yielded a rate of fusion equal to that of autologous bone graft alone [73]. It did not; however, meet the criteria as a graft substitute or enhancer. When added to the usual or a decreased amount of autologous bone, it failed to yield a higher fusion rate than autograft alone.

Martin et al. [69] investigated the effects of the newer formulations of Grafton DBM (flex and putty) on spine fusion. This study has shown that both the flex and putty forms act as graft substitutes and extenders. When used as a graft substitute the fusion rates were 100%, 83%, 58% and 73% for flex, putty, gel and autograft respectively. Fusion rates for enhancement of half the normal volume of autograft were 100%, 100%, 70%, and 33% for flex, putty, gel, and autograft respectively. The authors also studied the effects of guanidine devitalization. Guanidine extraction results in destruction of all osteoinductive potential, and the resultant product is purely an osteoconductive matrix.

The fusion rates in this study using devitalized flex, putty, and gel were 36%, 33%, and 0% respectively. It was concluded from these results that the increased fusion rates seen with the flex and putty forms of Grafton DBM were due to structural characteristics

[69]. The fibrous structure of these two products results in significantly greater osteoconductivity compared with the gel formulation and, hence, show an enhanced ability to serve as an osteoconductive graft substitute.

It is now evident that the formulation of DBM significantly influences fusion rate particularly in the case of animal models of spine fusion. There are no randomized clinical trials to show this in humans. However, the data from animal studies are compelling.

The next issue is graft orientation and its effect on bone formation and consequent fusion. It is obvious from the above discussion that the structural properties of DBM significantly affect osteoconductivity and overall fusion rate. Little is known about fiber orientation and its relationship to osteoconductivity. Fiber-based DBM products consist of randomly arranged collagen fibers resulting in a random matrix. It may be possible in the future to determine the effects of a more uniform arrangement of the fibers in DMB on osteoconductivity.

How Efficacious/Viable Is a Given DBM Product, and Should a Measure of Viability Be Provided by Manufacturers?

The issue of DBM viability is extremely important to the clinician and patient alike. Specific questions in relation to product, formulation and batch viability; however, are infrequently asked. The osteoinductive potential of a particular sample of DBM may not be known at the time of implantation. Several studies have assessed the osteoinductive potential of commercially available DBM and failed to show any viability using murine implantation [31–34] or rat spinal fusion models. Becker et al. [31] looked at DBM products from four different bone banks, Schwartz et al. [32] studied DBM from six different sources with a variety of processing and sterilization methods, and Garraway et al. [33] investigated several commercially available DBM products. No significant osteoinductive activity was found in any product in these studies.

Maddox et al. [74] found significant variability in DBM osteoinductive potential between individual batches from a single tissue bank. Wang et al. [34] presented a study at the North American Spine Society (15th Annual Meeting, 2000) that investigated the ability of three commercially available DBM products to induce posterolateral spine fusion in rats. The DBM products evaluated were: Dynagraft putty (Gen-Sci, Regeneration Laboratories, CA), Grafton putty (Osteotech, Inc. NJ), and Osteofil allograft bone paste (Regeneration Technologies, FL). Fusion occurred in 11/17 animals treated with Grafton putty, 14/18 treated with Osteofil paste, and 0/17 treated with Dynagraft putty. The authors concluded that although all the products claim to have osteoinductive potential, significant differences in their efficacy were shown.

As outlined previously, processing and sterilizing may have significant effects on DBM viability, and different products will therefore have different osteoinductive potential. Another influencing factor is donor-donor variability. Donor age has been shown to effect DBM viability [75–77]. Nonetheless, a recent study by the manufacturers of Grafton DBM suggest that graft osteoconductivity is unaffected for donors under 65 years of age [78].

Based on the review above, there appears to be considerable variation among various DBM products. Therefore, we must ask the question: should all manufacturers be compelled to provide a measure of viability for each batch of each DBM product? Should this be an in vitro or in vivo assay? Any measure of viability must be standardized. The implantation model of Edwards et al. is a well accepted in vivo measurement of DBM osteoinductivity [68]. To expect such a test to be performed for each batch of DBM may be excessive, but it would be reasonable to demand such an in vivo assay to be performed for each formulation by each manufacturer.

Adkisson et al. [79] have developed a reproducible, relatively rapid, bioassay that quantitatively correlates with the osteoinductive capacity of DBM. They correlated the proliferative effect of DBM in vitro on SaOs human osteosarcoma cells with the bone forming ability of the same DBM in an athymic rat implantation model. The in vitro assay correlated significantly with in vivo bone formation (r = 0.85, p<0.0005) [79]. Such an in vitro assay could potentially be used to quantify osteoinductive potential of all DBM products.

It may; however, be more accurate to assess the viability of a given DBM product by analyzing its BMP content rather than using an athymic implantation model, which may not mimic the human scenario very well. Interestingly, Li et al. [80] failed to identify BMP–2 and –4 in commercial demineralized freeze-dried bone allograft preparations.

Can the Efficacy of DBM Be Enhanced Using Autogenous Bone Marrow?

It would seem logical that the addition of osteoprogenitor cells to DBM should lead to increased efficacy. Bone marrow; however, contains osteoprogenitor cells in the order of 1 per 50,000 nucleated cells and thus the actual number of osteogenic cells per unit volume is relatively small [12]. Nevertheless, DBM in combination with autologous marrow has performed similarly to autograft bone in healing long-bone defects created in both lower and higher-order animals [81–84]. Results of this combination in human series have been reported. Tiedeman et al. [85] achieved a 61% success rate in 18 non-unions treated with DBM and autologous marrow, whereas Kakiuchi et al. [86] achieved only a 33% union rate with the use of DBM alone for non-unions. There were only 3 patients in this series.

There have been no spinal fusion studies using autologous bone marrow and DBM. There is no strong clinical evidence that bone marrow increases the clinical efficacy of DBM in humans, and prospective randomized controlled studies are required to clarify this.

Specific Clinical Applications for Which DBM Has Shown Efficacy

DBM has been used for a variety or orthopedic, craniofacial, and dental applications and the remainder of this section will deal with published evidence of efficacy for its use in humans.

DBM has been used extensively for packing cavitary defects following curettage or excision of bone cysts and tumors. Rates of complete defect repair ranging from 80–100% have been reported [54,55,85–90]. Most cases of failure were related to tumor recurrence. One of the largest series reported examined 73 patients available for long-term radiographic follow-up (mean 32 months) [86]. More than 90% of cases showed complete defect repair, 3 giant cell tumors, and 4 solitary bone cysts showed recurrence. DBM has been used to re-establish the cortical shell in large giant cell tumors initially managed with curettage and filled with polymethylmethacrylate cement. DBM was placed on the surface of the cement to fill the residual cortical defect. At 36 months' follow-up 10 of 10 patients had a reconstituted cortical shell [89].

The efficacy of DBM in the management of long-bone defects has been reported by several authors [85,86,90,91]. Kakiuchi et al. [86] treated 8 traumatic defects that required bone grafting with DBM. All fractures united; however, when DBM was used for the treatment of delayed unions by the same author, only a 33% union rate was achieved [86].

A composite of DBM and autologous bone marrow was used to treat 18 frank non-unions by Tiedeman et al. [85]; 11 (61%) achieved union. Johnson et al. [91] used a composite of DBM and human bone morphogenetic protein to treat 25 long-bone non-unions. In 10 patients additional internal fixation was used, and autologous bone graft was used in addition in 7 patients. Complete bony union was eventually achieved in 17 patients. Xiaobo et al. [90] treated 3 fractures, 7 delayed unions, and 7 non-unions of long-bones with DBM. Bony union was achieved in all patients.

Augmentation of spinal fusion is perhaps at present the most frequent application of DBM. This clinical scenario presents a significant challenge to DBM in its ability to enhance or generate a solid fusion. As outlined previously, significant differences exist between the various forms of DBM in their ability to generate spine fusion in animal models. This must be taken into account when analyzing the data from human studies as to date these studies have looked at gel-DBM only. No human studies using the fiber forms of DBM have been published. Mixed results have been reported in relation to the efficacy of DBM for spinal fusion in humans. Early reports by Urist and Dawson [92] indicated that DBM extract had similar efficacy to autograft in achieving posterolateral spine fusion. In contrast, Jorgenson et al. [56] reported significantly lower fusion rates (40% vs. 80%) with ethylene oxide sterilized DBM alone or with autograft when compared to autograft alone. This study involved the random allocation of different grafting materials to separate sides in 144 patients undergoing posterolateral spine fusion. The analytical methodology of this study has been questioned.

Lowery et al. [93] compared 54 patients treated with autograft (local and iliac crest) for posterolateral spine fusion with 36 patients treated with DBM and autograft composite. Fusion rate and quality were similar in both groups; however, the need for iliac crest graft harvest was significantly less in the DBM group.

Sassard et al. [94] retrospectively analyzed the fusion rates of 56 patients that underwent posterolateral spine fusion and received a composite of Grafton gel-DBM and local autologous bone graft obtained from the posterior elements. These patients were matched with 52 control patients that underwent similar procedures but in which iliac crest autograft was used. The fusion rates were 60% and 56% respectively. Fifteen control patients reported donor site pain. The use of DBM for anterior cervical fusion was reported by An et al. [95]. DBM and freeze-dried allograft were used in 39 patients, whereas 38 patients received autograft bone.

The pseudoathrosis rates in each group were 46% and 26% respectively. This did not reach statistical significance and there was no difference between the groups in terms of clinical outcome.

It would appear from the above studies that DBM combined with autograft gives similar posterolateral lumbar spine fusion rates. It is thus efficacious as a graft extender obviating the need for iliac crest graft when enough local autograft is available. It would seem that DBM alone is not as efficacious as autograft both in the lumbar and cervical spines. It must be pointed out that the newer formulations of DBM (flex and putty) may have graft-enhancing properties. Also in the study by Jorgenson et al. [56] ethylene oxide sterilized DBM was used either alone or in combination with autograft. The osteoinductive potential of this DBM must be questioned.

DBM has also been widely used in craniofacial, orbital, and dental reconstruction [96–99]. Reported success rates in mandibular and maxillary reconstruction are generally more than 90% where secondary interventions are taken as an indicator of failure [97,98]. High success rates have been reported with the use of DBM in closing skull defects [99]. Less encouraging results have been associated with the use of DBM implants for cosmetic facial augmentation with up to 50% resorption rates reported [100,101]. These implants were terminally sterilized with ethylene oxide.

SUMMARY

Allograft bone may be mineralized or demineralized. The properties of both may be significantly affected by different processing and sterilization techniques. The majority of mineralized allograft is osteoconductive with limited osteoinductive potential. Its antigenicity is dependent on post-harvesting processing. Demineralization of allograft bone unearths osteoinductive factors and the resultant DBM is both osteoconductive and osteoinductive. Osteoinductivity of DBM is significantly influenced by processing and sterilization and may vary from product to product and batch to batch. The osteoconductive properties of DBM are determined by its formulation.

There have been no adverse effects associated with the use of DBM; however, processing chemicals and additives may be potentially toxic if very large doses of DBM are used. Manufacturers should be required to disclose all additives and chemicals used. The risks of disease transmission by processed allograft are extremely low. Demineralization processing reduces this risk to essentially zero.

The clinical efficacy of DBM has been shown for a variety of applications in predominantly retrospective or non-controlled studies. Prospective randomized controlled trials are required to demonstrate efficacy particularly in posterolateral spinal fusion. At present information given by many manufacturers regarding DBM is far from satisfactory. We suggest that it should be mandatory that the following information be provided with each DBM product:

1. The type and quantity of each additive present in the product. This should also include residues of processing chemicals.
2. Safety profile of each additive.
3. Viral inactivation data.
4. Activity data. These data should be from human trials or higher animal trials that are site-specific. Human trials are preferable.

Data for biological activity ideally should be provided for every batch of DBM.

A standardized approach to activity assessment is needed, as are comparisons between products.

REFERENCES

[1]   Younger E. M. and Chapman M. W., "Morbidity at Bone Graft Donor Sites,"
      J Orthop Trauma, Vol. 3, 1989, pp. 192–195.
[2]   Boyce T., Edwards J., and Scarborough N., "Allograft Bone: The Influence of
      Processing on Safety and Performance," *Orthop Clin North Am*, Vol. 20, 1999,
      pp. 571–580.
[3]   Scarborough N. L., While E. M., Hughes J. V., Monrique S. T., and Poser J.
      W., "Allograft Safety, Viral Inactivation with Bone Demineralization,"
      Contemp Orthop, Vol. 31, 1995, pp. 257–261.
[4]   Buck B. E., Malinin T. I., and Brown M. D., "Bone Transplantation and Human
      Immunodeficiency Virus: An estimate of risk of acquired immunodeficiency
      syndrome (AIDS)," *Clin Orthop Rel Res,* Vol. 240, 1989, pp. 129–136.
[5]   Tomford W. W., "Transmission of Disease Through Transplantation of
      Musculoskeletal Allografts," *J Bone Joint Surg Am*, Vol. 77, 1995, pp. 1742–
      1754.
[6]   Centers for Disease Control, "Transmission of HIV Through Bone
      Transplantation: Case report and public health recommendations," *MMWR,*
      Vol. 39, 1988, pp. 597–599.
[7]   Simmonds R. J., Holmberg S. D., and Hurwitz R. L., "Transmission of Human
      Immunodeficiency Virus Type 1 From a Seronegative Organ and Tissue
      Donor," *N Engl J Med,* Vol. 326, 1992, pp. 726–732.
[8]   Stevenson S., "The Immune Response to Osteochondral Allografts in Dogs," *J
      Bone Joint Surg Am*, Vol. 69, 1987, pp. 573–582.
[9]   Stevenson S., Li X. Q., and Martin B., "The Fate of Cancellous and Cortical
      Bone after Transplantation of Fresh and Frozen Tissue-Antigen-Matched and
      Mismatched Osteochondral Allografts in Dogs," *J Bone Joint Surg,* Vol. 73,
      1991, pp. 1143–1156.
[10] Strong D. M., Friedlaender H. E., Tomford W. W., et al., "Immunologic
      Responses in Human Recipients of Osseous and Osteochondral Allografts,"
      Clin Orthop Rel Res, Vol. 326, 1996, pp. 107–114.
[11] Stevenson S. and Horowitz M., "The Response to Bone Allografts," *J Bone
      Joint Surg Am,* Vol. 74, 1992, pp. 939–950.
[12] Gazdag A. R., Lane J. M., Glaser D., and Forster R. A., "Alternatives to
      Autogenous Bone Graft: Efficacy and Indications," *J Am Acad Orthop
      Surgeons,* Vol. 3, 1995, pp. 1–8.
[13] Lubke C., Sittinger M., Burmester G. R., and Paulitschke M., "Cryo-
      preservation of Articular Cartilage: viability and functional examination after
      thawing," *Cells Tissues Organs,* Vol. 169, 2001, pp. 368–376.
[14] Rendel-Vazques M. E., Maneiro-Pampin E., Rodrigues-Cabarcos M., et al.,
      "Effect of Cryopreservation on Human Chondrocyte Viability, Proliferation and
      Collagen Expression," *Cryobiology*, Vol. 42, 2001, pp. 2–10.
[15] Kawabe N. and Yoshinaa M., "Cryopreservation of Cartilage," *Int Orthop*, Vol.
      14, 1990, pp. 231–235.

[16] Schachar N. S. and McGann L. E., "Investigations of Low Temperature Storage of Articular Cartilage for Transplantation," *Clin Orthop Rel Res,* Vol. 208, 1986, pp. 146–150.

[17] Borchers R. E., Gibson L. J., Burchardt H., et al., "Effects of Selected Thermal Variables on the Mechanical Properties of Trabecular Bone," *Biomaterials,* Vol. 16, 1995, pp. 545–551.

[18] Kagan R. J., Ed., "Standards for Tissue Banking," *Am Assoc Tissue Banks*, McLean, VA, 1998.

[19] Kang J. S. and Kim N. H., "The Biomechanical Properties of Deep Freezing and Freeze Drying Bones and Their Biomechanical Changes After In vivo Allograft," *Yonsei Med J,* Vol. 36, 1995, pp. 332–335.

[20] Hamer A. J., Strachan J. R., Black M. M., Ibbotson C. J., Stockley I., and Elson R. A., "Biomechanical Properties of Cortical Allograft Bone Using a New Method of Bone Strength Measurement: a comparison of fresh, fresh-frozen, and irradiated bone," *J Bone Joint Surg Br*, Vol. 78, 1996, pp. 363–368.

[21] Voggenreiter G., Ascheri R., Blumel G., et al., "Effects of Preservation and Sterilization on Cortical Bone Grafts: A scanning electron microscopic study," *Arch Orthop Trauma Surg,* Vol.113, 1994, pp. 294–296.

[22] Pelker R. R. and Friedlaender G. E., "Biomechanical Properties of Bone Allografts," *Clin Orthop Rel Res,* Vol. 174, 1983, pp. 54–57.

[23] Triantafyllou N., Sotiropoulous E., and Triantafyllou J. N., "The Mechanical Properties of Lyophilized and Irradiated Bone Grafts," *Acta Orthopaedica Belgica*, Vol. 41(Suppl 1), 1975, pp. 35–44.

[24] Conrad E. U., Ericksen D. P., Tencer A. F., et al., "The Effects of Freeze-drying and Rehydration on Cancellous Bone," *Clin Orthop Rel Res*, Vol. 290, 1993, pp. 279–284.

[25] Jerosch J., Granrath M., Clahsen H., et al., "Effects of Various Rehydration Periods on the Stability and Water Content of Bone Transplants Following Freeze-Drying, Gamma Sterilization and Lipid Extraction. [article in German]," *Z Orthop Ihre Grenzgeb,* Vol. 132, 1994, pp. 335–341.

[26] Currey J. D., Foreman J., Laketic I., et al., "Effects of Ionizing Radiation on the Mechanical Properties of Human Bone," *J Orthop Res,* Vol. 15, 1997, pp. 111–117.

[27] Godette G. A., Kopta J. A., and Egle D. M., "Biomechanical Effects of Gamma Irradiation on Fresh Frozen Allografts in Vivo," *Orthopedics,* Vol. 19, 1996, pp. 649–653.

[28] Buttermann G. R., Glazer P. A., and Bradford D. S., "The Use of Bone Grafts in the Spine," *Clin Orthop Rel Res*, Vol. 324, 1996, pp. 75–85.

[29] Sandhu H. S., Grewal H. S., and Parvataneni H., "Bone Grafting for Spinal Fusion," *Orthop Clin North Am,* Vol. 30, 1999, pp. 685–698.

[30] Bauer T. W. and Muschler G. F., "Bone Graft Materials. An Overview of the Basic Science," *Clin Orthop Rel Res,* Vol. 371, 2000, pp. 10–27.

[31] Becker W., Urist M. R., Tucker L. M., Becker B. E., and Ochsenbein C., "Human Demineralized Freeze-Dried Bone: Inadequate induced bone formation in athymic mice. A preliminary report," *J Periodontol*, Vol. 66, 1995, pp. 822–828.

[32] Schwartz Z., Mellonig J. T., Carnes D. L., De La Fontaine, et al., "Ability of Commercial Demineralized Freeze-Dried Bone Allograft to Induce New Bone Formation," *J Periodontol,* Vol. 67, 1996, pp. 918–926.

[33] Garraway R., Young W. G., Daley D., Harbrow D., and Bartold P. M., "An Assessment of the Osteoinductive Potential of Commercial Demineralized Freeze-Dried Bone in Murine Thigh Muscle Implantation Model," *J Periodontol,* Vol. 69, 1998, pp. 1325–1336.

[34] Wang J. C., Davies M., Kanim L. E. A., Ukatu C. J., Dawson E. G., and Lieberman J. R., "Prospective Comparison of Commercially Available Demineralized Bone Matrix for Spinal Fusion," Abstract- *Proceedings of the North American Spine Society; 15th Annual Meeting,* New Orleans, LA, 2000, pp. 35–36.

[35] Russell J. L. and Block J. E., "Clinical Utility of Demineralized Bone Matrix for Osseous Defects, Arthrodesis, and Reconstruction: Impact of processing techniques and study methodology," *Orthopedics,* Vol. 22, 1999, pp. 524–531.

[36] Urist M. R., Silverman B. F., Burning K., Dubuc F. L., and Rosenberg J. M., "The Bone Induction Principle," *Clin Orthop Rel Res,* Vol. 53, 1967, pp. 243–283.

[37] Reddi A. H. and Huggins C., "Biochemical Sequences in the Transformation of Normal Fibroblasts in Adolescent Rats," *Proc Natl Acad Sci, USA,* Vol. 69,1972, pp. 1601–1605.

[38] Urist M. R., "Bone: Formation by Autoinductive," *Science,* Vol. 150, 1965, pp. 893–899.

[39] Mellonig J. T., "Decalcified Freeze-dried Bone Allograft as an Implant Material in Human Periodontal Defects," *Int J Periodontics Restorat Dentist,* Vol. 4, 1984, pp. 40–55.

[40] Damien C. J. and Parsons J. R., "Bone Graft and Bone Graft Substitutes: a review of current technology and applications," *J Appl Biomater,* Vol. 2, 1991, pp. 187–208.

[41] Guo M. Z., Xia Z. S., and Lin L. B., "The Mechanical and Biological Properties of Demineralized Bone and Cortical Bone Allografts in Animals," *J Bone Joint Surg Br,* Vol. 73, 1991, pp. 791–794.

[42] Harakas N. K., "Demineralized Bone Matrix-induced Osteogenesis," *Clin Orthop Rel Res,* Vol. 18, 1984, pp. 239–251.

[43] Hosny M. and Sharawy M., "Osteoinduction in Rhesus Monkeys Using Demineralized Bone Powder Allografts," *J Oral Maxillofacial Surg,* Vol. 43, 1985, pp. 837–844.

[44] Urist M. R. and Iwata H., "Preservation and Biodegradation of the Morphogenetic Property of Bone Matrix," *J Theor Bio,* Vol. 38, 1973, pp. 155–167.

[45] Aspenberg P., Johnsson E., and Thomgren K., "Dose-dependent Reduction of Bone Induction Properties by Ethylene Oxide," *J Bone Joint Surg Br,* Vol. 72, 1990, pp. 1036–1037.

[46] Doherty M. J., Mollan R. A. B., and Wilson D. J., "Effect of Ethylene Oxide Sterilization on Human Demineralized Bone," *Biomaterials,* Vol. 14, 1993, pp. 994–998.

[47] Munting E., Wilmart J. F., Wijne A., Hennebert P., and Delloye C., "Effect of Sterilization on Osteoinduction: comparison of five methods in demineralized rat bone," *Acta Orthopaedica Scandanaviaca*, Vol. 59, 1988, pp. 34–38.

[48] Buring K. and Urist M. R., "Effects of Ionizing Radiation on the Bone Induction Principle in the Matrix of Bone Implants," *Clin Orthop Rel Res*, Vol. 55, 1967, pp. 225–234.

[49] Urist M. R. and Hemandez A., "Excitation Transfer in Bone: deleterious effects of cobalt 60 radiation-sterilization of bank bone," *Arch Surg*, Vol. 109, 1974, pp. 486–493.

[50] Ijiri S., Yamamuro T., Nakamura T., et al., "Effect of Sterilization on Bone Morphogenetic Protein," *J Orthop Res*, Vol. 12, 1994, pp. 628–636.

[51] Dahners L. E. and Hoyle M., "Chemical Sterilization of Bacterially Contaminated Bone without Destruction of Osteogenic Potential," *J Orthop Trauma*, Vol. 3, 1989, pp. 241–244.

[52] Hallfeldt K. K. J., Stutzle H., Puhlmann M., Kessler S., and Schweiberer L., "Sterilization of Partially Demineralized Bone Matrix: the effects of different sterilization techniques on osteogenetic properties," *J Surg Res*, Vol. 59, 1995, pp. 614–620.

[53] Moss S. D., Joganic E., Manwaring K. H., and Beals S. P., "Transplanted Demineralized Bone Graft in Cranial Reconstructive Surgery," *Ped Neurosurg*, Vol. 23, 1995, pp. 199–205.

[54] Upton J. and Glowacki J., "Hand Reconstruction with Allograft Demineralized Bone: 26 implants in 12 patients," *J Hand Surg Am*, Vol. 17, 1992, pp.704–713.

[55] Whiteman D., Gropper F. T., Wirtz P., and Monk P., "Demineralized Bone Powder: Clinical applications for bone defects of the hand," *J Hand Surg Br*, Vol. 18, 1993, pp. 487–490.

[56] Jorgenson S. S., Lowe T. G., France J., and Sabin J., "A Prospective Analysis of Autograft Versus Allograft in Posterolateral Lumbar Fusion in the Same Patient: a minimum of 1-year follow-up in 144 patients," *Spine*, Vol. 19, 1994, pp. 2048–2053.

[57] Cook S. D., Dalton J. E., Prewett A. B., and Whitecloud T. S., III, "In Vivo Evaluation of Demineralized Bone Matrix as a Bone Graft Substitute for Posterior Spinal Fusion," *Spine*, Vol. 20, 1995, pp. 877–886.

[58] Bostrum M. P. G., Yang X., Kennan M., Sandhu H., Dicarlo E., and Lane J. M., "An Unexpected Outcome During Testing of Commercially Available Demineralized Bone Graft Materials. How safe are the nonallograft components?" *Spine*, Vol. 26, 2001, pp. 1425–1428.

[59] Wang J. C., Kanim L. E. A., Hagakawa S., Yamane B. H., Vinters H. V., and Dawson E. G., "Dose-Dependent Toxicity of a Commercially Available Demineralized Bone Matrix Material," *Spine*, Vol. 26, 2001, pp. 1429–1436.

[60] Deichmann W., "Glycerol: Behavior in the animal organism," *Lancet*, Vol. 1, 1940, pp. 60–67.

[61] Kumana C., Chan G., Yu Y., et al., "Investigation of Intravascular Haemolysis During Treatment of Acute Stroke with Intravenous Glycerol," *Br J Clin Pharmacol*, Vol. 29, 1990, pp. 347–353.

[62] Backenroth R., "Glycerol-induced Acute Renal Failure Attenuates Subsequent HgCl$_2$-associated Nephrotoxicity: correlation of renal function and morphology," *Renal Failure*, Vol. 20, 1998, pp. 15–26.

[63] Zurovsky Y., "Models of Glycerol-induced Acute Renal Failure in Rats," *J Basic Clin Physiol Pharmacol*, Vol. 4, 1993, pp. 213–228.

[64] Uche E. M., Arowolo R. O., and Akinyemi J. O., "Toxic Effects of Glycerol in Swiss Albino Rats," *Res Commun Chem Pathol Pharmacol*, Vol. 56, 1987, pp. 125–128.

[65] Dickman C. A., "Osteoinductive Demineralized Bone: What's the risk?" Editorial, *Spine*, Vol. 26, 2001, pp. 1409–1410.

[66] Russell J. L., "Point of View," *Spine*, Vol. 26, 2001, pp. 1435–1436.

[67] Sandhu H. S., Khan S. N., Suh D. Y., and Boden S. D., "Demineralized Bone Matrix, Bone Morphogenetic Proteins, and Animal Models of Spine Fusion: an overview," *Eur Spine J*, Vol. 10, 2001, pp. S122–S131.

[68] Edwards J. T., Diegmann M. H., and Scarborough N. L., "Osteoinduction of Human Demineralized Bone: characterization in a rat model," *Clin Orthop Rel Res*, Vol. 357, 1998, pp. 219–228.

[69] Martin G. J., Boden S. D., Titus L., and Scarborough N. L., "New Formulations of Demineralized Bone Matrix as a More Effective Graft Alternative in Experimental Posterolateral Lumbar Spine Arthrodesis," *Spine*, Vol. 24, 1999, pp. 637–645.

[70] Boden S. D., Schimandle J. H., and Hutton W. C., "An Experimental Lumbar Intertransverse Process Spinal Fusion: radiographic, histologic, and biomechanical healing characteristics," *Spine*, Vol. 20, 1995, pp. 412–420.

[71] Boden S. D., Schimandle J. H., and Hutton W. C., "Lumbar Intertransverse Process Spine Arthrodesis Using a Bovine-derived Osteoinductive Bone Protein," *J Bone Joint Surg Am*, Vol. 77, 1995, pp. 1404–1417.

[72] Boden S. D., Schimandle J. H., and Hutton W. C., "1995 Volvo Award in Basic Sciences. The Use of an Osteoinductive Growth Factor for Lumbar Spinal Fusion. II. Study of Dose, Carrier, and Species," *Spine*, Vol. 20, 1995, pp. 2633–2644.

[73] Morone M. N. and Boden S. D., "Experimental Posterolateral Lumbar Spinal Fusion with a Demineralized Bone Matrix Gel," *Spine*, Vol. 23, 1998, pp. 159–167.

[74] Maddox E., Zhan M., Mundy G. P., Drohan W. N., and Burgess W. H., "Optimizing Human Demineralized Bone Matrix for Clinical Application," *Tissue Engineering*, Vol. 6, 2000, pp. 441–448.

[75] Jergesen H. E., Chua J., Kao R. T., et al, "Age Effects on Bone Induction by Demineralized Bone Powder," *Clin Orthop Rel Res*, Vol. 268, 1991, pp. 253–259.

[76] Nyssen-Behets C., Delaere O., Duchesne P. Y., et al., "Aging Effect on Inductive Capacity of Human Demineralized Bone Matrix," *Arch Orthop Trauma Surg*, Vol. 115, 1996, p. 303.

[77] Schwartz Z., Somers A., Mellonig J. T., Carnes D. L., et al., "Ability of Commercial Demineralized Freeze-dried Allograft to Induce New Bone

Formation is Dependent on Donor Age But Not Gender," *J Periodontol*, Vol. 69, 1998, pp. 470–478.

[78] Russel J. L., "Grafton Demineralized Bone Matrix: Performance Consistency, Utility and Value, *Tissue Engineering*, Vol. 6, 2000, pp. 435–440.

[79] Adkisson H. D., Strauss-Schoenberger J., Gillis M., Wilkins R., Jackson M., and Hruska K. A., "Rapid Quantitative Bioassay of Osteoinduction," *J Orthop Res*, Vol. 18, 2000, pp. 503–511.

[80] Li H., Pujic Z., Xiao Y., and Bartold P. M., "Identification of Bone Morphogenetic Proteins –2 and –4 in Commercial Demineralized Freeze-Dried Bone Allograft Preparations: pilot study," *Clin Implant Dental Related Res*, Vol. 2, 2000, pp. 110–117.

[81] Einhorn T. A., Lane J. M., Burstein A. H., Kopman C. R., and Vigorita V. J., "The Healing of Segmental Defects Induced by Demineralized Bone Matrix: a radiographic and biomechanical study," *J Bone Joint Surg Am*, Vol. 66, 1984, pp. 274–279.

[82] Tiedeman J. J., Strates B. S., Lippiello L., and Connolly J. F., "Enhanced Skeletal Healing by Percutaneous Injection of Bone Matrix and Bone Marrow," *Surgical Forum*, Vol. 39, 1988, pp. 523–526.

[83] Gebhart M. and Lane J. M., "A Radiographical and Biomechanical Study of Demineralized Bone Matrix Implanted into a Bone Defect of Rat Femurs with and Without Bone Marrow," *Acta Orthopedica Belgica*, Vol. 57, 1991, pp. 130–143.

[84] Tiedeman J. J., Connolly J. F., Strates B. S., and Lippielo L., "Treatment of Nonunion by Percutaneous Injection of Bone Marrow and Demineralized Bone Matrix: an experimental study in dogs," *Clin Orthop Rel Res*, Vol. 268, 1991, pp. 294–302.

[85] Tiedeman J. J., Garvin K. L., Kile T. A., and Connolly J. F., "The Role of a Composite, Demineralized Bone Matrix and Bone Marrow in the Treatment of Osseous Defects," *Orthopedics*, Vol. 4, 1995, pp. 1153–1158.

[86] Kakiuchi M., Hosoya T., Takaoka K., Amitani K., and Ono K., "Human Bone Matrix Gelatin as a Clinical Alloimplant: a retrospective review of 160 cases," *Int Orthop*, Vol. 9, 1985, pp. 181–188.

[87] Kado K. E., Gambelta L. A., and Perlman M. D., "Uses of Grafton for Reconstructive Foot and Ankle Surgery," *J Foot Ankle Surg*, Vol. 35, 1996, pp. 59–66.

[88] Iwata H., Hanamura H., Kaneko M., et al., "Chemosterilized Autolyzed Antigen-Extracted Allogeneic (AAA) Bone Matrix Gelatin for Repair of Defects from Excision of Benign Bone Tumors: a preliminary report," *Clin Orthop Rel Res*, Vol. 154, 1981, pp. 150–155.

[89] Pals S. D. and Wilkins R. M., "Giant Cell Tumor of Bone Treated by Curettage, Cementation, and Bone Grafting," *Orthopedics*, Vol. 15, 1992, pp. 703–708.

[90] Xiaobo H., Luniong Y., Chuanzin L., Schucheng W., and Yankun C., "Experimental and Clinical Investigations of Human Insoluble Bone Matrix Gelatin: a report of 24 cases," *Clin Orthop Rel Res*, Vol. 293, 1993, pp. 360–365.

[91] Johnson E. E., Urist M. R., and Finerman G. A. M., "Resistant Nonunions and Partial or Complete Segmental Defects of Long Bones: treatment with implants of a composite of human bone morphogenetic protein (BMP) and autolyzed, antigen-extracted, allogeneic (AAA) bone," *Clin Orthop Rel Res,* Vol. 277, 1992, pp. 229–237.

[92] Urist M. R. and Dawson E., "Intertransverse Process Fusion with the Aid of Chemosterilized Autolyzed Antigen-extracted Allogeneic (AAA) Bone," *Clin Orthop Rel Res,* Vol. 154, 1981, pp. 97–113.

[93] Lowery G. L., Maxwell K. M., Karasick D., Block J. E., and Russo R., "Comparison of Autograft and Composite Grafts of Demineralized Bone Matrix and Autologous Bone in Posterolateral Fusions: an interim report," *Innovat Technol Bio Med,* Vol. 16, 1995, pp. 1–8.

[94] Sassard W. R., Eidman D. K., Gray P. M., et al., "Augmenting Local Bone with Grafton Demineralized Bone Matrix for Posterolateral Lumbar Spine Fusion: Avoiding second site autologous bone harvest," *Orthopedics,* Vol. 23, 2000, pp. 1059–1065.

[95] An H. S., Simpson J. M., Glover M., and Stephany J., "Comparison Between Allograft Plus Demineralized Bone Matrix Versus Autograft in Anterior Cervical Fusion: a Prospective Multicenter Study," *Spine,* Vol. 20, 1995, pp. 2211–2216.

[96] Neigel J. M. and Ruzicka P. O., "Use of Demineralized Bone Implants in Orbital and Craniofacial Reconstruction and a Review of the Literature," *Ophth Plast Reconstr Surg,* Vol. 12, 1996, pp. 108–120.

[97] Mulliken J. B., Glowacki J., Kaban, L. B., Folkman J., and Murray J. E., "Use of Demineralized Allogeneic Bone Implants for the Correction of Maxillocraniofacial Deformities," *Ann Surg,* Vol. 194, 1981, pp. 366–372.

[98] Kaban L. B., Mulliken J. B., and Giowacki J., "Treatment of Jaw Defects with Demineralized Bone Implants," *J Oral Maxillofacial Surg,* Vol. 40, 1982, pp. 623–626.

[99] Moss S. D., Joganic E., Manwaring K. H., and Beals S. P., "Transplanted Demineralized Bone Graft in Cranial Reconstructive Surgery," *Ped Neurosurg,* Vol. 23, 1995, pp. 199–205.

[100] Ousterhout D. K., "Clinical Experience in Cranial and Facial Reconstruction with Demineralized Bone," *Ann Plastic Surg,* Vol. 15, 1985, pp. 367–373.

[101] Toriumi D. M., Larrabee W. F., Walike J. W., Millay D. J., and Eisele D. W., "Demineralized Bone Implant Resorption with Long-term Follow-up," *Arch Otolaryngol Head Neck Surg,* Vol. 116, 1990, pp. 676–680.

Musculoskeletal Allograft Tissue Banking and Safety

by Michael J. Joyce,[1] M.D. and David M. Joyce,[2] B.S.

INTRODUCTION

ALLOGRAFT MUSCULOSKELETAL TISSUES have been used successfully by orthopedic surgeons in the treatment of their patients over the decades. Allografts fill defects, provide structural support, including replacement of the large skeletal segments, and stimulate bone healing in the case of demineralized bone that has osteoinductive properties. The surgeon must evaluate the patient's orthopedic problem and determine the type of implant that will be most suitable. Will it be used for reconstruction or primarily to stimulate bone healing?

The array of allografts available include iliac crest wedges or fibulae, large long bone segments, osteoarticular grafts with cryopreserved cartilage, small segmental grafts including dowels, tendons with or without bone blocks, and demineralized bone matrix products that promote bone healing. This is contrasted with standard or custom metallic implants used to reconstruct large defects. Over the past decade, bone substitutes fashioned as scaffolds have been introduced to facilitate bone healing and to provide structural reconstitution. None of these bone substitute products have osteoinductive properties. To impact the osteoinductive aspect of bone healing, a number of manufacturers are creating device products that are seeded with bone morphogenic proteins. Manufacturers of these bone substitute osteoconductive products claim these products have an advantage over human tissue allografts by eliminating the theoretical risk of disease transmission associated with human tissue.

Despite these claims, the use of musculoskeletal allograft tissue has increased markedly over the last decade (Fig. 1). Although there has been a proliferation in the number and variety of bone substitute products, sales of allograft bone, demineralized bone matrix products and bone dowels have increased significantly to a level of more than 455 million dollars in annual gross revenue (Fig. 2).

[1]Cleveland Clinic Foundation, Orthopedic Surgeon; Past-President (1997–1999) American Association Tissue Banks; Associate Clinical Professor Orthopaedic Surgery: Case Western Reserve University, Cleveland, Ohio 44195.
[2]Case Western Reserve University, 10900 Euclid Ave., Cleveland, Ohio 44106.

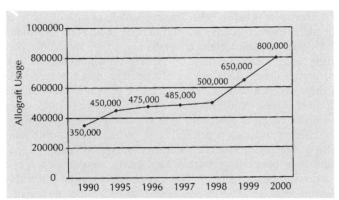

FIG. 1—Musculoskeletal allograft usage. Source: U.S. Census Bureau, Statistical Abstracts of US 2001.

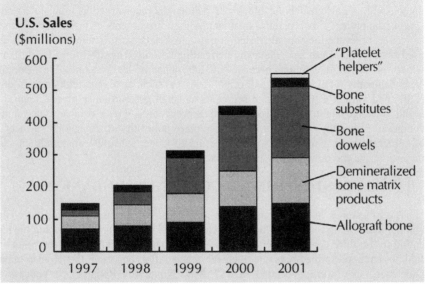

FIG. 2— U.S. sales of bone graft and bone substitutes. Source: Orthopedic Network News, industry estimates.

The orthopedic surgeon needs to become knowledgeable about both metallic implants and human tissue allografts. The latter requires at least a cursory understanding of standard tissue banking processes. The surgeon also has the responsibility to inform patients about the risks and benefits of various options and be able to discuss the biological and physiological aspects that relate to the specific uses of both allograft and bone substitute products.

Other issues related to the nature of healing or reconstructions that may represent varying degrees of difficulty for eventual success require the surgeon's consideration. A metaphyseal defect following elevation of a tibial plateau may easily permit the use of a bone substitute product, whereas other fracture healing or fusion problems may mandate the need for additive osteoinductive features to bring about bone formation.

Commonly used musculoskeletal allografts range from osteoinductive demineralized bone powders used with a variety of carriers to whole bone allografts used for reconstructive procedures. Bone can be processed as either bone powder, cortical, or cancellous chips, wedges, dowels, crests, struts, or pegs and can even be machined into screws and other shapes. Allografts can be provided as supporting segments or shafts. Large bone grafts range in size from a long bone with key soft tissue ligaments or insertions remaining intact to a hemipelvis or an acetabulum with surrounding bone support. Using dimethylsulfoxide (DMSO) as a type of cartilage cryopreservative, osteochondral long bone allografts can be used to reconstruct large joint segments especially following tumor removal. These large grafts can be combined with metallic joint implants to create an allograft-prosthetic composite for reconstructing a limb. Ribs, mandible, calvarial segments and ear ossicles are used in other reconstructive procedures.

The allograft split patellar ligament with a bone-tendon-bone construct and Achilles tendon with a calcaneal bone block are popular in reconstructing cruciate ligaments, sparing the patient's own patellar ligament. Allograft segments of fascia and rotator cuff as well as other tendons are also used in musculoskeletal soft tissue repair. Fascia lata is used as coverage. Both fascia lata and pericardium are used as substitutes for dura mater, which is in short supply, because of the concern for transmissible spongiform encephalopathy (TSE) associated prion diseases such as Creutzfeldt-Jackob disease (CJD) and variant CJD. Cartilage segments as small osteoarticular pieces, menisci and costal cartilage are used for reconstructive procedures. Fresh osteoarticular implants composed of healthy cartilage are used to replace unhealthy articular joint surfaces. Use of allograft bone would be vastly superior to bone substitute materials in certain reconstructive and bone healing procedures.

MILESTONES IN ALLOGRAFT TISSUE BANKING

The milestones in tissue banking are numerous. No discussion would be complete without mentioning the first reported musculoskeletal transplant [1] describing the legend dating to the third century when Cosmos and Damian, two Celician patron Saints were said to have performed unusual medical feats. After angering the Roman emperor Diocletian, they were beheaded in 287 A.D. Numerous Renaissance painters have depicted a purported fifth century posthumous miracle, which shows the two deceased Saints replacing a diseased limb of a church member with the lower extremity of a Moor who died earlier in the day (Fig. 3). The first human allograft transplant under aseptic conditions was reported in 1881 when two-thirds of a humeral shaft was restored [2]. Early reports of musculoskeletal tissue banking occurred in 1899 [3,4], focusing mainly on refrigeration of tissues. Alex Carrel [5] is credited with early studies of tissue banking performed in North America. Carrel proposed that cadaveric rather than amputated bone tissues could provide an almost limitless source of transplantable musculoskeletal tissue.

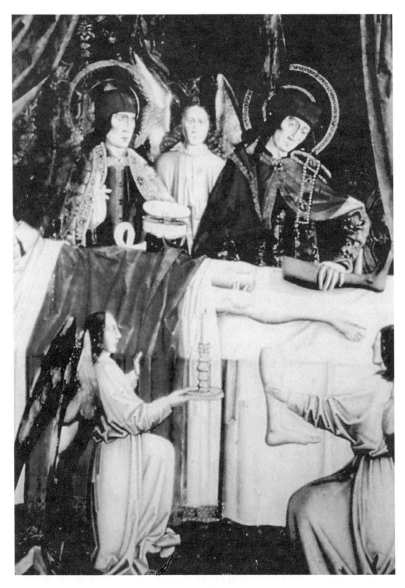

FIG. 3—Saints Cosmos and Damian in a 15th Century painting by an unknown artist. The twin brothers were famous for their medical skills in the third century. Posthumous miracles after their martyrdom in the early fourth century were attributed to them. Depicted is the act of limb transportation to a church member from a Moor. (Courtesy of Dr. Henry Mankin.)

F. H. Albee at New York Orthopedic Hospital [6] suggested that tissues should be refrigerated rather than frozen because of the potential for cellular damage. He raised concerns about the potential for disease transmission associated with the use of human tissue grafts. Eichlen in Havana, Cuba [7] is credited with establishing of the first formal bone bank, based on the concept developed earlier by Carrel and Albee. Bush at the New York Orthopedic Hospital in the 1940s [8,9] outlined special precautions necessary to minimize disease transmission. Deep freezing rather than refrigeration subsequently became the method for storage of a large number of grafts. In 1925, Lexer [10] reported a large series of allograft bone transplants with a 50% success rate.

In the late 1940s, George Hyatt [11–14], an orthopedic surgeon serving in the United States Navy, established the United States Navy Tissue Bank in Bethesda, Maryland. He organized a formal system for donor identification, recovery, processing, storage, and distribution of tissue grafts to various Navy and other medical facilities throughout the United States. Methods were developed to freeze dry bone and eventually most Navy Musculoskeletal Tissue Bank tissue was processed in this fashion. Hyatt established a system that required requesting permission from the next of kin and the review of donor history based upon the potential for disease transmission, in particular tuberculosis, syphilis, and hepatitis. In the 1960s and 1970s a number of early reports concerning the successful use of allograft tissues were generated. Ottolenghi [15] reported the use of long bone osteoarticular allograft segments. Work accomplished at a number of centers, in particular Case Western Reserve University by Herndon and Chase [16] and Curtiss et al. [17] supported earlier work of Bonfiglio et al. [18] that reported freezing seemed to reduce the antigenicity of these allografts.

Parrish at M.D. Anderson Hospital in Houston, Texas [19,20] reported favorable results using large long bone allografts and articular replacements in the late 1960s and 1970s. Following these reports, Mankin established the Musculoskeletal Tissue Bank at the Massachusetts General Hospital in 1971 and in 1983 he reported the review of his first 200 large bone allografts, the largest series reported to date at the time [21].

Mankin expressed concern regarding the effects of freeze-drying on the strength of long bones. Allografts used in large reconstructive long bone procedures subsequently have usually been accomplished using deeply frozen long bones. Methods to preserve chondrocytes in articular cartilage were initiated using glycerol but subsequently the use of 10% DMSO as a preservative has evolved. Some programs retrieve fresh, non-frozen osteocartilagenous segments, keeping the cartilage viable in media until early transplantation.

One of the most important stimuli to the growth of musculoskeletal tissue banking in the United States was the development of the American Association of Tissue Banks (AATB) in the late 1970s. Informal association meetings and exchange of information evolved into the formal establishment of the AATB in 1976. The organization published the first Standards for Tissue Banking in 1984. A voluntary inspection and accreditation program was initiated in 1986 and a program of training and certification for tissue bank specialists began in 1989. The AATB Standards are reviewed yearly with current published Standards 2002 in effect [22].

Because of concerns by the federal government regarding the importation of poorly screened cadaveric tissue, the FDA promulgated the Interim Rule on Human Tissue Intended for Transplantation on December 14, 1993, which became effective immediately. With publication of this regulation, FDA implemented the auditing of tissue banks. The Interim Rule was modified and became the Final Rule on Human Tissue Intended for Transplantation effective on January 26, 1998. During the past eight years, FDA has required a number of banks to modify their procedures and to initiate the recall of tissue. In 1994 the voluntary AATB Inspection and Accreditation Program began using trained former FDA compliance officers. Currently there are approximately 75 accredited tissue banks that comply with the requirements of the voluntary accreditation program of the AATB (listing on website www.aatb.org).

GOVERNMENTAL REGULATIONS

In 1969 the Uniform Anatomical Gift Act was passed to facilitate the act of donation and to provide protection to those who perform retrieval from the allegation of violation of the statutes of assault and battery/physical abuse of a corpse. Over time each state adopted similar statutes.

In 1984 the National Organ Transplant Act was passed by Congress establishing the organ procurement system as we know it today and establishing Medicare reimbursement for renal transplantation.

With the recognition of the human immunodeficiency virus (HIV) as a threat to human health in the early 1980s, the FDA promptly worked with pharmaceutical manufacturers to develop and license the HIV antibody test for potential donors of blood products. FDA licensure was accomplished in March of 1985.

Within weeks, the tissue banking community had adopted HIV antibody testing. As risk factors for HIV became recognized, scrutiny of donor screening was further intensified not only for HIV risks but also for hepatitis risks. The United States Public Health Service (USPHS) issued a number of guidance documents for screening for risk factors in donors of blood and blood products. As with HIV testing, these too were rapidly adopted by tissue banks for use in screening potential tissue donors.

Hepatitis C (HCV) was identified in the 1980s as the agent for transmission of what was formerly known as non-A, non-B hepatitis. HCV antibody testing, first generation, was licensed by the FDA for blood products in 1990. Sensitivity and specificity of this first generation test was recognized as being problematic and a second generation HCV antibody test was licensed in 1992 for blood products. These tests were incorporated immediately in tissue banking.

Emphasis on more rigid donor screening was heightened in the early 1990s when the FDA reported that inadequately screened tissue from foreign countries was being imported into the United States and released for human use. Because of concerns regarding this inadequate donor screening and testing, FDA published the Interim Rule on Human Tissue Intended for Transplantation in December 14, 1993. The rule was effective immediately and FDA inspection of tissue banks was initiated. FDA published the Final Rule on Human Tissue Intended for Transplantation in 1997, which then became effective months later on January 26, 1998. This regulation was accompanied by a number of guidance parameters.

The Joint Commission for Accreditation of HealthCare Organization (JCAHO) recognized that many hospitals operated surgical tissue banks (banking and storage of femoral heads from patients following total hip replacement surgery) and that blood banks were one of the chief distribution centers of tissue in hospitals. In 1995 JCAHO began providing oversight of these hospital-based banks. The level of oversight and inspection varies according to the amount of time JCAHO inspectors allot to hospital-based tissue banking operations.

To help determine whether human tissues should be regulated as devices, biologicals or a separate category of "human tissues," the FDA promulgated the "Proposed Approach to Regulation of Cellular and Tissue-Based Products" on February 28, 1997.

In 1998, the Center for Medicare and Medicaid Services (CMS—formally HCFA) provided requirements for hospital participation in organ and tissue donation (Conditions of Participation). This law requires all hospitals to report deaths to the local organ procurement organization (OPO). Medicare reimbursement to the hospital is predicated on hospital compliance with this rule.

In 1999, the FDA promulgated the "Proposed Rule for Donor Suitability Determination for Tissue Donation" and in 2001 the "Proposed Rule for Good Tissue Practices." Comments were solicited on both proposed regulations. The emphasis on good tissue practices (GTPs) is on quality assurance and quality control with validation of tissue processing practices.

In 2001, the FDA published the "Human Cells, Tissues, and Cellular & Tissue Based Products; Establishment Registration and Listing." This regulation required all tissue establishments to register with the agency.

Throughout the 1980s and 1990s the Public Health Service (PHS) and both FDA and the Center for Disease Control and Prevention (CDC) published a number of guidelines and other guidance documents related to screening and testing for HIV, HBV, and HCV. Those documents are tabulated in Table 1.

TISSUE BANKING

Through the efforts of hospital educational programs and the efforts of the OPO in the community, hospital nursing personnel and physicians are made aware of procedures to identify potential organ and tissue donors.

With the 1998 CMS requirement for hospital participation in organ and tissue donation, a potential donor is identified and request for potential donation is initiated. This is often done with the hospital and the organ procurement personnel working together as a team. Specific parameters are established concerning eligibility of the potential donor. Hospitals develop contractual arrangements with the OPO and also may designate tissue banks with whom they choose to work. Some OPOs are also tissue banks or have contracts with established tissue banks or tissue recovery programs. In many areas of the United States, OPOs work with established tissue banks that may be local or national in scope and may concentrate in ocular, cardiovascular, musculoskeletal, and/or skin tissue.

Once an extensive detailed inquiry into the potential donor's medical, social, and sexual history is made, provisional clearance for donation is given and informed consent is obtained. Consent can be obtained by hospital personnel, OPO coordinators or the coordinator of the tissue recovery team. Informed consent is accomplished according to the applicable Anatomical Gift Acts and federal, state and/or local laws and regulations. The consenting person can be a) the potential donor, b) the individual empowered legally to grant consent according to law, or c) the potential donor's next of kin in order of legal

TABLE 1—Guidance documents.

1983	Centers for Disease Control: Prevention of acquired immunodeficiency syndrome (AIDS): Report of inter-agency recommendations. *MMWR*, Vol. 32, 1983, pp. 101–103.
1984	Centers for Disease Control: Update: acquired immunodeficiency syndrome (AIDS) in persons with hemophilia. *MMWR*, Vol. 33, 1984, pp. 589–591.
1985	Centers for Disease Control: Provisional Public Health Service inter-agency recommendations for screening donated blood and plasma for antibody to the virus causing acquired immunodeficiency syndrome. *MMWR*, Vol. 34, 1985, pp. 1–5.
1988	Centers for Disease Control: Transmission of HIV through bone transplantation: case report and public health recommendations. *MMWR* Vol. 37, 1988, pp. 597–599.
1988	Centers for Disease Control: Licensure of screening tests for antibody to human T-lymphotropic virus type 1. *MMWR*, Vol. 37, 1988, pp. 736–740.
1991	Centers for Disease Control: Public Health Service Inter-Agency Guidelines for Screening Donors of Blood, Plasma, Organs, Tissues and Semen for Evidence of Hepatitis B and Hepatitis C. *MMWR*, Vol. 40(RR–4), 1991, pp. 1–17.
1994	Centers for Disease Control: Guidelines for preventing transmission of human immunodeficiency virus through transplantation of human tissue and organs. *MMWR*, Vol. 43(RR-8), 1994, pp. 1–17.
1997	Guidance for Industry, screening and testing Donors of Human Tissue Intended for Transplantation, HHS, FDA, (CBER) (July) pp. 1–11, 1997.
1998	Center for Disease Control: Recommendations for Prevention and Control of Hepatitis C Virus (HCV) Infection and HCV-Related Chronic Disease. *MMWR*, Vol. 47(RR-19), 1998.
2002	Federal Register, FDA: Guidance for Industry: Validation of Procedures for Processing of Human Tissues Intended for Transplantation; Vol. 67, March 13, 2002.

Interim Rule: Human Tissue Intended for Transplantation; FDA Interim Rule: Opportunity for public comment. *Fed Regist*, Vol. 58, 1993, pp. 65514–65521.

Final Rule: Human Tissue Intended for Transplantation; FDA Final Rule-21 CFR Parts 16 and 1270. *Fed Regist,* Vol. 62, 1997, pp. 40429–40447.

precedence. Permission must be documented. Consent may also be obtained through telephone, facsimile, or electronic transmission. There are established guidelines for obtaining consent using these methods. Consent should outline the specific tissues and areas of the body from which tissue will be recovered and whether the tissues may or may not be used for research or tissue engineering. The consenting person may establish the parameters for tissue retrieval. The Association of Organ Procurement Organizations (AOPO), National Funeral Directors Association (NFDA) and AATB have formulated a statement outlining parameters for best practices for organ and tissue donation covering issues of notification, disclosure, consent, recovery, reimbursement, communication, education and support (Appendix I).

DONOR SCREENING

A detailed review of the documented medical history and inquiry of the patient's next of kin or significant other is made and documented. During donor screening a specific review determines that there is no history of:
- Recent active infection or sepsis
- Systemic viral illness (hepatitis, HIV, West Nile, others)
- Untreated syphilis, active tuberculosis, leprosy
- Autoimmune disease
- Ingested toxic substances that would be ultimately harmful in tissue transplantation (arsenic, lead, mercury, etc.)
- Rheumatoid arthritis, systemic lupus erythematosis, polyarteritis nodosa, sarcoidosis, myasthenia gravis
- Clinically significant metabolic bone disease
- Clinically significant malignancy
- Dementia, history of dura mater transplantation or use of human derived pituitary growth factor (because of concerns of spongiform disease e.g., CJD)
- Risk factors for HIV as established by the USPHS

Key aspects in donor screening include scrutiny that there is no evidence of:
- Active infection including viral, bacterial, or fungal
- Physical evidence of risk of sexually transmitted disease such as genital ulcers, herpes simplex, syphilis, chancroid
- Needle tracts that would be nonmedical and tattoos within the past 12 months
- Lymph node enlargement especially disseminated lymphadenopathy
- Jaundice, yellow sclera, or enlargement of the liver
- Blue or purple spots consistent with Kaposi's sarcoma (often times a marker for HIV infection)
- Evidence of anal intercourse manifested by perianal condylomata
- Oral thrush
- Local open wounds, especially over areas from which tissues are to be retrieved, as well as clinically significant skin lesions

Most organizations provide established donor screening forms that allow a coordinator to uniformly review not only the hospital medical records and the physician records but also to use in questioning family members in detail about specific risk factors. The AATB Medical Advisory Committee has established a suggested questionnaire for use in donor screening (Appendix II). Eastlund [24] has emphasized how the risk of transmission of disease can be reduced with quality donor screening.

Donor screening also includes review of autopsy findings if an autopsy is accomplished. Based on careful donor screening, which includes medical history, social history, physical examination, and quality serological testing, most contraindications for donation and use of tissue for transplantation should be recognized initially. Autopsy findings help to document the cause of death, identify and qualify pneumonias, differentiate between viral hepatitis and ischemia hepatic problems, identify sepsis and confirm the diagnoses of covert malignancies. An expert pathologist can frequently determine if lymph node enlargement is caused by inflammation or HIV [25]. The autopsy report is reviewed by the tissue bank medical director before release of tissue for transplantation. The estimated risk of acquired immunodeficiency syndrome from HIV in bone transplantation was stated to be 1:1,667,600 by Buck et al. [26] in 1989 if rigorous quality donor screening, autopsy by a qualified pathologist looking for subtle HIV findings and negative serology (antibody and antigen) were accomplished.

SEROLOGICAL TESTING

The FDA requires that serological tests be performed by laboratory certified under the Clinical Laboratory Improvement Amendments of 1988 (CLIA). These FDA-required tests are: HIV 1/HIV 2 antibody, HB_sAg, and HCV antibody (1270 Final Rule). Hepatitis-B core antibody testing is a general New York State requirement for all donors. AATB-accredited tissue banks are also required to test for HTLV-I/HTLV-II antibody, syphilis and hepatitis-B core antibody for living donors. Tissue banks often do additional testing in the form of HIV antigen testing, HIV PCR testing, cytomegalovirus (CMV) testing and NAT (nucleic acid amplification test) testing for hepatitis, none of which is currently required by the FDA for screening tissue donors.

All serology tests are predicated on issues of sensitivity and specificity. In order for an antigen test to be positive, sufficient antigen needs to be present. Antibody formation to an antigen does not occur immediately in an individual who is potentially infectious. This creates a window period, the period of time it takes for a sufficient amount of antibody to develop so that it can be detected by the antibody test. A report in 1996 [27] using data from 586, 507 blood donors estimated the risk of the infectious window to be 1:493,000 for HIV; 1:63,000 for HBV; 1:103,000 for HCV using the licensed tests at that time for blood donors. The reported residual risk for the standard tests in which the test is negative but the donor may be infectious is HIV 1/HIV 2 antibody (residual risk 1:689,655), HB_sAg (residual risk 1:77,220), HCV antibody (residual risk 1:19, 850) [GAO/HEHS – 98-205 Blood Plasma Safety].

Nucleic acid amplification test (NAT) testing can further reduce the period of time between which a donor becomes infectious and the time when the virus becomes detectable by screening tests. The window period, using an FDA licensed test for HIV antibody, is 22 days; for HCV antibody 70 days; and for HBV (HB_sAg) 56 days. Using NAT testing, the HIV window can be reduced to 7–12 days, HCV 10–29 days and HBV to 41–50 days [28]. The window period during which a patient may be asymptomatic but infectious while serological tests indicate negative results is outlined in Table 2. The residual risk as outlined previously is predicated on using the current standard FDA-licensed tests for banks that do not include NAT testing. Starting in 1999, nucleic acid amplification testing has been used to directly detect viral genetic material. According to the American Association of Blood Banks' Website, www.aabb.org, the estimated risk of the infectious window is 1:900,000 for HIV, 1:137,000 for hepatitis B, and 1:1,000,000 for HCV using screening and licensed tests at this time for blood donors. The current stated incidence in the literature from the Retrovirus Epidemiology Donor Study [29] of the rate of risk for the window period model for blood donors in the United States using NAT testing 2000-2002 is HIV 1:2,000,000; HBV 1:250,000; and HCV 1:2,000,000.

TABLE 2—Period between infection and time virus is detectable by screening tests.

Window Period Period between infection and time virus is detectable by screening tests.			
	Virus		
	HIV	HCV	HBV
Window Period using FDA Licensed Tests	22 days (anti HIV$_{1,2}$)	70 days (anti HCV)	56 days (HB$_s$Ag)
Window Period using NAT* Testing	7-12 days**	10-29 days	41-50 days
*Nucleic Acid Test ** p24 testing between 12 and 22 days Source: Busch MP and Kleinman SH, Transfusion 40:143-146, 2000.			

HIV antigen and HIV PCR testing are not licensed for screening donors of human tissue.

The serological tests over the years have been predicated on blood donor screening parameters using FDA licensed tests for living blood donors. Only in recent years has there been an FDA licensed test authorized for use to screen samples from cadaveric donors. Many tests lack sensitivity and specificity when performed using cadaveric serum, resulting in a number of false positives. Currently the only FDA-licensed tests using cadaveric serum samples are HIV 1/HIV 2 and HCV [30].

Dilution of a donor's blood volume by infusion of blood or other fluids has raised concerns regarding the sensitivity of serological testing. Ideally, a pre-transfusion blood specimen would be made available for serologic testing. The FDA requires the tissue bank have in place an algorithm that evaluates the volumes administered in the 48 hours before the collection of the blood specimen to ensure that there has not been plasma dilution sufficient to affect serology test results.

TISSUE RETRIEVAL

With the demand for allograft tissue and improved access to tissue donors, the number of musculoskeletal procurements have increased over the years (Fig. 4). The vast

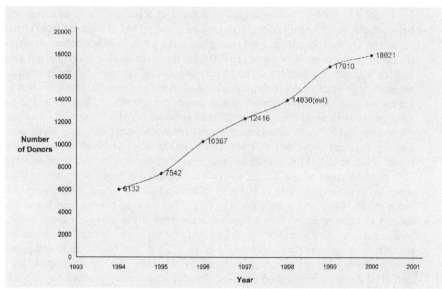

FIG. 4—U. S. trends of musculoskeletal tissue donors: donors recovered by AATB accredited tissue banks.

majority of tissue recovered is by AATB accredited banks with only two major tissue processors not accredited.

Ideally, tissues are surgically excised using aseptic conditions with airflow specifications similar to an operating room environment. Adhering to aseptic principles reduces the potential for contamination. Good tissue practices according to AATB Standards require that musculoskeletal tissues be procured within 24 hours postmortem or within 12 hours postmortem if the body has not been refrigerated.

Some tissue retrieval takes place in environments such as morgues where surgical drapes are employed and adherence to sterile technique is used. Allografts retrieved under these conditions usually are processed using subsequent sterilization techniques such as irradiation, ethylene oxide or other validated process. Grafts such as cryopreserved osteochondral grafts or fresh osteoarticular grafts that cannot be disinfected or sterilized must be retrieved using the rigid sterile techniques similar to those of an operating room to reduce the risk of bacterial contamination.

There is discussion as to whether musculoskeletal grafts can ever be called sterile unless industrial sterilization procedures are implemented similar to those defined by FDA for metallic devices or pharmaceuticals. "Sterile" is defined as a state in which there is one in a million (1×10^{6}) chance of a viable organism's being present after irradiation or other sterilization process. It is important to know the biology of the organism and the level of contamination. The bioburden (number of organisms) must be known to accurately predict the log reduction attainable by the sterilization technique employed (i.e., ability to achieve 1×10^{6} risk of contamination). Therefore most tissue banks and all AATB accredited banks do pre-processing cultures to ascertain whether the tissue is contaminated prior to processing.

Tissue can become contaminated as a result of a bacteremia or unrecognized sepsis before death, or as a result of tissue degradation and spread of bacteria from an associated colonized viscus (bowel) or organ (lung) or open wounds either before death or during the tissue retrieval process (poor sterile technique, poor quality room air and air flow, or contact with bowel, bladder or lung). Pre-processing cultures can be accomplished by vigorous multi-surface swabbing of individual tissue pieces with the swabs that are either plated on agar plates for aerobic and/or anaerobic growth evaluation and/or placed in broth media with or without the inclusion of anaerobic media.

Studies have shown that culture results have a higher predictive value when small tissue pieces are immersed in broth media rather than swabbed on the surface of the tissue. Veen et al. [31] demonstrated that results of cultures ranged from an incidence of 92% positive when whole fibular pieces were cultured in broth compared to 9% positive when cultures from surface swabs were placed on plates. When swabs were cultured in broth media, there was a 36% positive rate. The value of postmortem blood cultures is subject to interpretation. It is difficult to determine if the positive culture resulted from contamination during culturing or from hematogenous spread of micro-organisms premortem or postmortem. Vehmeyer et al. [32] in the Netherlands compared blood, bone marrow, and tissue swab cultures in 95 cadaveric bone donors. The review described eight positive blood cultures, three of which were positive for both blood and marrow. In only one donor were both the blood culture and the marrow culture positive for the same organism whereas the tissue swabs tested negative. In nine donors, identical organisms were noted on a swab culture of at least one tissue at procurement as compared to either the marrow or blood culture. Eight of nine times the organism was coagulase negative staphylococcus. Deijkers et al. [33] analyzed bacterial contamination of 2000 cultures from 200 cadaveric donors retrieved under sterile operating room conditions. Grafts were swab cultured after being rinsed with antibiotic solutions (polymyxin B and bacitracin) for the initial 150 donors and with saline for the latter 50 donors. Low virulence or low pathogenic organisms (predominately skin flora) were noted on 50% of the grafts and high pathogenic organisms (predominately staphylococcus aureus and gram negatives) on 3% of the grafts. The risk of contamination for low risk pathogens increased by a factor of 1.6 for each added member of the procurement team. The risk of contamination with high-risk pathogenic organisms was 3.4 times greater in traumatic deaths and 5.2 times higher when blood cultures were positive. Organ procurement, when preceding the tissue procurement, did not significantly influence the risk of contamination. Antibiotic wash was not an effective means of reducing contamination and may have masked an even higher potential positive culture rate. Additionally, classifying an organism such as coagulase negative staphylococcus as a low pathogenic organism may indeed be an understatement when one considers the devastating infection that may occur if the graft is used for an allograft-prosthetic composite or as a strut in revision total hip joint surgery. Vehmeyer et al. [34] also showed the inadequacy of simple swab cultures for tissues. Two donors with postmortem positive cultures of both blood and heart valve yielded a 25% positive rate for the same organism when an entire piece of tissue was cultured in broth and was positive only infrequently when tissue swabs were used. The results confirmed the limited sensitivity of swab culturing techniques.

Forsell [35] analyzed positive microbiological cultures from a review of 1036 donors of multiple banks and identified statistically significant increases in bacteriologic bioburden after certain types of recovery. Significant increases in bioburdens were seen with recovery after autopsy; length of time taken for recovery; and size of recovery team. It was interesting how little effect time after death and location of tissue donor recovery (morgue/funeral home compared to operating room) had on changes in bioburden.

TISSUE PROCESSING

Years ago the standard practice was to surgically remove a femoral head from a patient undergoing a total hip replacement, place it in a sterile glass or plastic container, store it in a deep freezer and use it for eventual transplantation as a bone graft or for structural support in another patient. Over the years, as the practice has evolved and improved, tissue processing facilities follow the more rigidly prescribed good tissue practice guidelines (GTPs) proposed by the FDA. Tissue processing facilities may be stand-alone or multi-service providers. Tissues are shipped to processing facilities in a wet cold state or frozen state. After careful donor screening and serological testing review, tissue is processed in a clean air room. Attempts are made to remove or reduce cellular and tissue debris that could harbour bacteria and viruses. It is believed that these mechanical debridements and washes significantly reduce the potential for disease transmission. Various proprietary bacteriological and virucidal washes are available. As stated earlier, most tissue banks evaluate the bacteriological bioburden before processing using pre-processing cultures to evaluate contamination. Discard of tissue from a potential donor lot may be predicated on certain types of bacteriological contamination. As indicated by these pre-processing cultures, treatment with 1.2–1.8 Mrads (~12–18 kilogray) may also be used to reduce bacteriological and viral bioburden before processing. Some banks irradiate (1.5 to 3.5 Mrads or ~15–35 kilogray) tissue at the end of the processing sequence, helping to eliminate contaminants after processing and final packaging. Final product microbiological testing for bacterial contamination either by destructive testing or swab culturing is routine. Techniques and methods used in tissue processing are validated using strict quality control (QC) and quality assurance (QA) measures. Tissue processing facilities are required to have separate QC and QA programs with responsibilities accomplished by individuals not directly involved in tissue processing. All of these practices are audited by the facility. Tissues are processed as freeze-dried or frozen grafts. Before the tissue release, the tissue bank medical director (licensed physician) reviews donor screening medical history, serology testing and processing records before release of tissue for distribution for eventual use in transplantation.

Some tissues are sterilized with either ethylene oxide, gamma, or electron beam irradiation. A sterilization dose for bacteria of 1.5–2.0 Mrads (~ 15–25 kilogray) can be used for bone products. For structural grafts, including soft tissues, higher amounts of gamma radiation may impact unfavorably on the integrity of the tissue, particularly cartilage. Gamma irradiation historically has been validated using *Bacillus* spores. Penetration of bone by gamma irradiation is not a significant problem.

Ethylene oxide (ETO) is used for sterilization both in hospitals and in manufacturing. Adequacy of depth of penetration of ETO for large bone allograft segments and soft tissues is a consideration. Therefore, ETO is used mostly for freeze-dried grafts and most freeze-dried products are sterilized using ETO. When ETO is used, breakdown by-products are released and may be retained on the product as ETO residuals. These residuals are examined and quantitated so that remaining levels conform to required

Environmental Protection Agency and FDA standards. These residuals in certain large amounts are considered carcinogenic and toxic. Ethylene oxide residuals may also cause a potential inflammatory response after implantation [36].

Several processors have tried to address the risk of disease transmission of both viruses and bacteria using proprietary techniques that employ high pressure purging of marrow and cells, virucidal and bacteriologic washes with surfactants, alcohol, and iodine, and use of irradiation and/or ethylene oxide. For maintenance of tissue integrity, it is important that proteins are not denatured and that demineralized bone retains its osteoinductive properties. The integrity of cancellous chips used for osteoinduction is less impacted because these are not osteoinductive and usually are not required to maintain structural strength. Some allografts cannot be processed in this manner without an adverse affect on the integrity of the graft. An example would be the use of alcohol baths and high pressure washing causing damage to soft tissue allografts.

Several investigators have evaluated the radiosensitivity of the human immunodeficiency virus. Spire et al. [37] reported that 10 kilogray (~1 Mrad) was sufficient to inactivate the virus. Others perceive viral inactivation as a logarithmic reduction based on viral bioburden. Conway et al. [38,39] calculated that 36 kilogray was necessary to sterilize tissue from an infected donor. Kitchen et al. [40] showed that an even slightly higher dose was necessary to inactivate the virus in the blood of infectious patients. Campbell et al. [41] recommended that a dose of at least 25 kilogray was necessary for bone that had a viral load adequate enough to cause infection in the laboratory setting. Campbell et al. [42] in a later publication documented the dose-response relationship for frozen allograft bone. The irradiation dose required to inactivate the HIV bioburden was 35 kilogray and the dose required to achieve a sterility assurance level of 10^6 was 89 kilogray. Fideler et al. [43,44] showed that the irradiation dosage needed to be increased to 30–40 kilogray before viral DNA could not be detected in frozen human bone-patellar ligament-bone grafts obtained from infected cadavera. Whether the presence of detectable viral DNA following irradiation will lead to an infectious state is unclear. Smith et al. [45] also showed that gamma irradiation 1.5–2.5 Mrad (~15–25 kilogray) did not constitute a virucidal dose for HIV type I. The number of viral particles in tissue from two different infectious donors may be different, with the higher bioburden of one donor requiring a higher level of irradiation to effect viral inactivation. In contrast to the effectiveness of lower doses of irradiation against bacteria, these lower doses of irradiation have not been proven effective against viruses when there is a higher titer concentration.

Nor is irradiation completely harmless to the tissue. Investigators have shown that irradiation of demineralized freeze-dried products at levels of 25 kilogray reduces the amount of new bone formation induced by the demineralized product when compared to non-irradiated controls [46,47,48]. Low-dose irradiation up to 20 kilogray seemed not to affect cytokine activity in demineralized bone [49]. Wientroub and Reddi [50] reported in 1988 that a dose of 25 kilogray did not affect the osteoinductive properties of bone matrix. Dziedzic–Goclawski et al. [51], using 35 and 50 kilogray gamma irradiation, demonstrated that lyophilized decalcified bone matrix irradiated at room temperature did not induce osteogenesis in a muscle heterotopic model whereas new bone formation was induced with irradiated deeply frozen (-72°C) demineralized bone matrices. They proposed that the preservation of osteoinductive capacity of irradiated deeply frozen demineralized matrix may depend on the presence of water and the temperature during irradiation. Ijiri et al. [52] studied the effect of 25 kilogray gamma irradiation on partially purified bone morphogenetic protein and type I collagen. Osteoinduction was reduced considerably in both compared to controls but was less affected when accomplished with ethylene oxide at 29°C compared to 37°C. Collagen was far more labile than bone morphogenetic protein when gamma irradiated. Studies by Moreau et al. [53] on irradiated bone cores from human femoral heads at 25 kilogray when compared to non-irradiated frozen cores demonstrated a two to three fold increase in peroxidated lipids. When slices of these bone cores were transferred to confluent osteoblast-like cell layers, cell death was dramatically increased around the gamma- irradiated slices. Defatted slices that had been gamma irradiated did not induce cell death. A suggestion was made that defatting procedures should be added when preparing bone allografts if the grafts are irradiated.

Pelker and Friedlaender [54–56] demonstrated doses of more than 30 kilogray adversely affected the bending and torsional strength of large cortical grafts. Currey et al. [57] evaluated the effects of ionizing irradiation of four paired femora using 17 kilogray, 29.5 kilogray and 94.7 kilogray. Young's modulus was unchanged by any level of irradiation but significantly reduced bending strength, work to fracture, and impact energy absorption; in each case, the severity of the effect increased as the dosage increased. Even at low doses, irradiation caused the bone to become more brittle and reduced the energy absorbing capacity. Bright and Burchardt [58] reported adverse effects in bone that was freeze-dried before irradiation. Anderson et al. [59] using proximal tibial cancellous bone segments, performed mechanical compression tests on fresh frozen specimens irradiated at 10, 31, 51, and 60 kilogray compared to non-irradiated controls. Significant differences in normalized failure stress and normalized elastic modulus were found only in the 60 kilogray specimens. Zhang et al. [60] compared frozen and freeze dried iliac crest bone wedges irradiated at 2.0–2.5 Mrad (~20–25 kilogray). They were unable to show significant differences in mechanical and material properties using uniaxial compression testing when compared to non-irradiated wedges. Jinno et al. [61] demonstrated that a preprocessing lower dose gamma irradiation of 1.5 Mrad (~15 kilogray) did not consistently or significantly affect the incorporation of syngeneic or allogeneic mid femoral shaft cortical grafts in a rat model. Studies of pull out strength of screws in processed human tibial allograft bone were performed by Simonian et al. [62]. Cortical sections of processed tibial bone with irradiation (1.57–1.87 Mrad), freeze-drying or ethylene oxide were compared to control specimens. The hydrated freeze-dried specimens required significantly less force for screw pull out. The screw pull out force for irradiated specimens and ethylene oxide did not significantly differ from the controls. Voggenreiter et al. [63] showed a deleterious effect of 25 kilogray and 50 kilogray on "autograft" irradiated reimplanted rat tibial cortical segments. The 50 kilogray specimens had fractured at three weeks at over a 60% rate and the 25 kilogray irradiated grafts showed 50% reduction of incorporation compared to controls and 1 or 5 kilogray groups. Hamer et al. [64] investigated the effect of irradiation 6.8, 28.5 and 60 kilogray at room temperature alone, and irradiation with freezing of human cadaveric femoral rings. Simple freeze thawing to −70° C had no effect on the gradient of the elastic region of the samples. There was no effect on elastic behavior but there was a reduction in strength to 64% compared to non-irradiated controls after irradiation to 28.5 kilogray. There was a dose-dependent reduction in strength and the ability of the samples to absorb work before failure. Hamer et al. [65] also found that bone iradiated with 30.2 kilogray at -78° C was less brittle and had less collagen damage than when irradiated at room temperature. Sequential dependence of freeze-drying coupled with irradiation sterilization on biomechanical properties was demonstrated by Randall et al. [66] with a femoral rat model. After various treatment of specimens (irradiated at room temperature; freeze-dried; irradiated then freeze-dried; freeze-dried then irradiated room temperature), microfractures were demonstrated in more than 90% of specimens either freeze-dried alone or with irradiation. A mechanical trend was noted that the freeze-dried then irradiated bones were weaker when compared with freeze-dried bones alone.

Loty et al. [67] reviewed both biologic properties of allografts and a clinical series of 150 massive allografts that had been sterilized with 25 kilogray gamma irradiation. Biologically there was a 20% decrease in strength of the allograft after irradiation. The clinical results demonstrated a low infection rate with an approximately 80% satisfactory result. Hernigou et al. [68] reviewed the clinical French experience from 1984–1988 of 127 massive allografts, which had received 25 kilogray by linear acceleration (electron beam) while in a deeply frozen state. There were seven (5.5%) nonunions and eight fractures (6%). When patients (84) received chemotherapy or radiation therapy, the rate of infection was 13%. The rates of complications did not seem to differ with other reported clinical non-irradiated large graft series. Lietman et al. [69] reviewed the clinical outcome (average 5 year follow-up) of irradiated (10 kilogray to 30 kilogray) massive structural allografts from the Massachusetts General Hospital series 1987–1991 with a comparable non-irradiated control group. The outcome differed significantly only in the incidence of fracture with irradiated grafts associated with an increased fracture rate compared to non-irradiated grafts. The rate of infection did not significantly differ.

Soft tissue allografts may also be adversely affected by irradiation. Fideler et al. [70] studied in-vitro testing of bone-tendon-bone patellar ligament grafts to tensile failure, reported a 15% reduction in strength following irradiation to 20 kilogray compared to fresh-frozen controls. Rasmussen et al. [71] compared pairs of frozen human patellar tendon-bone ligament allografts that were either non-irradiated or 4 Mrad (~40 kilogray) of gamma irradiation. Irradiation shortened the tendon 0.6 mm but did not significantly alter static or cyclic creep. Irradiation produced the greatest changes during failure testing, reducing the graft linear stiffness and maximum force. They acknowledged that the in-vitro study does not describe how a graft may perform during early healing and later collagen remodelling in-vivo. Butler et al. [72] reported doses of 20 kilogray did not adversely affect outcome of irradiated grafts for anterior cruciate reconstruction in the goat model at six months. Goertzen et al. [73] evaluated cryoperserved irradiated bone-anterior cruciate-bone allografts using the dog model. The grafts treated with 25 kilogray with argon gas protection were able to sustain loads similar to non-irradiated controls. Gibbons et al. [74] showed deleterious reduced stress, strain and strain energy density in the midportion of goat allograft patellar ligaments, which had received 30 kilogray. Bettin et al. [75] studied freeze-dried 26 kiloray irradiated sheep medial collateral liagments. Maximum load was decreased 24%, elongation 7%, and a decrease in stress 20%. Recommendations were made to study doses of 15 to less than 26 kilogray. Studies on irradiated menisci by Yahia [76] showed that simple freezing caused no change in failure but irradiation to 25 kilogray caused significant reduction in elastic properties.

Research is being conducted regarding irradiation damage that is dependent on target size and density as well as the nonselective free radical damage to proteins and nucleic acids. Dose rate, water content, oxygen level, temperature, and the use of irradiation stabilizers/protectants indeed effect the impact that irradiation has on demineralized bone, soft tissue and bone allografts. Animal studies and human clinical outcome studies are needed. Additionally, the surgeon may decide that a reduction in biomechanical performance is insignificant when compared to the clinical application.

TISSUE STORAGE

Freeze-dried musculoskeletal tissues can be stored in vacuum bottles or impervious foil packages at room air temperatures on a shelf. Deeply frozen grafts are usually stored in freezers at temperatures between minus 60 to 70°C. This reduces the growth of the slowly forming ice crystals during prolonged storage and should inactivate proteolytic enzymes that may harm the integrity of the graft. Some banks store frozen grafts at temperatures below minus 120°C with the use of specially designed cryogenic mechanical freezers using liquid nitrogen.

Once bone or soft tissue is deeply frozen, all attempts are made to keep the tissue frozen continuously, including during transport of tissue on dry ice when shipped for distribution and clinical use. This tissue remains deeply frozen until the time of clinical use in transplantation.

DISTRIBUTION

Facilities that process tissues may also distribute tissues or may return the processed allograft tissue to the bank that recovered the tissue. Distribution of tissue is then instituted by the tissue bank. Tissues can be processed as demineralized bone products, either as powders or with various carriers such as glycerol or hyaluronate. The use of carriers with these demineralized bone products previously had not changed their status of regulation by FDA as human tissue products and not medical devices. The agency does not require premarket approval for release of the human tissue product on the market and has established a Tissue Reference Group to evaluate the designation of tissue-containing products either as a tissue or device. For demineralized bone products, to date there are no established parameters to demonstrate efficacy, or safety, or bone formation properties. Recently, the agency has notified manufacturers of demineralized bone products that if a carrier is used with the product and the product cannot meet the criteria of minimal manipulation, the product will be re-evaluated and most likely reclassified as a device. However, the decision is not final and the approach is being questioned by the AATB.

Tissue products may be freeze-dried in sterile jars with vacuum packaging, vacuum packaged in impervious plastics or foils or packaged frozen as large segments of bone transported on dry ice and kept frozen until the time of transplantation. Tissue banks attempt to track tissue from donor retrieval to distribution and implantation in the patient. However, there are no federal requirements for hospitals to provide information about the use of the tissue including the patient in whom the tissue was implanted. Attempts have been made using self-addressed postcards provided with the allograft to be returned to the tissue bank; these document the physician, date, and specific use of the transplantable tissue. JCAHO hospitals are required to maintain a registry for tissue implant uses. However, as alluded to earlier, this requirement is enforced with varying degrees of vigor.

DISEASE TRANSMISSION

Over the past decade more than 5 million musculoskeletal tissue allografts have been implanted safely in the United States. There have been relatively few reported instances of disease transmission associated with allograft tissue although operating room infections are fairly common. Last year the CDC reported 500,000 infections related to non-allograft surgical procedures alone [77]. There have been some reports of allograft related infections. Most of these infections are not related to the allograft but to problems of the soft tissue envelop that lead to a secondary bacterial infection that is often nosocomial in nature. There have been several recent reports where the allograft has been implicated as being the cause of infection. A current investigation conducted by AATB with the assistance of the CDC and FDA is ongoing. AATB-accredited banks are required to maintain an adverse reactions file. AATB and FDA inspectors review these files at the time of the on-site inspection.

Review of the literature shows that tuberculosis has been associated with tissue implantation. James et al. [78] in 1953 reported four cases of tuberculosis related to transplantation of ribs following thoracoplasty. Tomford et al. [79] in 1981 reported an attempt to identify infections related to procedures using freeze-dried allograft bone from the Navy Tissue Bank. He identified only one bacterial infection among 303 bone implants that was probably related to the allograft (positive culture of graft at time of implantation matched the culture of the infection but results of post processing culture at the tissue bank were negative). In 1988, Lord et al. [80] published a large series of 283 massive bone allografts including osteoarticular and segmental grafts in which three bacterial infections were related directly to the frozen bone allograft. In 1990, Tomford et al. [81] further reviewed the experience with frozen allografts and reported no infections in 134 cases involving cadaveric femoral heads, small bone segments, and soft tissue grafts. Of the 287 patients in whom a bone allograft was used, an infection developed in thirteen (5%). The allograft was implicated as the source of bacterial infection in three of 324 implants. The three cases originated from the same donor and all were culture positive for *Serratia marcescens*. These grafts had not been processed beyond being sterilely wrapped at the time of retrieval and subsequently deeply frozen.

The CDC reported in Morbidity and Mortality Report (MMWR) December 2001 [82] five incidents that are currently under investigation. One report, a clostridial infection, was associated with a fresh osteoarticular graft. The recipient eventually died. Upon further review by the processor, cultures of several other grafts that had not been distributed were positive for clostridia. Two other reports of two infections each from a single donor of bone-tendon-bone tissue used in allograft ligament reconstruction during arthroscopy were included in this same MMWR. In the first two cases where tissue was retrieved from a common donor from the same Florida tissue bank, quality control review documented that the tissue was to have been terminally sterilized with gamma irradiation before release but was inadvertently not irradiated. Organisms identified were *Citrobacter werkmanii/youngae* and *group B beta hemolytic streptococcus* in one patient and *Klebsiella oxytoca* and *Hafnia alvei* in the other patient. These species were present on donor tissue cultures during the time of processing. In the second two cases, *Pseudomonas aeruginosa* infections of the same genotypic pattern was isolated in two separate patients undergoing knee arthroscopic allograft reconstruction in 2000. These two patients had surgery three days apart by different surgeons at the same surgical facility using irradiated tissue from the same knee of a common donor. One of the infections was polymicrobial. The tissue had been terminally irradiated using 1.6–2.0 Mrads (~16 - 20 kilogray). Lookback identified that no pre-processing cultures or blood cultures were performed by the bank on this 63-year-old donor. It was confirmed that the tissue indeed had been irradiated and that cultures of representative co-processed tissues from the knee and bacillus spore testing were negative following irradiation prior to release of this tissue for human use. It is unclear whether the tissue allograft was the causative factor responsible for these two latter infections. A limited epidemiological report of the surgical center regarding the incidence of infection showed no other postoperative infections among 1,000 anterior cruciate reconstructions over the preceding 4 years. A complete review would necessitate scrutiny of the freestanding surgical center's practices regarding sterile technique and arthroscopy equipment maintenance and sterilization (usually done chemically with disinfectants).

A more recent MMWR report [83] in March 2002 solicited and tabulated additional cases of allograft associated bacterial infections including the ones reported three months earlier. Twenty-six cases under review are possibly associated with allograft tissue. Two of these cases of bacterial infection occurred in 1986. Thirteen clostridial infections were identified. A majority of these clostidial infections were associated with tissue supplied by the same non-AATB accredited tissue processor.

Hepatitis has been reported to be transmitted through musculoskeletal tissue. Shukin [84] reported serum hepatitis assumed to be hepatitis B associated with an allograft in 1954. Eggen and Nordbo [85] reported, as an editorial comment in Lancet 1992, transmission of hepatitis C through transplantation of an unprocessed frozen femoral head.

In 1995, Conrad et al. [86] reported a unique epidemiological study that documented two cases of hepatitis C transmission associated with a frozen non-irradiated bone allograft. The original first-generation HCV (HCV 1.0) test was licensed in May 1990. A more sensitive hepatitis C second-generation test (HCV 2.0) was licensed 22 months later in March 1992. Tissue banks usually store serum from donors in order to protect stored inventory. If additional FDA-licensed tests are developed, the agency could require use of the newer serology screening test before tissue in inventory is released for human implantation. This inventoried serum sample provided the tissue bank the opportunity to perform a lookback of 470 donors, identifying donors (<1%) that were HCV antibody negative using the first-generation test but positive for the HCV 2.0 test using the stored specimen. During the same time, based on negative serology for the hepatitis C first-generation test, some tissue from two cadaveric donors, which subsequently tested positive for HCV 2.0 upon retesting approximately 2 years later, previously had been used for allograft transplantation. Attempts were made to track recipients and perform the second-generation HCV 2.0 test. Sera from five of six recipient patients who received tissue from the first donor were negative. One patient who tested positive had associated risk factors (sexual partner with hepatitis C). All these tissues had been irradiated with 1.7 Mrads (~17 kilogray). The second donor yielded five recipients of which four out of five were HCV positive. One had risk factors for HCV. Three recipients who were subsequently HCV positive had the use of non-irradiated frozen bone-patellar ligament-bone (two) or a proximal femoral allograft. On further testing the hepatitis C genome in two recipients were identical to that of the donor of the allograft.

A more recent case of transmission of hepatitis C virus has been reported [87] in both organs and tissues from a 40-year-old donor who died in 2000 of an intracranial hemorrhage in Oregon. The anti-HCV antibody by ELA 2.0 was confirmed negative, but the donor was in retrospect positive for HCV RNA (NAT test). The donor was the source of 82 tissues, seven organs, and two corneas. There were forty recipients in 14 states and two countries. The transplanted tissues and organs were the probable vehicle of HCV transmission in at least six recipients including a patellar ligament allograft. The CDC is providing epidemiological review of this donor case that was recovered during the serological negative hepatitis antibody window but infectious state.

HIV has been shown to be transmissible through blood and blood products. As in the case of hepatitis transmission related to tissue, the cause of HIV transmission is most probably the blood that has been retained in the tissue graft. In 1988, CDC documented the first case of HIV transmission related to tissue that occurred in 1984 [88]. This incident occurred before HIV testing had been adopted (first licensed HIV antibody test March 1985) and involved a 52-year-old male donor whose femoral head was removed and stored by deep freezing −80° C following a total hip replacement. The femoral head was subsequently used in a spinal fusion in a female recipient in 1984 who had no risk factors for HIV, including no blood transfusions. She subsequently developed AIDS in 1988. In a retrospective review, the donor's history indicated lymph node enlargement at the time of donation and a lymph node biopsy a few months before the donation of the femoral head. History also included intravenous drug abuse but this information was not elicited at the time of donation. The donor developed *Pneumocystis carinii* in July of 1986 and was documented to be HIV positive. Based solely on donor screening exclusion parameters in effect since 1984, this man would not have been considered a potential tissue donor either in 1984 or today even if he had been HIV- antibody-negative.

In 1992, Simonds et al. [89] reported in the *New England Journal Medicine* an episode of three HIV cases that resulted following a tissue allograft from a common donor that was retrieved in 1985. The 22-year-old donor had eventually died of a gunshot wound to the head; thirty-two hours after the incident both organs and tissues were retrieved. Donor screening revealed no risk factors, prospectively and retrospectively. Results of serological testing performed at tissue retrieval were negative on two separate tests, using first-generation HIV antibody testing, the only test licensed for donor screening at the time. Kidneys, heart, and liver were transplanted. Four frozen musculoskeletal allografts and 48 bone and soft tissue processed freeze-dried allografts were banked. All organ recipients subsequently seroconverted to being HIV positive. Initially, it was surmised that, at least in some of these organ recipients, blood transfusions had been the cause of the HIV infection. The fact that these patients had seroconverted was not reported to the organ procurement agency that had also retrieved the tissue. It was not until 1991, after a femoral head from this donor was implanted in a 72-year-old female patient in 1985 who subsequently became HIV-positive which was recognized in 1991, that the donor organs and tissue were suspected as the cause of the seroconversion. The tissue bank had retained stored donor lymphocytes from the spleen; this cell sample was tested in 1991 by polymerase chain reaction (PCR) testing. The results were positive for HIV, using this sophisticated test licensed for diagnosis only. No serum was available to declare if newer generation HIV antibody or antigen testing would have provided a positive result. The tissue bank immediately initiated a recall. Hospitals and other facilities to which six pieces of freeze-dried tissue had been sent were unable to determine the disposition of the tissue. Forty-eight recipients were identified of which 41 were tested for HIV. Thirty-four recipients of tissue tested non-reactive for HIV: two corneas recipients, three recipients of freeze-dried tissue, 25 recipients of ethanol-treated bone, and three recipients of irradiated dura mater. However, three tissue recipient cases were identified as seropositive for HIV after transplantation. Two had received an unprocessed frozen femoral head allograft and one case an unprocessed frozen bone-tendon-bone allograft. These three were associated with the transmission of HIV. The other frozen graft, a proximal femoral allograft from which the marrow was thoroughly washed, was implanted and the recipient shows no evidence of HIV infection to date.

This particular case, that graphically shows the window period when the donor is infectious but serologically antibody negative on testing, has been cited repeatedly in the literature. Presentation of this case has promoted dialogue that needs to take place between and among OPOs, tissue banks and physicians, so that results of serological testing can be shared among all recovery groups. Adverse transplant recipient outcomes must be reported promptly to respective OPOs, tissue banks, and eye banks.

In addition to standard processing techniques, demineralized bone products are treated in acid to attain demineralization. To date, disease transmission associated with demineralized bone products has never been reported.

Emerging diseases such as CDJ variant (mad cow disease) and West Nile Virus (which has been implicated in transmission of disease to organ recipients [90]) will provide future challenges to the safety of transplantable tissues.

SUMMARY

More than 850,000 musculoskeletal tissue allografts were distributed in the United States in 2001. Reports of disease transmission over the past decade are indeed very rare. There are no reports of disease transmission using demineralized bone products. Conventional sterilization techniques typically used to sterilize metallic implants may adversely affect functional, biological and mechanical properties of certain musculoskeletal tissue allografts. Use of 25 kilogray or higher of gamma irradiation has been shown to have some adverse effect on tissue allografts.

Allograft tissue can be treated with 12–20 kilogray to eliminate bacterial contamination and reduce viral bioburden. This range often is used to minimize the negative effect of higher doses of gamma irradiation.

Effectiveness of irradiation or any sterilization technique is dependent upon both the level of bioburden of the bacterial or viral contamination and the dosage level. A dose of 12–36 kilogray is not effective in eliminating spongiform disease caused by prions.

Safety of a musculoskeletal tissue allograft is based on FDA proposed good tissue practices (GTPs), which are patterned on AATB Standards and predicated on donor screening and physical examination, careful processing techniques with attention to detail towards quality control and quality assurance validation measures. The American Association of Tissue Banks publishes the only tissue banking standards that are universally recognized. These standards, initially published in 1984, are reviewed and revised annually. AATB also operates the only accreditation program that exists. In 1993 the federal government converted some of these voluntary standards into the Interim Rule Human Tissue Intended for Transplantation and began to audit banks. As a result of FDA's action, certain banks were closed, some tissue was destroyed and the practices of most other banks were modified. Tissue banks may not report or advertise that they have been FDA-inspected. FDA audits and comments are in the public domain and are available under the Freedom of Information Act. However, the process of public retrieval of this information may take significant time. The FDA warning letters to a bank from the Agency are available on the FDA website.

Reporting of adverse episodes to a central agency that can subsequently provide investigation and documentation of the adverse episode needs to be implemented. The federal government has recommended the reporting of infections involving allograft tissue to the tissue banks, tissue processors, FDA's Medwatch System, and CDC. Most infections are not caused by the tissue allograft. However, to anticipate emerging problems in tissue banking, review and scrutiny of adverse episodes must be accomplished to protect future transplant recipients.

Outcome studies are needed to improve safety, document efficacy, and expand our knowledge of musculoskeletal tissue products. To date there are limited reports outlining the potential benefit of tissue implants and limited reports outlining the benefit of bone substitute products. Not all clinical situations are the same. One situation may require osteoconduction and the use of a scaffold. Other situations may require osteoinductivity to facilitate healing.

It is imperative that surgeon and patient interaction occurs with a discussion outlining the options as well as risks and benefits of various implants. It is very important to have a basic understanding of musculoskeletal tissue banking. Just as the surgeon may need to provide information about which metallic implant will be used, the surgeon needs basic information regarding an allograft implant. Some tissue banks allow the surgeon easy access to such information through the package insert. Often times this information must be solicited from the tissue bank. In all instances, the orthopedic surgeon needs to know preexisting parameters that the tissue bank uses to determine or help assure the quality of the allografts.

Finally it is most important to recognize that the use of human allograft tissue is predicated on the gracious altruistic act of the donor/donor family. Tissue transplantation would not be possible except for this generous donation.

Acknowledgment

The authors express their deepest appreciation for the editorial assistance of Jeanne Mowe, Executive Director AATB, James Forsell, Ph.D., Martell Winters and secretarial assistance from Carolyn Evans.

REFERENCES

[1] Mankin H. J., Dopplet S. H., and Tomford W. W., "Clinical Experience with Allograft Implantation: The first 200 cases," *Clin Orthop Rel Res,* Vol. 174, 1983, pp. 69–86.

[2] MacEwen W., "Observations Concerning Transplantation of Bone: Illustrated by a case of inter-human osseous transplantation, whereby over two-thirds of the shaft of a humerus was restored," *Proc R Soc Lond,* Vol. 32, 1881, pp. 232–247.

[3] Grohe B., "Die vita propria der zellen des periostes," *Arch Pathol Anat Physiol Klin Med,* Vol. 155, 1899, pp. 428–464.

[4] Morpurgo B., "Die vita propria der zellen des periosts," *Arch Pathol Anat Physiol Klin Med,* Vol. 157, 1899, pp. 172–183.

[5] Carrel A., "The Preservation of Tissues and Its Application in Surgery," *J Am Med Assoc,* Vol. 59, 1912, pp. 523–527.

[6] Albee F. H., "The Fundamental Principles Involved in the Use of the Bone Graft in Surgery," *Am J Med Sci,* Vol. 149, 1915, pp. 313–325.

[7] Albee F. H., Discussion of Carrel A., "The Preservation of Tissues and its Application in Surgery," *J Am Med Assoc,* Vol. 59, 1912, pp. 527–528.

[8] Bush L. F., "The Use of Homogenous Bone Grafts: A preliminary report on the bone bank," *J Bone Joint Surg,* Vol. 29, 1947, pp. 620–628.

[9] Bush L. F. and Garber C. Z., "The Bone Bank," *J Am Med Assoc,* Vol. 137, 1948, pp. 588–594.

[10] Lexer E., "Joint Transplantation and Arthroplasty," *Surg Gynecol Obstet,* Vol. 40, 1925, p. 782.

[11] Hyatt G. W., "Fundamentals in the Use and Preservation of Homogenous Bone," *U.S. Armed Forces Med J,* Vol. 1, 1950, pp. 841–852.

[12] Hyatt G. W., "Storage," *Transplant Bull,* Vol. 1, 1954, pp. 159–160.

[13] Hyatt G. W., Turner T. C., Bassett C. A. L., Pate J. W., and Sawyer P. N., "New Methods for Preserving Bone, Skin and Blood Vessels," *Postgrad Med,* Vol. 12, 1952, pp. 239–254.

[14] Hyatt G. W. and Butler M.C., "Bone Grafting: The procurement, storage, and clinical use of bone homografts," *Instructional Course Lectures* XIV, R. B. Raney, Ed., American Academy of Orthopedic Surgeons, J. W. Edwards, Ed., Ann Arbor, MI, 1957, pp. 343–373.

[15] Ottolenghi C. E., "Massive Osteo and Osteo-articular Bone Grafts: Techniques and results of 62 cases," *Clin Orthop Rel Res,* Vol. 87, 1972, p. 156.

[16] Herndon C. H. and Chase S. W., "The Fate of Massive Autogenous and Homogenous Bone Grafts Including Articular Surfaces," *Surg Gynecol Obstet,* Vol. 273, 1954, pp. 98.

[17] Curtiss P. H., Jr, Powell A. E., and Herndon C. H., "Immunological Factors in Homogeneous-bone Transplantation. III. The Inability of Homogeneous Rabbit Bone to Induce Circulating Antibodies in Rabbits," *J Bone Joint Surg Am,* Vol. 41, 1959, p. 1482.

[18] Bonfiglio M., Jeter W. S., and Smith C.L., "The Immune Concept: Its relation to bone transplantation," *Ann N.Y. Acad Sci,* Vol. 59, 1955, p. 417.

[19] Parrish F. F., "Treatment of Bone Tumors by Total Excision and Replacement with Massive Autologous and Homologous Grafts," *J Bone Joint Surg Am*, Vol. 48, 1966, p. 968.

[20] Parrish F. F., "Allograft Replacement of All or Part of the End of a Long Bone Following Excision of a Tumor: report of twenty-one cases," *J Bone Joint Surg Am*, Vol. 55, 1973, pp. 1–22.

[21] Mankin H. J., Dopplet S. H., and Tomford W. W., "Clinical Experience with Allograft Implantation: The first 200 cases," *Clin Orthop Rel Res*, Vol. 174, 1983, pp. 69–86.

[22] *AATB–Standards for Tissue Banking 2002*, American Association of Tissue Banks Publishers, McLean, VA.

[23] *AATB Newsletter*, Vol. 24, July 2001.

[24] Eastlund T., "Infectious Disease Transmission Through Tissue Transplantation. Reducing the Risk Through Donor Selection," *Cell Transplant*, Vol. 4, 1995, pp. 455–477.

[25] Butler J. J. and Osborne B. N., "Lymph Node Enlargement in Patients with Unsuspected Human Immunodeficiency Virus Infections," *Hum Pathol*, Vol. 19, 1988, pp. 849–854.

[26] Buck B. E., Malinin T. I., and Brown M. D., "Bone Transplantation and Human Immunodeficiency Virus: an estimate of risk of acquired immunodeficiency syndrome (AIDS)," *Clin Orthop Rel Res*, Vol. 240, 1989, pp. 129–136.

[27] Schreiber G. B., Busch M. P., Kleinman S. H., and Korelitz J. J., "The Risk of Transfusion–transmitted viral infections," *N Engl J Med*, Vol. 334, 1996, pp. 1685–1690.

[28] Busch M. and Kleinman S. H., "Nucleic Acid Amplification Testing of Blood Donors for Transfusion—transmitted infectious diseases," *Transfusion*, Vol. 40, 2000, pp. 143–146.

[29] Glynn S. A., Kleinman S. H., Wright D. J., Busch M. P., "International Application of the Incidence Rate/Window Period Model," *Transfusion*, Vol. 42, 2000, pp. 966–972.

[30] CBER, "Guidance for Industry, Availability of Licensed Donor Screening Tests Labeled for Use with Cadaveric Blood Specimens," June 2000.

[31] Veen M. R., Bloem M. D., and Petit P. L. C., "Sensitivity and Negative Predictive Value of Swab-cultures in Musculoskeletal Allograft Procurement," *Clin Orthop Rel Res*, Vol. 300, 1994, pp. 259–263.

[32] Vehmeyer S. B. W., Bloem R. M., Deijkers R. L. M., Veen M. R., and Petit P. L. C., "A Comparative Study of Blood and Bone Marrow Cultures in Cadaveric Bone Donation," *J Hosp Inf*, Vol. 43, 1999, pp. 305–308.

[33] Deijkers R. L. M., Bloem R. M., Petit P. L. C., Vehmeyer S. B., and Veen M. R., "Contamination of Bone Allografts: Analysis of incidence and predisposing factor," *J Bone Joint Surg Br*, Vol. 79, 1997, pp. 61–166.

[34] Vehmeyer S. B. W., Bloem R. M., and Petit P. L. C., "Microbiology Screening of Post-Mortem Bone Donors – Two Case Reports," *J Hosp Inf*, Vol. 47, 2001, pp. 193–197.

[35] Forsell J. H. and Liesman J., "Analysis of Potential Causes of Positive Microbiological Cultures in Tissue Donors," *Cell and Tissue Banking,* Vol. 1, 2000, pp. 111–115.

[36] Jackson D. W., Windler G. E., and Simon T. M., "Intraarticular Reaction Associated with the Use of Freeze-dried, Ethylene Oxide-sterilized Bone-patella Tendon-Bone Allografts in the Reconstruction of the Anterior Cruciate Ligament," *Am J Sports Med*, Vol. 18, 1990, pp. 1–11.

[37] Spire B., Dormont D., Barre-Sinoussi F., Montagnier L., and Chermann J. C., "Inactivation of 7 Lymphadenopathy-associated Virus by Heat, Gamma Rays, and Ultraviolet light," *Lancet*, Vol. 1, 1985, pp. 188–189.

[38] Conway B., Tomford W. W., Hirsch M. S., Schooley R. T., and Mankin H. J., "Effects of Gamma Irradiation on HIV-1 in a Bone Allograft Model," *Trans Orthop Res Soc*, Vol. 15, 1990, p. 225.

[39] Conway B., Tomford W., Mankin H. J., Hirsch M. S., and Schooley R. T., "Radiosensitivity of HIV-1 – Potential Application to Sterilization of Bone Allografts [letter]," *AIDS*, Vol. 5, 1991, pp. 608–609.

[40] Kitchen A. D., Mann G. F., Harrison J. F., and Zuckerman A. J., "Effect of Gamma Irradiation on the Human Immunodeficiency Virus and Human Coagulation Proteins," *Vox Sang*, Vol. 56, 1989, pp. 223–229.

[41] Campbell D. G., Li P., Stephenson A. J., and Oakeshott R. D., "Sterilization of HIV by Gamma Irradiation. A Bone Allograft Model," *Internat Orthop*, Vol. 18, 1994, pp. 172–176.

[42] Campbell D. G. and Li P., "Sterilization of HIV with Irradiation: relevance to infected bone allografts," *Australian and New Zealand J Surg,* Vol. 69, 1999, pp. 517–521.

[43] Fideler B. M., Vangsness C. T., Jr., Moore T., Li Z., and Rasheed S., "Effects of Gamma Irradiation on the Human Immunodeficiency Virus. A Study in Frozen Human Bone-patellar Ligament-bone Grafts Obtained from Infected Cadavera," *J Bone Joint Surg Am*, Vol. 76, 1994, pp. 1032–1035.

[44] Fideler B. M., Vangsness C. T. Jr., Lu B., Orlando C., and Moore T., "Gamma Irradiation: effects on biochemical properties of human bone-patellar tendon-bone allografts," *Am J Sports Med*, Vol. 23, 1995, pp. 643–646.

[45] Smith R. A., Ingels J., Lochemes J. J., Dutkowsky J. P., and Pifer L. L., "Gamma Irradiation of HIV-1," *J Orthop Res*, Vol. 19, 2001, pp. 815–819.

[46] Burwell R. G., "Studies in the Transplantation of Bone. VIII. Treated Composite Homografts-Autografts of Cancellous Bone: an analysis of inductive mechanisms in bone transplantation," *J Bone Joint Surg Br*, Vol. 48, 1966, pp. 532–566.

[47] Buring K. and Urist M. R., "Effects of Ionizing Radiation on the Bone Induction Principle in the Matrix of Bone Implants," *Clin Orthop Rel Res*, Vol. 55, 1967, pp. 225–234.

[48] Urist M. R. and Hernandez A., "Excitation Transfer in Bone. Deleterious Effects of Cobalt 60 Radiation-sterilization of Bank Bone," *Arch Surg*, Vol. 109, 1974, pp. 486–493.

[49] Puolakkainen P. A., Ranchalis J. E., Strong D. M., and Twardzik D. R., "The Effect of Sterilization on Transforming Growth Factor Isolated from Demineralized Human Bone," *Transfusion*, Vol. 33, 1993, pp. 679–685.

[50] Wientroub S. and Reddi A. H., "Influence of Irradiation on the Osteoinductive Potential of Demineralized Bone Matrix," *Calcif Tissue Int*, Vol. 42, 1988, pp. 255–260.

[51] Dziedzic-Goclawska A., Ostroski K., Stachowicz W., Michalik J., and Grzesik W., "Effect of Radiation Sterilization on the Osteoinductive Properties and Rate of Remodeling of Bone Implants Preserved by Lyophilization and Deep-freezing," *Clin Orthop Rel Res*, Vol. 272, 1991, pp. 30–37.

[52] Ijiri S., Yamamuro T., Nakamura T., Kotani S., and Notoya K., "Effect of Sterilization on Bone Morphogenetic Protein," *J Orthop Res*, Vol. 12, 1994, pp. 628–636.

[53] Moreau M. F., Gallois Y., Basie M. F., and Chappard D., "Gamma Irradiation of Human Bone Allografts Alters Medullary Lipids and Release Toxic compounds for Osteoblast-like Cells," *Biomaterials*, Vol. 21, 2000, pp. 369–376.

[54] Pelker R. R., Friedlaender G. E., and Markham T. C., "Biomechanical Properties of Bone Allografts," *Clin Orthop Rel Res*, Vol. 174, 1983, pp. 54–57.

[55] Pelker R. R. and Friedlaender G. E., "Biomechanical Aspects of Bone Autografts and Allografts," *Orthop Clin North Am*, Vol. 18, 1987, pp. 235–239.

[56] Pelker R. R. and Friedlaender G. E., "Biomechanical Aspects of Bone Autografts and Allografts," *Bone & Cartilage Allografts*, G. E. Friedlaener, V. M. Goldberg, Eds., American Academy of Orthopedic Surgeons, 1991.

[57] Currey J. D., Foreman J., Laketic I., Mitchell J., Pegg D. E., and Reilly G. C., "Effects of Ionizing Radiation on the Mechanical Properties of Human Bone," *J Orthop Res*, Vol. 15, 1997, pp. 111–117.

[58] Bright R. and Burchardt H., "The Biomechanical Properties of Preserved Bone Grafts,"*Osteochondral Allografts: biology, banking, and clinical applications*, G. E, Friedlaender, H. J. Mankin, K. W. Sell, Eds., Boston, Little, Brown and Co., 1983, pp. 241–247.

[59] Anderson M. J., Keyak J. H., and Skinner H. B., "Compressive Mechanical Properties of Human Cancellous Bone after Gamma Irradiation," *J Bone Joint Surg Am*, Vol. 74, 1992, pp. 747–752.

[60] Zhang Y., Homsi D., Gates K., and Wolfinbarger L., "A Comprehensive Study of Physical Parameters, Biomechanical Properties, and Statistical Correlations of Iliac Crest Bone Wedges Used in Spinal Surgery. IV. Effect of Gamma Irradiation on Mechanical and Material Properties," *Spine*, Vol. 19, 1994, pp. 304–308.

[61] Jinno T., Miric A., Feighan J., Kirk S. K., Davy D. T., and Stevenson S., "The Effects of Processing and Low Dose Irradiation on Cortical Bone Grafts" *Clin Orthop Rel Res*, Vol. 375, 2000, pp. 275–285.

[62] Simonian P. T., Conrad E. U., Chapman J. R., Harrington M. S., and Chansky H. A., *Clin Orthop Rel Res*, Vol. 302, 1994, pp. 290–296.

[63] Voggenreiter G., Ascheri R., Blumel G., and Schmit-Neurerburg K. P., "Extracorporeal Irradiation and Incorpation of Bone Grafts. Autogeneic Cortical Grafts Studied in Rats,"*Acta Orthop Scand*, Vol. 67, 1996, pp. 583–588.

[64] Hamer A. J., Strachan J. R., Black M. M., Ibbotson C. J., Stockley I., and Elson R. A., "Biomechanical Properties of Cortical Allograft Bone Using a New Method of Bone Strength Measurement: A comparison of fresh, fresh-frozen and irradiated bone," *J Bone Joint Surg Br*, Vol. 78, 1996, pp. 363–368.

[65] Hamer A. J., Stockley I., and Elson R. A., "Change in Allograft Bone Irradiated at Different Temperatures," *J Bone Joint Surg Br*, Vol. 81, 1999, pp. 342–344.

[66] Randall L. R., Pelker R. R., Friedlaender G. E., Goldsmith S. L., and Panjabi M. M., "Sequential Dependence of Freeze-Drying and Irradiation on Biomechanical Properties of Rat Bone," *Am J Orthop*, Vol. 3, 2002, pp. 129–134.

[67] Loty B., Courpied J. P., and Tomeno B., "Bone Allografts Sterilized by Irradiation: Biological Properties, Procurement and Results of Massive Allografts," *Internat Orthop*, Vol. 14, 1990, pp. 237–242.

[68] Hernigon P., Delephine G., Goutallier D., and Julierson, "Massive Allograft Sterilized by Irradiation," *J Bone Joint Surg Br*, Vol. 75, 1993, pp. 904–913.

[69] Lietman S. A., Tomford W. W., Gebhardt M. C., Springfield D. S., and Mankin H. J., "Complications of Irradiated Allografts in Orthopedic Tumor Surgery," *Clin Orthop Rel Res*, Vol. 375, 2000, pp. 214–217.

[70] Fideler B. M., Vangsness C. T., Jr, Moore T., Li Z., and Rasheed S., "Effects of Gamma Irradiation on the Human Immunodeficiency Virus. A Study in Frozen Human Bone-patellar Ligament-bone Grafts Obtained from Infected Cadavera," *J Bone Joint Surg Am*, Vol. 76, 1994, pp. 1032–1035.

[71] Rasmussen T. J, Feder S. M., Butler D. L., and Noyes F. R., "The Effects of 4 Mrad Gamma Irradiation on the Initial Mechanical Properties of Bone-patellar Tendon-Bone Allografts," *Arthroscopy*, Vol. 10, 1994, pp. 188–197.

[72] Butler D. L., Oster D.M., Feder S. M., Grood E. S., and Noyes F. R., "Effects of Gamma Irradiation on the Biomechanics of Patellar Tendon Allografts of the ACL in the Goat," *Trans Orthop Res Soc*, Vol. 16, 1991, p. 205.

[73] Goertzen M. J., Clahsen H., Burrig K. F., and Schulitz K. P., "Anterior Cruciate Ligament Reconstruction Using Cryopreserved Irradiated Bone-ACL-bone Allograft Transplants," *Knee Surg Sports Traumat Arthrosc*, Vol. 2, 1994, pp. 150–157.

[74] Gibbons M. J., Butler D. L., Grood E. S., Bylski-Austrow D. I., Levy M. S., and Noyes F. R., "Effects of Gamma Irradiation on the Initial Mechanical and Material Properties of Goat Bone – Patellar Tendon – Bone Allograft," *J Orthop Res*, Vol. 9, 1991, pp. 209–218.

[75] Bettin D., Rullkotter V., and Polster J., "Primary Biomechanical Influences of Different Sterilization Methods on Freeze-dried Bone-ligament Transplantation," *Arch Ortho P Trauma Surg (Germany)*, Vol. 119(3–4), 1994, pp. 236–240.

[76] Yahia L. H., Drouin G., and Zukor D., "The Irradiation Effect on the Initial Mechanical Properties of Meniscal Grafts" *Biomed Mater Eng*, Vol. 3, 1993, pp. 211–221.

[77] Nicols, R. L., "CDC: Emerging Infectious Diseases – Preventing Surgical Site Infections: A Surgeons Perspective," *CDC*, Vol. 7, April 2001, pp. 1–11.

[78] James J. I. P., "Tuberculosis Transmitted by Banked Bone," *J Bone Joint Surg Br*, Vol. 35, 1953, p. 578.

[79] Tomford, W. W., Starkweather R. J., and Goldman M. H., "A study of the Clinical Incidence of Infection in the Use of Banked Allograft Bone," *J Bone Joint Surg Am*, Vol. 63, 1981, pp. 244–248.

[80] Lord C. F., Gebhardt M. C., Tomford W. W., and Mankin H. J.,"Infection in Bone Allografts: Incidence, nature, and treatment," *J Bone Joint Surg Am*, Vol. 70, 1988, pp. 369–376.

[81] Tomford W. W., Thongphasuk J., Mankin H. J., and Ferraro M. J., "Frozen Musculoskeletal Allografts: A study of the clinical incidence and causes of infection associated with their use," *J Bone Joint Surg Am*, Vol. 72, 1990, pp. 1137–1143.

[82] Centers for Disease Control, "Unexplained Deaths Following Knee Surgery– Minnesota 2001," *MMWR*, Vol. 50, 2001, p. 1080.

[83] Centers for Disease Control, "Allograft – Associated Bacterial Infections – United States 2002," *MMWR*, Vol. 51, 2002, pp. 207–210.

[84] Shutkin N. M., "Homologous-serum Hepatitis Following the Use of Refrigerated Bone-bank Bone: Report of a case," *J Bone Joint Surg Am*, Vol. 36, 1954, pp. 160–162.

[85] Eggen B. M. and Nordbo S. A., "Transmission of HCV by Organ Transplantation [letter]," *New Eng J Med*, 1992, pp. 326:411.

[86] Conrad E. U., Gretch D. R., Obermeyer K. R., Moogk M. S., Sayers M., Wilson J. J., et al., "Transmission of the Hepatitis-C Virus by Tissue Transplantation," *J Bone Joint Surg Am*, Vol. 77, 1955, pp. 214–224.

[87] Tugwell, B. D., Patel, P., Williams, I. T., Thomas, A. R., Homan, H., Hedbeg, K., and Ciesiak, P. R., "Hepatitis C Virus (HCV Transmission to Tissue and Organ Recipients from an Antibody-Negative Donor," *Presentation to American Society of Microbiology Annual Meeting 2002*, United States, 2002.

[88] Centers for Disease Control, "Transmission of HIV Through Bone Transplantation: Case report and public health recommendations," *MMWR*, Vol. 37, 1988, pp. 587–598.

[89] Simonds R. J., Holmberg S. D., Hurwitz R. L., et al., "Transmission of Human Immunodeficiency Virus Type 1 From a Seronegative Organ and Tissue Donor," *N Eng J Med*, 1992, Vol. 326, pp. 726–732.

[90] Centers for Disease Control, "MMWR Update: Investigations of West Nile Virus Infections in Recipients of Organ Transplantation and Blood Transfusion," *MMWR*, Vol. 51, 2002, pp. 833–836.

The reader is directed to additional excellent references:

[1] Friedlaender G. D., "Appropriate Screening for Prevention of Infection Transmission by Musculoskeletal Allografts," *AAOS Instructional Course Lectures*, Vol. 49, 2000, pp. 615–619.

[2] Czitrom A., Winkler H. (Eds.), *Orthopedic Allograft Surgery*, Springer-Verlag, Vienna, NY, 1996.

[3] Tomford, W. W., "Current Concepts Review: Transmission of Disease through Transplantation of Musculoskeletal Allografts," *J Bone Joint Dis*, Vol. 77A, 1995, pp. 1742–1754.

[4] William W. T. (Ed.), *Musculoskeletal Tissue Banking*, Raven Press 1993.

[5] Czitrom A., Gross A. E. (eds), *Allografts in Orthopedic Practice*, Williams & Wilkins, Baltimore, M. D., 1992.

[6] Malinin, T., "Acquisition and Banking of Bone Allografts." *Bone Grafts & Bone Substitutes*, M. B. Habel, A. H. Reddi (Eds)., W.B. Saunders Company, Philadelphia PA, 1992.

[7] Friedlaender G. E., Goldberg V. M., (eds), *Bone and Cartilage Allografts: Biology and Clinical Applications*. Park Ridge, IL, American Academy of Orthopedic Surgeons, 1991.

APPENDIX I

AATB-AOPO-NFDA

Best Practices for Organ and Tissue Donation

In order to facilitate the organ/tissue donation process and accommodate the specific requirements of a funeral service and burial, the American Association of Tissue Banks (AATB) and the Association of Organ Procurement Organizations (AOPO) [hereafter referred to as "recovery agency(ies)] and the National Funeral Directors Association (NFDA) have adopted the following "Best Practices."

Mutual support and recognition of the roles each organization plays in the donation process is imperative in order for any of these "Best Practices" to succeed. In achieving the goals outlined in these "Best Practices," we not only strengthen our individual organizations, but we form together a strong cord that will better serve the families that we mutually share and, ultimately, each recipient in the transplant communities.

Each organization will promote and educate its members, state associations and others on its contents. This effort is essential if funeral directors, tissue banks and organ procurement organizations are to successfully meet the goals of the federal government's initiative to increase organ and tissue donation throughout the United States.

1. **NOTIFICATION**

   a. **The recovery agency(ies) should notify the funeral director handling the funeral arrangements for the donor family as soon as details of the anticipated recovery are known. This notification should follow the consent process for the donation. In the event that a funeral home is not known at the time of consent, this notification will take place as soon as the donor family has determined a funeral home.**

   b. The recovery agency(ies) handling the donation should, at the time of the initial contact, notify the funeral director of the following:

      i. The nature of the donation;
      ii. The geographic location of the donation recovery;
      iii. The anticipated timing of the donation recovery;
      iv. A contact person or number for the funeral director to call for updates, questions or concerns; and
      v. Next of kin information.

   c. **Further, the recovery agency(ies) should contact the funeral director as the situation**

develops or changes, especially as it relates to the pick-up time and/or location of the donor body. This is especially important when a donor body is to be transported to a medical examiner/coroner for tissue recovery, autopsy or other purpose.

d.   The recovery agency's representative will ensure that the medical examiner/coroner has the name and phone number of the funeral director/home (if known), and that the funeral director should be notified when the body is ready for pick-up.

e.   Finally, the recovery agency(ies) should contact the funeral director/home when the body is ready for pick-up.

2.   **DISCLOSURE**

a.   Once a donor has been medically qualified, the recovery agency's representative who interviews the donor family should inform them that there are many factors that may impact the timing of the funeral, including the timing of the recovery procedure and/or autopsy that need to be completed.

b.   The consent process discussion, or the consent form where applicable, should also include an explanation regarding the impact that the donation process may have on burial arrangements and on the appearance of the body. The family will be encouraged to discuss any particular needs in relation to the timing of the funeral, clothing preferences, and other related issues with their funeral director.

c.   Any consent for anatomical gift form signed by a family should be specific in describing the organs/tissues/eyes to be recovered.

3.   **RECOVERY PROCEDURES**

To facilitate the embalming and preparation process, the following procedures are recommended:

a.   All involved major arteries should be ligated to ensure the integrity of the vascular system;

b.   Replace all recovered bones with prostheses;

c.   Contact the funeral director to determine the preferred type of incision closure prior to the completion of the recovery;

d.   Consider using a U or Y chest incision rather than a midline opening for the chest;

e.   Elevate the head with a head block especially with eye recovery or a prolonged recovery process; and

f.   No facial bone recovery if a viewing (private or public) is planned.

4.   **REIMBURSEMENT**

Every recovery agency should establish a policy regarding compensation of funeral directors if additional time and materials are required to prepare a donor body for embalming and/or viewing. The funeral home should not assess the donor family any additional charges, resulting from the donation.

5. **COMMUNICATION/EDUCATION**

The most important and essential aspect of a successful relationship between funeral directors and recovery agencies is communication and a better understanding by each of the operational aspects of the other. Therefore, to ensure and facilitate successful organ and tissue donation and the funeral and burial processes for the families we all serve, it is imperative that funeral directors and recovery agencies reach out to each other and establish those lines of communication. By doing so, the issues and concerns of each can be addressed and resolved. This outreach should also include actual visits by each to the other's place of business. These visits may promote a greater appreciation for each entity's role and contribute to a strong, lasting relationship.

6. **SUPPORT**

The NFDA will publicly support, and encourage its members to support the concept of donation. The funeral director should respect the family's wishes to donate, and use his/her relationship with the donor family to facilitate the donation recovery process. If the funeral director takes exception to a specific donation, he/she should communicate his/her concerns to the tissue bank/OPO before expressing them to the donor family. Ideally, the funeral director will view donation as an integral part of the donor family's efforts to deal with the loss, and as an aid in the progression of the grieving process.

All recovery agency members have an obligation to be cognizant of the manner in which donation and its' effects on the donor body are discussed with families. The recovery agency(ies) should refrain from telling families that absolutely no change to the donor's appearance is guaranteed. The recovery agency(ies) should also be aware of the timing of the donation process and its' effect on the funeral service itself.

Adopted March 11, 2001

APPENDIX II

Sample Questionnaire for Potential Tissue Donors
Medical History and Behavioral Risk Assessment

Page 1

Donor Name/I.D.#UNOS I.D.# (if Organ Donor): _____ DOB _____

Person Interviewed A: _____ Relationship to potential donor: _____

Person Interviewed B: _____ Relationship to potential donor: _____

Place of interview: _____ Date of interview: _____

Person Conducting Interview _____
and Completing Form: (Print Name)   (Title)

Signature: _____

To be asked of the interviewee(s):
Do you feel that you knew the potential donor well enough to answer questions regarding medical/behavioral history?

❏ Yes ❏ No

The interviewee should be instructed to answer all questions, "to the best of your knowledge." The interviewer should comment and elaborate on all questions answered "yes."

1. Has the potential donor:		
a. Been treated by a physician in the past two years or have a family physician?	❏ No	❏ Yes, physician name and contact info _____
b. Been hospitalized in the past two years? Why and When?	❏ No	❏ Yes, hospital_____
c. Been treated in a psychiatric facility in the past two years?	❏ No	❏ Yes, facility _____
2. Did the potential donor have any serious illnesses, infections or surgical procedures in the past? If yes, please list.	❏ No	❏ Yes
3. Did the potential donor take any medications, vitamins or supplements on a regular basis or recently? Please list.	❏ No	❏ Yes
4. Did the potential donor use tobacco products?	❏ No	❏ Yes
a. Cigarettes?	❏ No	❏ Yes packs per day_____ for _____years
b. Other?	❏ No	❏ Yes _____
c. Quit using tobacco products?	❏ No	❏ Yes _____ When?_____
5. Did the potential donor drink alcohol? How much and how long? What type?	❏ No	❏ Yes

This uniform donor assessment record may be helpful for screening potential tissue donors. While, ultimately, it is the responsibility of each tissue bank to determine what procedures are necessary to help ensure the safety of transplantable tissues, this document should be viewed as presenting guidelines that have widespread acceptance.

Sample Questionnaire for Potential Tissue Donors

Medical History and Behavioral Risk Assessment

Page 2

6. Did the potential donor ever use non-prescribed drugs or other substances, e.g. cocaine, marijuana, steroids, inhalants?	❑ No	❑ Yes
What, how much and when? By what route?		
7. Has the potential donor ever been exposed to toxic substances, e.g. lead, pesticides or other? When?	❑ No	❑ Yes
What was the potential donor's occupation?	Occupation	
8. In the past three years has the potential donor traveled outside of the United States (except Canada)? Describe where and when.	❑ No	❑ Yes
a. Been diagnosed or treated for malaria or Chagas disease?	❑ No	❑ Yes
b. Taken anti-malarial drugs?	❑ No	❑ Yes
c. Been in a malaria endemic area in the past year?	❑ No	❑ Yes
9. Has the potential donor ever received blood transfusions or blood products?	❑ No	❑ Yes
When?		
10. Was the potential donor? a. Ever refused as a blood donor or told not to donate?	❑ No	❑ Yes
Why? When? b. Ever a blood donor?	❑ No	❑ Yes
11. Did the potential donor ever receive a human or animal organ or tissue transplant, e.g., bone, cornea, skin, heart, kidney, dura mater?	❑ No	❑ Yes
What kind and when?		
12. In the past 12 months did the potential donor have any of the following?		
a. Tattoo?	❑ No	❑ Yes
b. Ear/body piercing?	❑ No	❑ Yes
c. Acupuncture?	❑ No	❑ Yes
d. Accidental needle stick?	❑ No	❑ Yes
e. A bite in the past 6 months from an animal suspected of rabies?	❑ No	❑ Yes
If yes, provide details such as body site, when, by whom and how many?		
For a, b or c, were needles shared?	❑ No	❑ Yes
13. In the past 12 months was the potential donor: a. Vaccinated or immunized for any reason?	❑ No	❑ Yes
b. Any in the past 4 weeks? What vaccinations?	❑ No	❑ Yes
c. When?	❑ No	❑ Yes
Was the potential donor vaccinated for hepatitis B?	❑ No	❑ Yes
14. Was the potential donor ever given human pituitary derived growth hormone?	❑ No	❑ Yes

Interviewer's initials_____   Date_____   Donor ID#_____

Rev 1/1/02

Sample Questionnaire for Potential Tissue Donors
Medical History and Behavioral Risk Assessment

Page 3

15. Did the potential donor have any history of:		
a. Heart disease?	❑ No	❑ Yes_____
b. High blood pressure? For how long?	❑ No	❑ Yes_____ years
c. Chest pain?	❑ No	❑ Yes_____
d. Poor circulation especially in the legs?	❑ No	❑ Yes_____
e. Leg ulcers?	❑ No	❑ Yes_____
f. Taking medication for heart or blood pressure problems? If so, what?	❑ No	❑ Yes_____

16. Did the potential donor:		
a. Have any type of liver disease or hepatitis?	❑ No	❑ Yes_____
b. Have any history of jaundice?	❑ No	❑ Yes_____
c. Ever have a positive test for hepatitis?	❑ No	❑ Yes_____
d. Live with or have sexual relations with persons diagnosed with viral hepatitis in the past 12 months?	❑ No	❑ Yes_____

17. Did the potential donor have:		
a. Any kidney related diseases?	❑ No	❑ Yes_____
b. Kidney stones?	❑ No	❑ Yes_____
c. Frequent infections?	❑ No	❑ Yes_____
d. Kidney dialysis treatments? When and how long?	❑ No	❑ Yes_____

18. Did the potential donor have a history of:		
a. Digestive or intestinal problems?	❑ No	❑ Yes_____
b. Bloody stools?	❑ No	❑ Yes_____
c. Intestinal surgery or intestinal cancer?	❑ No	❑ Yes_____
d. Recent weight loss? How much? Reason?	❑ No	❑ Yes_____
Height _____ Weight _____		

19. Did the potential donor:		
a. Have a history of diabetes ?	❑ No	❑ Yes_____
b. If yes, did he/she require medication? name of medication? length of treatment?	❑ No	❑ Yes_____
c. Have a history of gestational diabetes?	❑ No	❑ Yes_____

20. Did the potential donor have any history of:		
a. Lung disease?	❑ No	❑ Yes_____
b. Asthma?	❑ No	❑ Yes_____
c. Emphysema?	❑ No	❑ Yes_____
d. A positive skin test for tuberculosis? If yes, was there follow-up?	❑ No	❑ Yes_____
e. Treatment for tuberculosis (TB)? When?	❑ No	❑ Yes_____

21. Has the potential donor:		
a. Ever had cancer? What type? When?	❑ No	❑ Yes_____
b. Ever received radiation therapy or drugs for cancer?	❑ No	❑ Yes_____
number of years free of cancer _____years		
date of last check up _____		

22. Did the potential donor have a history of any of the following autoimmune diseases:		
a. Rheumatoid arthritis?	❑ No	❑ Yes_____
b. Systemic lupus erythematosus?	❑ No	❑ Yes_____
c. Polyarteritis nodosa?	❑ No	❑ Yes_____
d. Sarcoidosis?	❑ No	❑ Yes_____
e. Other?	❑ No	❑ Yes_____

Sample Questionnaire for Potential Tissue Donors

Medical History and Behavioral Risk Assessment

Page 4

23. Did the potential donor suffer from any type of neurologic or brain disease such as:		
a. Alzheimer's?	❏ No	❏ Yes_____
b. Seizures?	❏ No	❏ Yes_____
c. Periods of confusion or recent memory loss?	❏ No	❏ Yes_____
d. History of brain tumor?	❏ No	❏ Yes_____
e. Polio or degenerative neurological disease?	❏ No	❏ Yes_____
f. Encephalitis?	❏ No	❏ Yes_____
Has the potential donor or any of the donor's blood relatives had Creutzfeldt-Jakob Disease (CJD)?	❏ No	❏ Yes_____
Or been told they were at risk for CJD?	❏ No	❏ Yes_____
24. Did the potential donor have any history of bone or joint disease?	❏ No	❏ Yes_____
a. Rheumatoid arthritis?	❏ No	❏ Yes_____
b. Other arthritis?	❏ No	❏ Yes_____
c. Osteoporosis?	❏ No	❏ Yes_____
d. Osteomyelitis?	❏ No	❏ Yes_____
e. Broken bones?	❏ No	❏ Yes_____
25. Did the potential donor have a history of skin infections such as leprosy, eczema, dermatitis or inflammatory skin diseases?	❏ No	❏Yes_____
CURRENT CRITERIA FOR HIGH RISK BEHAVIOR		
26. In the past twelve months has the potential donor had or been treated for any sexually transmitted disease such as syphilis, gonorrhea, genital herpes or venereal warts?	❏ No	❏Yes_____
Or had sexual relations with such an individual?	❏ No	❏Yes_____
27. Has the potential donor recently exhibited or experienced:		
a. Unexplained weakness, fatigue or flu-like symptoms such as persistent cough, cold, shortness of breath, swollen lymph nodes for greater than one month	❏ No	❏Yes_____
b. Nausea, vomiting, persistent diarrhea	❏ No	❏ Yes_____
c. Night sweats or fever >100.5° F. for greater than 10 days?	❏ No	❏ Yes_____
d. Blue or purple spots on the skin or mucous membranes?	❏ No	❏ Yes_____
e. Significant weight loss or opportunistic (unusual) infections?	❏ No	❏ Yes_____
28. Has the potential donor ever had a positive test for HIV?	❏ No	❏ Yes_____
Has the potential donor been tested for HIV?	❏ No	❏ Yes
When? Result?		
29A. Male Donors: Has the potential donor had sexual relations with another male in the past 5 years or ever?	❏ No ❏ Female	❏ Yes_____
29B. Female Donors: Has the potential donor had sexual relations with males who have had sex with other males in the past 5 years or ever?	❏ No ❏ Male	❏ Yes_____

Interviewer's initials_____   Date_____   Donor ID#_____

Rev 1/1/02

Sample Questionnaire for Potential Tissue Donors
Medical History and Behavioral Risk Assessment   Page 5

30. Has the potential donor ever used a needle to inject drugs into the vein, muscle, or under the skin for nonmedical use?	❑ No	❑ Yes ❑ When _____
Or had sexual relations with such an individual in the past 12 months?	❑ No	❑ Yes_____
31. Has the potential donor received human-derived clotting factor concentrates for hemophilia or related clotting disorders?	❑ No	❑ Yes_____
Or had sexual relations with such an individual in the past 12 months?	❑ No	❑ Yes_____
32. Has the potential donor engaged in sex in exchange for money or drugs in the past 5 years?	❑ No	❑ Yes_____
Or had sexual relations with such an individual in the past 12 months?	❑ No	❑ Yes_____
33. Was the potential donor exposed to known or suspected viral hepatitis or HIV-infected blood through accidental needlestick or through contact with an open wound, non-intact skin, or mucous membrane in the past 12 months?	❑ No	❑ Yes_____
Or had sexual relations with such an individual in the past 12 months?	❑ No	❑ Yes_____
34. Has the potential donor had sex in the past 12 months with any person known or suspected to have viral hepatitis or HIV infection?	❑ No	❑ Yes_____
35. Has the potential donor:		
a. Ever been in jail? When? How long?	❑ No	❑ Yes
b. Ever been an inmate of a correctional system or jail or mental institution for more than 72 hours in the past 12 months?	❑ No	❑ Yes_____
c. Ever been released from a correctional system, jail or mental institution in the past 12 months?	❑ No ❑ No	❑ Yes_____ ❑ Yes_____
PEDIATRIC DONORS		
36. A. Was the child 18 months of age or less?	❑ No	❑ Yes_____
36. B. If under 5 years of age, was the child breast fed within the past 12 months? **If the answer to either question 36A or 36B is yes, to determine if a pediatric donor was born to a mother with or at risk for HIV or viral hepatitis infection, a separate Medical History and Behavioral Risk Assessment questionnaire must be completed for the mother.**	❑ No	❑ Yes_____
EYE DONORS		
37. Did the potential donor have a history of diseases, infections, or surgeries involving the eyes?	❑ No	❑ Yes_____

a. Glaucoma?
    b. Cataracts?
    c. Corneal disease?
    d. Laser surgery?
    e. Radial keratotomy?
	❑ No
	❑ No
	❑ No
	❑ No
	❑ No
		❑ Yes_____
		❑ Yes_____
		❑ Yes_____
		❑ Yes_____
		❑ Yes_____

Did the potential donor have an eye physician?	❑ No	❑ Yes_____

Sample Questionnaire for Potential Tissue Donors

Medical History and Behavioral Risk Assessment

Page 6

ALL DONORS	
38. Having answered many questions about medical diseases and behavioral risk-factors, do you now have any concerns that it might not be safe to proceed with organ or tissue donation?	❏ No ❏ Yes_____

Are there other individuals that may provide additional information regarding any of these questions? ❏ Yes   ❏ No

NAME_____ **TELEPHONE**_____

RELATIONSHIP_____

ADDITIONAL COMMENTS: (please refer to question numbers where applicable)

_____

_____

_____

_____

_____

_____

_____

_____

_____

_____

_____

_____

Interviewer's initials_____   Date_____   Donor ID#_____

Rev 1/1/02

Clinical Perspectives on the Use of Bone Graft Based on Allografts*

by Scott Hofer, [1] *D.O., Seth S. Leopold,* [2] *M.D., and Joshua J. Jacobs,* [3] *M.D.*

INTRODUCTION

ALLOGRAFT BONE AND BONE GRAFT substitutes based on human allograft are widely used in orthopedic surgery. Some of the more common indications for the use of human bone allograft and its derivatives include the use of large structural allografts in tumor reconstructions, morcellized cancellous grafts for a variety of joint arthroplasty and trauma applications, as well as demineralized bone matrix (DBM) products to augment arthrodesis procedures in the hand, foot, spine, and elsewhere.

Bone allografts were used clinically as early as 1909 by Macewen [102]. Today, revision hip arthroplasty consumes more donor bone than does primary hip replacement or other areas within orthopedic surgery [52], and demineralized bone matrix and other bone graft substitute are seeing wider use [2,50,76,81,85,115,134,138,142,158–160,168, 169]. However, large prospective studies still have not been done to evaluate many common indications.

Advantages of using allograft bone, compared to autograft, include decreases in operative time, blood loss, donor site complications, postoperative pain, and (in some series) length of hospital stay [45,146,176,177]. The potential risks of allograft include transmission of infectious diseases, fracture of structural grafts, and nonunion [9,43,74]. Since the institution of strict donor screening and tissue testing there have been only two reported incidences of HIV transmission from allografts [23,151].

The means of preparation of the graft material has been shown to affect graft performance in certain settings [14,181,182], and the type of graft selected (cortical, cancellous, or bone-graft substitute) affects the rate of healing and the strength of the site receiving the graft [74]. Broadly, any material used for bone grafting will provide one or more of the following properties: osteoconductive scaffolding, osteoinductive stimulation of new bone formation, and/or osteogenic potential for the growth and differentiation of bone cell lines [8,12,14,55,132,163]. Cortical bone grafts also provide a measure of initial structural strength that is useful in certain applications, particularly in the spine, hand,

[1]Major, United States Army Medical Corps, Orthopaedic Surgery Service, William Beaumont Army Medical Center, El Paso, TX 79920.
[2]Department of Othopaedic Surgery and Sports Medicine, University of Washington School of Medicine, Seattle, WA 98195.
[3]Orthopedic Surgery, Rush-Presbyterian-St. Luke's Medical Center, Chicago, IL 60612.
*Mandatory disclaimer: The views expressed in this article are those of the authors and do not reflect the offical policy of the Department of Defense or the U. S. Government.

and foot [73,78,91,105,119,125,127,139,140,154,165,171,173]. The present review summarizes the contemporary clinical literature on the use of allograft and allograft-based bone graft substitutes for non-trauma applications within clinical orthopedics.

BASIC SCIENCE FOR CLINICIANS

Bone allograft materials have several different properties that can be used to assist in surgical reconstructions: osteoconductivity, osteoinductivity, osteogenic potential, and varying amounts of initial structural strength or capacity to bear load [12,55,132]. The process of graft preparation may affect all of these factors. Fresh allografts, in theory, offer a finite but non-zero number of viable cells; as such, these grafts have the highest osteogenic potential. These grafts also offer an osteoconductive scaffolding, osteoinductive growth factors, and, depending on how much cortical bone is used, good initial strength for load-bearing reconstructions. However, fresh grafts have a high degree of immunogenicity, and carry a risk of disease transmission; because of those disadvantages, fresh bulk allografts are rarely used in the clinical setting. Fresh-frozen allografts are maintained at temperatures below –60°C to diminish enzymatic degradation, maintain the graft's structural properties, and decrease immunogenicity. Fresh-frozen grafts are valuable in composite osteochondral allografts, which are used in tumor reconstructions and sports medicine applications [1,18,25,27,28,31,32,60,106,108, 154]; both of those settings take advantage of the availability of viable cartilage cells at the joint surface. Fresh-frozen cancellous allografts are preferred for a revision technique used in hip replacement surgery called impaction grafting [1,18,25,27,28,31,32,60,106, 108,154]; in that technique, the favorable compliance properties of the graft, once thawed to room temperature, permit packing cancellous bone tightly without the morcellized graft crumbling. Lyophilization, or freeze drying, involves the removal of water from the tissue which, when combined with vacuum packing, can lead to extended shelf life at room temperature. This process decreases anitigenicity and maintains the graft's osteoconductive properties, but destroys the osteoprogenitor cells and thus eliminates any osteogenic or osteoinductive properties [8,55]. A product derived from allograft bone tissue, called demineralized bone matrix, is produced by acid demineralization of donor bone. The process destroys the osteoconductive properties but maintains osteoinductive factors, and decreases antigenicity and risk of infectious disease transmission [55].

Allograft bone incorporates differently depending on the type of bone that composes the graft specimen. Structural grafts consisting largely of cortical bone such as intercalary allografts typically are replaced by creeping substitution [43,44,55,105,132]. In time, such grafts undergo substantial resorption, and offer a good measure of initial structural integrity, but can weaken as the creeping substitution takes place. Cancellous allografts offer only minimal structural support, but actually increase in strength as osteoblastic new bone formation takes place within the trabeculae of the graft.

STRUCTURAL ALLOGRAFTS FOR ONCOLOGICAL INDICATIONS

Bulk allografts have been used for decades in tumor reconstructions with good results [31,43,56,73, 91,105–108,154,175]. In view of the increased emphasis on limb-salvage procedures over amputations in the past quarter-century, long-term follow-up series are beginning to be published on techniques employing bulk allografts. Retrieval studies, including work by Enneking and others [43,44,108], have shown incomplete incorporation of the graft at 5 years, and other authors have shown that remodeling continues as late as 9 years after surgery [165]. Rates of osseous union at the graft-host junction are in the range of 85–90% in many series [25,43,44,105–108]. Nonunions may be related to infection, surgical technique, problems with immunogenicity, or other causes [44,100]. Other reported complications have included fracture (in 7–38% percent of cases), which often occurs more than two years after surgery. The mechanism likely involves weakening of the bone as remodeling and vascularization occur; and may be treated surgically with open reduction internal fixation [9, 43, 108].

The use of osteoarticular allografts have had only mixed results, and are not widely favored as a primary reconstructive technique by all investigators [43,44,60,83,106]. Retrieval studies by Enneking et al. found no viable chondrocytes in those grafts [43,44], whereas other authors have reported long-term survival, with evidence of metabolic activity in the chondral matrix [27]. Despite overall complication rates as high as 38–69% in some series, many patients with osteoarticular allografts and other bulk grafts for oncological indications have achieved satisfactory, durable results [9,25,32,43,56,91, 100,105–108,154,175,180]. When osteoarticular allografts become symptomatic with arthrosis, collapse at the joint surface, or instability, it is frequently possible to perform total knee arthroplasty (TKA) to reconstruct the failed joint. Although fraught with complications (including a 46% rate of revision in one series [118], this technique is available to help maintain a previously successful attempt at limb salvage for oncological indications.

STRUCTURAL ALLOGRAFTS IN THE SPINE

The use of structural cortical grafts for anterior cervical spinal fusions is well accepted in both the orthopedic and neurosurgical literature [2,12,16,20,21,46,47,59,62, 96,99,119,135,140,157,164,167,172,173,176]. Initially, the widely practiced Smith-Robinson technique was advocated for use with tricortical bone graft harvested from the patient's own iliac crest. However, the donor-site morbidity associated with harvesting autograft is non-trivial: in one series, 5.6% of patients developed a wound infection or dehiscence, and 3% required a return to the operating room to treat a local complication at the donor site [146]. In view of those findings, several authors have investigated the use of allograft. Although studies have arrived at different conclusions regarding the use of autograft versus allograft for anterior cervical fusions [2,167], the data from these studies seldom show statistically significant differences between treatment groups. This may be a function of the characteristically small sample sizes included in these reports.

The technique of meta-analysis offers a potential way around the problem of small sample size; a meta-analysis performed by Floyd et al. [47] found that autograft showed a higher rate of union and a lower incidence of graft collapse when used for anterior cervical arthrodesis. However, despite apparently improved radiographic results, no statistically significant clinical differences were found in groups of patients treated with either type of graft. Of note, that meta-analysis reviewed nearly 400 manuscripts and found only four that met the inclusion criteria, which were based on soundness of study design. The non-union rate for multiple-level cervical fusions seems to rise disproportionately in patients treated with allograft compared to those treated with autograft [178]. As a result, some practitioners believe that either autograft or allograft may be used for single-level fusions, but that autograft is preferable for the more demanding multiple-level procedures.

Nearly every type of lumbar spine arthrodesis procedure may likewise be performed with either allograft or autograft. Several reports have shown excellent results using allograft for anterior lumbar arthrodesis [141], pseudarthrosis repair [26], and scoliosis surgery [59], among other procedures. As with the cervical spine techniques, advocates of lumbar spine interventions that use allograft cited the reduction in donor site morbidity and recuperative times as principal reasons for choosing this technique. Also similar to the literature on the cervical spine, large randomized prospective trials comparing allograft and autograft in the lumbar spine have yet to be done.

STRUCTURAL ALLOGRAFTS IN JOINT REPLACEMENT

Acetabular Reconstruction

The use of whole-acetabulum transplants in hip reconstruction is indicated in the most severe cases of bone loss following failed total hip arthroplasty (THA) [15,125,126]. Acetabular transplants provide immediate stability, restoration of the normal hip center, and, in theory, reconstitution of acetabular bone stock in the most severely bone-deficient patients. These grafts are typically fixed to the remaining host pelvis with multiple screws; the prosthetic acetabular socket is then cemented into the bulk acetabular allograft, sometimes using a reconstruction cage [125]. Intermediate-term follow-up has provided promising results; however, it must be mentioned that all of those series are in the hands of high-volume revision arthroplasty surgeons who are familiar with this technically demanding approach [15,125,126].

Bulk allografts, using either shaped segments of distal femoral condyles or femoral heads have been in use for decades (Fig. 1). Although their use remains controversial, several points appear to emerge consistently in the published literature: (1) Cementless sockets should not be used with large acetabular allografts; (2) The likelihood of failure of a bulk allograft increases with the percentage of coverage that the graft is providing over the acetabular implant, with components less than 30% covered by allograft performing well, and components with more than 50% coverage doing poorly; (3) Acetabular reconstruction cages should be used in many or most cases in which bulk grafting of the acetabulum is performed [13, 149].

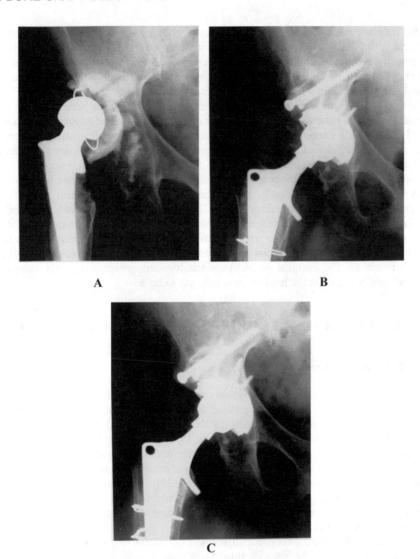

FIG. 1—Radiographs of a patient in whom a bulk allograft was used in acetabular revision surgery. (a) Preoperative radiograph of a failed right acetabular component that had been inserted with cement. There is severe superolateral loss of bone. (b) Radiograph made six weeks after revision with a cementless porous-coated acetabular component and a femoral head allograft secured with cancellous bone screws. (c) Radiograph made 55 months after revision, showing incorporation of the bulk femoral head allograft. (From Padgett, D. E., Kull, L., Rosenberg, A., Sumner, D. R. and Galante, J. O., "Revision of the Acetabular Component without Cement after Total Hip Arthroplasty," *J Bone Joint Surg Am,* 1993, Vol. 75, pp. 663–673.)

FEMORAL RECONSTRUCTION IN THA

So-called allograft-prosthetic composites, which consist of a cemented femoral stem within a large segment of allograft proximal femur that together are joined to host femur during a revision THA, remain an uncommon procedure to treat the most severe cases of femoral bone loss following hip replacement. Potential indications for this procedure include circumferential defects greater than 5 cm in length, severe endosteal bone loss in the metaphysis and diaphysis of the upper femur, and certain patterns of femoral discontinuity [8,63,127]. The principal advantages of this technique are good initial stability of the construct in the presence of bone deficiency, and the possibility of maintaining the restored bone stock over the longer term. Fixation has been achieved by a number of methods, including step cuts stabilized by fluted stems, cement, or plates, onlay grafts with cerclage wires, or insertion of the entire allograft-prosthetic composite within the ectatic host proximal femur [24,113] (Fig. 2). Results at short to intermediate-term follow-up have been somewhat mixed, with cases of early functional success being compromised by later infections, fractures, or dislocations. When possible, most revision arthroplasty surgeons prefer extensively coated long-stemmed cementless implants [3, 38,87,92,93,101,124,128].

Cortical strut allografts, affixed with cerclage cables or wires, are commonly used to reinforce the structurally deficient femur during revision THA [37,61,66–71,123]. This type of graft is particularly useful to bridge a non-circumferential defect—such as an intra-operative perforation, or an area of markedly thinned cortical bone near the tip of a loose stem—and union of the structural graft to host bone is predictably good, although slow. Other revision techniques, such as cancellous impaction allografting with cement, often use cortical struts as an adjunctive technique to increase the initial and ultimate strength of the construct [94, 110, 114].

Revision Total Knee Arthroplasty

Just as in THA, bulk allografts [40–42,57,84,130,161] and allograft-prosthetic composites are used to restore the severely bone-deficient knee at the time of revision total knee replacement (TKA). Bulk allografts for load-bearing applications at the time of revision TKA seem to provide durable results [130]. That histological study of both autopsy retrieval and revision arthroplasty specimens found new bone formation at the periphery of large allografts, no signs of graft collapse, and a durable prosthesis-cement-graft interface, but no signs of revascularization within the grafts themselves. Autograft specimens within that series show viable bone [130]. Durable clinical results have been published using bulk allografting techniques by several groups of investigators [41,155, 161].

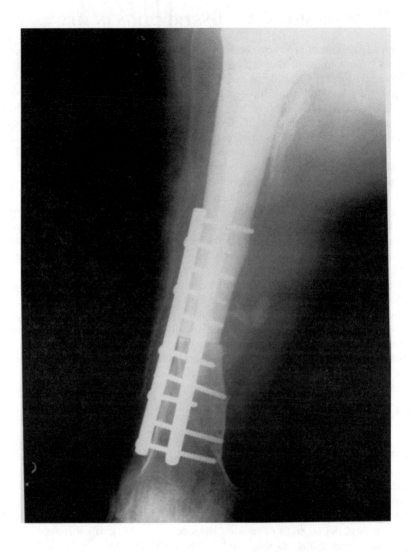

FIG. 2—Radiographs of a patient in whom an allograft-prosthetic composite was used to reconstruct massive proximal femoral bone loss in total hip revision surgery. (a) Immediate postoperative radiograph of a whole-segment proximal femoral allograft stabilized to the host distal femur with a compression plate. The long-stem femoral component has been cemented to the allograft only.

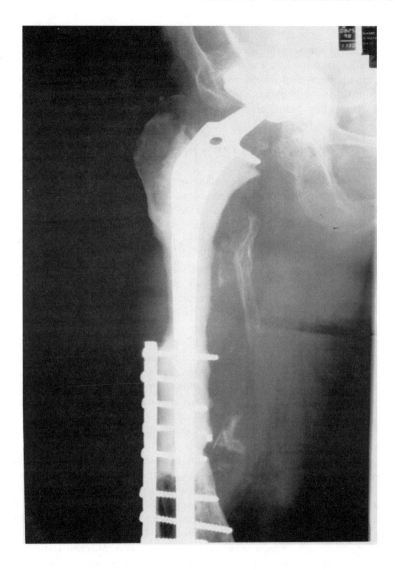

FIG. 2—(b) Radiograph made 56 months after revision demonstrating osseous union at the allograft/host bone junction. Extensive remodeling is also shown in the allograft as evidenced by the thinning of the lateral cortex just proximal to the compression plate.

Allograft-prosthesis composites are one option for the most severely bone-deficient revision TKA patients. This technique involves preparing a whole-segment (i.e., distal femur) allograft to receive cemented TKA components, and performing osteosynthesis to obtain union at the host-graft junction. Although this technique also has a high rate of complications, is quite technically demanding, and fairly time-consuming, it is associated with satisfactory short- to intermediate-term clinical results [24,64,65]. The alternative to this technique is to implant a segmental or modular oncology prosthesis (rotating hinge TKA); intermediate-term results using such devices have similar survivorship to the allograft-prosthesis composites [6,166]. To date, there have been no clinical studies directly comparing allograft-prosthesis composites and rotating hinge TKAs.

DEMINERALIZED BONE MATRIX (DBM)

Urist first recognized the osteoinductive properties of bone 35 years ago when transplanting human demineralized bone into muscle pouches of animals and saw the formation of ectopic bone [163]. Research has since shown that the active components of DBM are low molecular weight glycoproteins including bone morphogenic proteins [116]. Since that time autograft has been the primary source of osteoinduction in orthopedic surgery. In the past decade clinical trials [81,85,138,159,162,169] have shown that when demineralized bone matrix is used in arthrodeses or for treatment of bone cysts in children (often as bone graft extender or in conjunction with cancellous allograft), similar fusion rates to autogenous graft were achieved without the added morbidity of graft harvest [81,115,142,162,169].

Varied applications of allograft bone matrix in hand surgery have included the use of DBM to reconstruct benign tumorous conditions and traumatic or congenital defects with equal, or better results, to those treated with conventional autogenous bone grafting [162, 168]. Other investigators reporting on the usage of DBM for other skeletal tumorous conditions report similar healing rates as those seen with conventional autogenous bone grafting [81,85,158–160,162,168,169]. In the area of facilitating/augmenting arthrodeses in the spine, prospective studies [2,79] have shown the statistical superiority of autograft over DBM in terms of fusion integrity and graft collapse, although studies have failed to show a convincing superiority of autogenous grafting over the use of demineralized bone matrix in terms of overall results. In terms of assisting in fusions in the appendicular skeleton, several authors [80,115] reported excellent results in foot/ankle arthrodeses with DBM. Another study [29] found no advantage in its use when arthrodesis is performed arthroscopically. DBM's definitive role in skeletal fusions therefore has yet to be defined. There has been some concern as to the consistency of DBM as various donors have various quality of bone to harvest and process [138]. Although there are no large randomized prospective studies defining the efficacy of DBM, and DBM has not been specifically evaluated in any rigorous clinical studies within the field of adult reconstructive orthopedics (hip or knee replacement), its potential advantages nevertheless make it an exciting topic currently under evaluation.

CANCELLOUS BONE GRAFT IN REVISION THA

More allograft bone is used for revision hip arthroplasty than for any other purpose [52]; most of the allograft bone used in THA revisions is cancellous. Accordingly, the remainder of this review will cover in greater depth the clinical results obtained with cancellous grafting in revision hip surgery.

Acetabulum

Cancellous Allograft and Cementless Cups

Cementless hemispherical acetabular components implanted without structural grafting provide the best results for acetabular revision when bone stock permits this type of reconstruction [33,77,90,95,121,156,174]. Large series over intermediate- to long-term periods of follow-up have shown that cementless reconstruction without bulk allograft provides high success rates even when large segmental or combined cavitary/segmental defects are present, provided that component stability can be obtained with remaining posterior column and weight-bearing dome bone stock [90,95,174].

Although most acetabular revisions do not need bulk grafting, a large majority—79–86% in recent revision series [90,95,121]—require morselized cancellous allograft for contained bone defects. The natural history of cancellous grafting of contained columnar defects and even uncontained medial wall defects is well studied and favorable [4,36,53, 90,95,122,174]. This kind of graft is associated with radiographically improved bone stock, in particular with respect to reconstitution of an osseous medial acetabular wall (Fig. 3). Limited histological data are available from post-mortem retrieval to indicate that bone healing and graft incorporation indeed occur [72].

Radiolucencies are common in patients who have had morselized bone graft placed in conjunction with a cementless cup [33,90,112,122] but these lucencies are typically thin and non-progressive [90,95]. Although these lucencies probably represent areas of resorption or of porous coating that are not bone-ingrown [33,112], cups with non-progressive radiolucencies have not been associated with a higher incidence of migration or loosening [112, 121].

Although the American Academy of Orthopedic Surgeons (AAOS) grading system of acetabular bone-stock deficiency is based, at least in part, on a distinction between so-called segmental (AAOS Type I) and cavitary (AAOS Type II) defects [30], this system does not account for the size of defects nor does it effectively distinguish certain important anatomic differences from among the possible locations of segmental or cavitary deficiency. For instance, a massive combined segmental and cavitary defect (AAOS Type III) that destroys the entire anterior column and most of the medial wall is still reconstructible with a hemispherical cementless cup and morselized graft [77,90,94, 122]. On the other hand, an isolated segmental defect that renders the posterior column structurally unsound might require a large structural allograft or even an acetabular transplant [61,129].

To date, no clinical studies have directly compared autogenous cancellous graft with allograft or with any technique involving DBM in cementless acetabular revisions, though several that have employed both autograft and allograft have commented that no differences were observed with the numbers available [89,112,122,174]. Likewise, no differences have been observed in clinical series to date among the various forms of morselized allograft, such as freeze-dried, fresh-frozen, or irradiated.

Grafting of Osteolytic Defects and Cementless Component Retention

Osteolysis is an important potential mode of failure following total hip arthroplasty [94,104,144,183], which, disturbingly, is often asymptomatic until it compromises component stability and leaves massive peri-acetabular bone defects [103,104,143].

Early detection of this insidious problem is perhaps the most important reason for annual screening of the asymptomatic arthroplasty patient.

Patterns of bone loss differ depending on the mode of fixation. Cemented all-polyethylene cups tend to develop linear radiolucencies, which often represent the progressive resorption of bone leading to aseptic loosening [145,183]. In contrast, lysis around well fixed cementless acetabular components tends to be localized and expansile. This type of osteolysis causes loosening only when massive periprosthetic bone loss has resulted, which significantly compromises the eventual revision [103,104,143,183].

Historically, this problem has been treated by revising the acetabular component, with or without grafting the lytic defects [104]. Certainly, where cemented acetabular components are concerned, this is likely to be needed, since significant osteolysis around these components typically heralds aseptic loosening [145, 183]. But more recently, investigators have examined curettage with or without cancellous allografting of osteolytic lesions around well-fixed cementless acetabular components *without* component revision [103,143]. The technique involves obtaining circumferential acetabular exposure, verifying solid component fixation, debridement of all pseudocapsule, curettage of osteolytic defects either from the cup margin inwards or through screw-holes, impaction of morselized allograft into the osteolytic areas, and finally, exchange of the worn polyethylene bearing surface.

To date, three studies have evaluated so-called lesional treatment of peri-acetabular osteolysis adjacent to cementless cups [103,104,143]. All have concluded, based on 2–5-year follow-up, that curettage and polyethylene exchange consistently arrests the progression of peri-acetabular osteolysis without the need for revision of well-fixed components [103,104,143]. Although bone grafting was not required to halt or reverse the bone loss, when it was used, radiographic incorporation of the graft was consistent and appeared to help reconstitute peri-acetabular bone [103,143]. Although the long-term results using this approach are not yet known, curettage and cancellous allografting of lytic lesions adjacent to well-fixed cementless cups that have modular polyethylene liners appears justified.

Cancellous Allograft and Acetabular Reconstruction Rings/Cages

Many of the clinical series that investigated the use of acetabular reconstruction rings or cages used bulk structural allograft in addition to cancellous graft [54,137,179]. Because bulk allografting itself has been associated with inconsistent results, with failure rates between four and 47% depending on the technique and follow-up duration [88, 127], it is probably not possible to determine the effect of the cancellous graft itself on composite reconstructions that used both morselized and structural allograft.

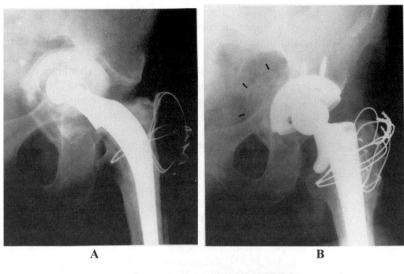

A   B

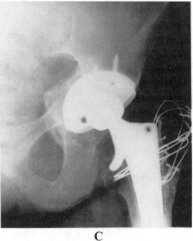

C

FIG. 3 —Radiographs of a patient in whom a non-contained medial graft was used in acetabular revision surgery. (a) Preoperative radiograph of a failed left acetabular component that had been inserted with cement. There is disruption of the iliopubic column. (b) Radiograph made six weeks after revision with morselized cancellous allograft and a cementless porous-coated acetabular prosthesis. (c) Radiograph made 41 months after revision. The characteristic consolidation and incorporation of the medial bone graft can be seen. (From Padgett, D. E., Kull, L., Rosenberg, A., Sumner, D. R. and Galante, J. O., Revision of the Acetabular Component without Cement after Total Hip Arthroplasty, *J Bone Joint Surg Am*, Vol. 75, 1993, pp. 663–673.)

On the other hand, there are several series that used reconstruction rings or cages exclusively with morselized allograft and cemented sockets, without any bulk grafting [10,51,133,179]. This technique was used most commonly for AAOS Type III acetabula (combined segmental and cavitary bone deficiency), with the longest series to date reporting at a mean of seven years [179]. Failure rates were somewhat high, even in the shorter-term studies, ranging from 10% fair/poor hip scores [51] to 24% combined aseptic/septic loosening [10]. In the only study with intermediate-term follow-up (mean seven years) [179], the incidence of significant component migration was 44%, and the revision rate was more than 20%. Somewhat better results were obtained in sub-cohorts within studies that were selected for contained cavitary defects (AAOS Type II) rather than segmental or combined defects (AAOS Types I or III, respectively) [54]. Similarly, another study of cancellous grafting and reconstruction cages showed a sixfold increase in revision rate when combined cavitary and segmental defects were compared to cavitary defects alone [179]. No differences were shown between allograft and autograft in any of these series, with the numbers available.

Several factors render interpretation of these results somewhat unreliable. First, pre-operative grading of acetabular bone deficiency remains unsettled, as numerous grading systems are in common use [15,30,61], though none of them have been independently validated. In addition, there is considerable disagreement over when to use acetabular reconstruction cages or rings at all. Many studies support the cementless hemispherical cup as the gold standard acetabular revision technique, even in cases with combined cavitary and segmental defects [33,77,90,94,121,150,156,174], provided that there is an intact posterior column and weight-bearing dome. When those structures are compromised, it is likely that any reconstruction will fail—even a reconstruction cage or ring—unless the posterior column and weight-bearing dome are reconstructed with bulk graft [22,129,179]. On the other hand, there is general agreement that reconstruction cages—with or without pelvic reconstruction plates—can be used to bridge pelvic dissociations (AAOS Type IV), and cancellous allografting can help defects of this type to remodel, once the reconstruction cage has provided rigid internal fixation.

Acetabular Impaction Allografting with Cement

Although considerable interest has been given to impaction allografting for femoral reconstruction [34,35,58,94,109,114], it is not widely known that published results on acetabular cancellous impaction grafting with cement preceded those reports on the femoral side by almost a decade [153]. By incorporating wire mesh or small bone block grafts into the reconstruction, the technique has been used to reconstitute segmental and cavitary defects in acetabular revision surgery [5,147,152]. The basic science support for impaction allografting includes animal models as well as human biopsy and retrieval specimens. These studies showed that bone graft revascularization, new bone formation, and bone stock reconstitution all were achieved when allograft was impacted into place and stabilized with polymethylmethacrylate bone cement [19,120,136,152].

Briefly, the technique [147,152,153] involves debridement and assessment of remaining acetabular bone stock, followed by converting any (medial or peripheral) segmental defects into contained cavitary defects using metal mesh. Morselized allograft then is impacted firmly into the cavitary defects, and the graft is covered with a second layer of wire mesh; an all-polyethylene cup then is cemented directly into this construct. Interpretation of the available results of this technique [147,152,153], and its variations [5,86] is limited by differences in surgical methodology, clinical evaluation methods, and inclusion criteria, which in one series restricted use of the technique to contained cavitary defects [86].

Based on radiographic criteria, the bone grafts appeared to unite and remodel, but clinical and radiographic failure rates have varied widely, from 11–31% [5,147,152]. The study with the longest follow-up published on the technique had five revisions and five additional radiographic failures in a cohort of 60 patients at a mean of 11.8 years [147]. These failure rates are higher—in some cases considerably higher—than the failure rates generally observed with cementless component revisions at 8–12 years [90,95,148]. Failures of acetabular impaction grafting were associated with component malposition, combined cavitary and segmental defects (AAOS Type III), and use of allograft rather than autograft [86]. The latter was the only study of any application of cancellous grafting for hip revision that suggested allograft may be inferior to autograft. In view of the fact that three or four femoral heads may be needed for one revision with this technique [5,147,152], it may be difficult to make clinical use of this finding. Despite its limitations, acetabular impaction grafting may be indicated as a method of reconstituting bone stock for later revisions, and it may have a role in patients with severe osteopenia and certain patterns of cavitary bone loss, in whom cementless fixation might be unsatisfactory.

Acetabular Allografts with Bipolar Endoprosthesis

The bipolar endoprosthesis is used most often to treat displaced femoral neck fractures [7]. Some investigators broadened the indications for its use, with the intention of using it as a temporary spacer in a two-stage procedure—along with cancellous allograft—intended to reconstitute bone stock [148]. Subsequent conversion to a traditional fixed acetabular total hip revision was planned in these cases, but early results suggested this was not necessary [111], because patients seemed satisfied with the function and relief of pain the bipolar provided in the short-term.

Unfortunately, at longer-term follow-up, it became evident that use of the bipolar endoprosthesis and bone grafting for acetabular deficiency resulted in an unacceptably high rate of failure. Socket migration, instability, progressive bone loss, and pain all were reported as mechanisms of failure with this technique [17,170]. Other investigators found that bone grafts tended to resorb and did not prevent progressive medial and superior migration of the bipolar socket [170]. Contained, central defects were effectively treated with this approach in one study [170]. However, that pattern of bone loss is easily addressed with numerous more reliable techniques; accordingly, the bipolar endoprosthesis has been largely abandoned as a method of reconstituting the bone-deficient acetabulum.

Femur

Lesional Treatment of Osteolysis with Cancellous Grafting

Although cancellous grafting has been used with cementless acetabular components to treat pelvic osteolysis, as has been described earlier in this review, relatively little work has been done using allograft chips in the treatment of femoral osteolysis [75]. One report found that femoral osteolysis halted or regressed in patients after placement of a stable cementless revision stem, whether or not the lesions were treated with cancellous allograft. On the basis of those limited data, it is difficult to comment on the use of morselized allografting in the setting of cementless femoral revision.

Femoral Impaction Allografting with Cement

Cancellous impaction allografting for femoral component revision, as currently practiced, is a modification of a technique initially used for acetabular reconstruction in the setting of protrusio acetabuli [150]. It was first used for femoral reconstruction in 1985, without cement, by a group in England [98]; but 2 years later, because of early failures, the originators of the technique began to use cement [58]. Interestingly, despite that unhappy experience, cementless impaction allografting was attempted in one other series, quite recently [131]. This group also reported unsatisfactory results with the technique. The standard technique for impaction allografting, which was initially described by Gie et al. [58], therefore includes the use of methacrylate bone cement [34, 35,94,109,114].

Follow-up studies of patients who have undergone a procedure substantially similar to that described by Gie et al. [58] now have been published by numerous other groups [34,35,94,110,114]. Not withstanding the high incidence of major complications (8–28%) [35,94,114]; impaction allografting remains appealing because it seems to restore bone stock in a majority of patients, according to several clinical series [35,58,114].

Several centers have reported short-term (minimum 18–24 months) follow-up using cancellous impaction grafting with cement for femoral component revision, using polished, tapered, collarless stems [34,35,58,114]. Advocates of the technique using these devices state that subsidence does not automatically lead to clinical loosening because the stem's wedge-shaped geometry may allow restabilization within the cement mantle as subsidence occurs [35,58]. Cold flow of the cement mantle [48] may help the stem to subside without becoming symptomatically loose. Subsidence of the wedge-shaped stem also may provide a beneficial compressive load to the bone graft [97,120].

However, other authors have raised concerns about the supposed benign nature of stem subsidence [34,49,109,114], and impaction allografting has been performed using stems that resist subsidence. Implants with a rough surface finish [82] and polymethylmethacrylate precoating [11,94] have been chosen by some investigators for this reason.

When evaluating the published reports on impaction allografting, three important issues limit comparisons among clinical series. The most evident limitation is the inconsistent use of inclusion criteria in those papers. Although several series have attempted to limit inclusion to patients with more advanced stages of femoral bone-stock deficiency [94,109,114], sometimes using accepted grading criteria such as the AAOS

Classification for Femoral Abnormalities [30,94,110,114], other studies have specifically excluded such complex reconstructions [58,98]. Series of unselected, consecutive femoral revisions also have been presented [35,82], and still other studies do not define their inclusion criteria at all [34]. Another important limitation to consider when comparing clinical reports on this technique is the impressive number of variables that may affect the outcome in these cases. Published series have differed with respect to stem geometry, cement, allograft material, surgical approach, and aftercare, and many other factors. Although some of these issues have been investigated [11,110], the effects of most of these variables are not known. Specifically, the use of bone-graft substitutes and derivatives—such as demineralized bone matrix—has not been studied in the context of impaction allografting. Finally, methods of patient analysis, including clinical and radiographic assessment and follow-up duration, have differed markedly among published reports, with predictable effects on the apparent outcomes.

Major complications are unfortunately common with impaction allografting, and include intraoperative and postoperative femoral fractures, prosthetic dislocations, and a high incidence of trochanteric nonunion—between 33% and 50% [94,114]—when trochanteric osteotomies are used. The importance of stem subsidence remains a controversial issue, with some investigators hypothesizing that subsidence is necessary or beneficial for graft incorporation [35,58], and others implicating it as the cause of serious complications, including thigh pain, cement mantle fracture, and hip dislocation [34,49, 109,114].

Although the differences in inclusion criteria, surgical technique, and clinical assessment make analysis of the published results somewhat difficult, the short-term to intermediate-term results with this technique are promising. Series that used severe bone deficiency as the indication to perform impaction allografting had failure rates ranging from 9–12% at 2- to 4-year minimum follow-up [94,114]. Not surprisingly, this failure rate was higher than was observed in series that excluded some of the more severe cases of bone loss [58], or those in which the procedure was performed in a group of consecutive patients undergoing femoral revisions [35, 82].

Although femoral impaction allografting has the potential to restore bone-stock, which is appealing in the multiply revised femur, substantial questions remain about its durability and high rate of complications [34,49,109]. Studies of cementless revision with extensively porous-coated stems have shown excellent durability, relatively few complications, and good clinical results over the long-term [3,39,93,117] although concerns about stress shielding of the proximal femur persist as these patients enter the second decade following revision. Nevertheless, using these devices appears to halt the progression of osteolysis, whether or not morselized allograft is used [75]. For those reasons, extensively coated femoral stems probably should be used for most femoral revisions.

CONCLUSION

Human allograft bone is used in nearly every subspecialty within orthopedic surgery, although high-quality comparative studies between allograft and autograft, or between allograft and a bone-graft derivative such as DBM, have not been performed for most common indications. Both basic science and clinical research will continue to guide surgeons toward the most appropriate uses of these products.

REFERENCES

[1]   Alleyne K. R. and Galloway M. T., "Management of Osteochondral Injuries of the Knee," *Clin Sports Med*, Vol. 20, 2001, pp. 343–364.

[2]   An H. S., Simpson J. M., Glover J. M. and Stephany J., "Comparison Between Allograft Plus Demineralized Bone Matrix Versus Autograft in Anterior Cervical Fusion. A Prospective Multicenter Study," *Spine*, Vol. 20, 1995, pp. 2211–2216.

[3]   Aribindi R., Barba M., Solomon M. I., Arp P., and Paprosky W., "Bypass Fixation," *Orthop Clin North Am*, Vol. 29, 1998, pp. 319–329.

[4]   Avci S., Connors N., and Petty W., "2- to 10-year Follow-up Study of Acetabular Revisions Using Allograft Bone to Repair Bone Defects," *J Arthroplasty*, Vol. 13, 1998, pp. 61–69.

[5]   Azuma T., Yasuda H., Okagaki K., and Sakai K., "Compressed Allograft Chips for Acetabular Reconstruction in Revision Hip Arthroplasty," *J Bone Joint Surg Br*, Vol. 76, 1994, pp. 740–744.

[6]   Barrack R. L., Lyons T. R., Ingraham R. Q., and Johnson J. C., "The Use of a Modular Rotating Hinge Component in Salvage Revision Total Knee Arthroplasty," *J Arthroplasty*, Vol. 15, 2000, pp. 858–866.

[7]   Bateman J. E., "Single-Assembly Total Hip Prosthesis--Preliminary Report," 1974, *Clin Orthop Rel Res*, Vol. 251, 1990, pp. 3–6.

[8]   Behairy Y. and Jasty M., "Bone Grafts and Bone Substitutes in Hip and Knee Surgery," *Orthop Clin North Am*, Vol. 30, 1999, pp. 661–671.

[9]   Berrey B. H., Jr., Lord C. F., Gebhardt M. C., and Mankin H. J., "Fractures of Allografts. Frequency, Treatment, and End-results, " *J Bone Joint Surg Am*, Vol. 72, 1990, pp. 825–833.

[10] Berry D. J. and Muller M. E., "Revision Arthroplasty Using an Anti-protrusio Cage for Massive Acetabular Bone Deficiency," *J Bone Joint Surg Br*, Vol. 74, 1992, pp. 711–715.

[11] Berzins A., Sumner D. R., Wasielewski R. C., and Galante J. O., "Impacted Particulate Allograft for Femoral Revision Total Hip Arthroplasty. In Vitro Mechanical Stability and Effects of Cement Pressurization," *J Arthroplasty*, Vol. 11, 1996, pp. 500–506.

[12] Boden S. D. and Schimandle J. H., "Biologic Enhancement of Spinal Fusion," *Spine*, Vol. 20, 1995, pp. 112–123.

[13] Bohm P. and Banzhaf S., "Acetabular Revision with Allograft Bone. 103 Revisions with 3 Reconstruction Alternatives, Followed for 0.3–13 Years," *Acta Orthop Scand*, Vol. 70, 1999, pp. 240–249.

[14] Boyce T., Edwards J., and Scarborough N., "Allograft Bone, The Influence of Processing on Safety and Performance," *Orthop Clin North Am*, Vol. 30, 1999, pp. 571–581.

[15] Bradford M. S. and Paprosky W. G., "Acetabular Defect Classification: a Detailed Radiographic Approach," *Sem Arthroplasty*, Vol. 6, 1995, pp. 76–85.

[16] Brantigan J. W., "Pseudarthrosis Rate After Allograft Posterior Lumbar Interbody Fusion with Pedicle Screw and Plate Fixation," *Spine*, Vol. 19, 1994, pp. 1271–1279; discussion, p. 1280.

[17] Brien W. W., Bruce W. J., Salvati E. A., Wilson P. D., Jr. and Pellicci P. M., "Acetabular Reconstruction with a Bipolar Prosthesis and Morseled Bone Grafts," *J Bone Joint Surg Am*, Vol. 72, 1990, pp. 1230–1235.

[18] Bugbee W. D. and Convery F. R., "Osteochondral Allograft Transplantation," *Clin Sports Med*, Vol. 18, 1999, pp. 67–75.

[19] Buma P., Lamerigts N., Schreurs B. W., Gardeniers J., Versleyen D., and Slooff T. J., "Impacted Graft Incorporation after Cemented Acetabular Revision. Histological Evaluation in 8 Patients," *Acta Orthop Scand*, Vol. 67, 1996, pp. 536–540.

[20] Buttermann G. R., Glazer P. A., Hu S. S., and Bradford D. S., "Anterior and Posterior Allografts in Symptomatic Thoracolumbar Deformity," *J Spinal Disord*, Vol. 14, 2001, pp. 4–66.

[21] Buttermann G. R., Glazer P. A., Hu S. S., and Bradford D. S., "Revision of Failed Lumbar Fusions. A Comparison of Anterior Autograft and Allograft," *Spine*, Vol. 22, 1997, pp. 2748–2755.

[22] Cabanela M. E., "Reconstruction Rings and Bone Graft in Total Hip Revision Surgery," *Orthop Clin North Am*, Vol. 29, 1998, pp. 255–262.

[23] Centers for Disease Control, "Semen Banking, Organ and Tissue Transplantation, and HIV Antibody Testing," *MMWR*, Vol. 37, 1988, pp. 57–58.

[24] Clatworthy M. G. and Gross A. E., "The Allograft Prosthetic Composite: When and How," *Orthopedics*, Vol. 24, 2001, pp. 897–898.

[25] Clohisy D. R. and Mankin H. J., "Osteoarticular Allografts for Reconstruction after Resection of a Musculoskeletal Tumor in the Proximal End of the Tibia," *J Bone Joint Surg Am*, Vol. 76, 1994, pp. 549–554.

[26] Cohen D. B., Chotivichit A., Fujita T., Wong T. H., Huckel, C. B., Sieber A. N., et al., "Pseudarthrosis Repair. Autogenous Iliac Crest Versus Femoral Ring Allograft," *Clin Orthop Rel Res*, Vol. 371, 2000, pp. 46–55.

[27] Convery F. R., Akeson W. H., Amiel D., Meyers M. H., and Monosov A., "Long-Term Survival of Chondrocytes in an Osteochondral Articular Cartilage Allograft. A Case Report," *J Bone Joint Surg Am*, Vol. 78, 1996, pp. 1082–1088.

[28] Convery F. R., Meyers M. H., and Akeson W. H., "Fresh Osteochondral Allografting of the Femoral Condyle," *Clin Orthop Rel Res*, Vol. 273, 1991, pp. 139–145.

[29] Crosby L. A., Yee T. C., Formanek T. S., and Fitzgibbons T. C., "Complications Following Arthroscopic Ankle Arthrodesis," *Foot Ankle Int*, Vol. 17, 1996, pp. 340–342.

[30] D'Antonio J. A., Capello W. N., Borden L. S., Bargar W. L., Bierbaum B. F., Boettcher W. G., et al., "Classification and Management of Acetabular Abnormalities in Total Hip Arthroplasty," *Clin Orthop Rel Res*, Vol. 249, 1989, pp.126–137.

[31] Davis A., Bell R. S., Allan D. G., Langer F., Czitrom A. A., and Gross A. E., "Fresh Osteochondral Transplants in the Treatment of Advanced Giant Cell Tumors," *Orthopade*, Vol. 22, 1993, pp. 146–151.

[32] DeGroot H., III, and Mankin H., "Total Knee Arthroplasty in Patients Who Have Massive Osteoarticular Allografts," *Clin Orthop Rel Res*, Vol. 373, 2000, pp. 62–72.

[33] Dorr L. D. and Wan Z., "Ten Years of Experience with Porous Acetabular Components for Revision Surgery," *Clin Orthop Rel Res,* Vol. 319, 1995, pp. 191–200.

[34] Eldridge J. D., Smith E. J., Hubble M. J., Whitehouse S. L., and Learmonth I. D., "Massive Early Subsidence Following Femoral Impaction Grafting," *J Arthroplasty,* Vol. 12, 1997, pp. 535–540.

[35] Elting J. J., Mikhail W. E., Zicat B. A., Hubbell J. C., Lane L. E., and House B., "Preliminary Report of Impaction Grafting for Exchange Femoral Arthroplasty," *Clin Orthop Rel Res,* Vol. 319, 1995, pp. 159–167.

[36] Emerson R. H., Jr., Head W. C., Berklacich F. M., and Malinin T. I., "Noncemented Acetabular Revision Arthroplasty Using Allograft Bone," *Clin Orthop Rel Res,* Vol. 249, 1989, pp. 30–43.

[37] Emerson R. H., Jr., Malinin T. I., Cuellar A. D., Head W. C. and Peters P. C., "Cortical Strut Allografts in the Reconstruction of the Femur in Revision Total Hip Arthroplasty. A Basic Science and Clinical Study," *Clin Orthop Rel Res,* Vol. 285, 1992, pp. 35–44.

[38] Engh C. A., Culpepper W. J., II, and Kassapidis E., "Revision of Loose Cementless Femoral Prostheses to Larger Porous Coated Components," *Clin Orthop Rel Res,* Vol. 347, 1998, pp. 168–178.

[39] Engh C. A., Glassman A. H., Griffin W. L., and Mayer J. G., "Results of Cementless Revision for Failed Cemented Total Hip Arthroplasty," *Clin Orthop Rel Res,* Vol. 235, 1988, pp. 91–110.

[40] Engh G. A., and Ammeen D. J., "Bone Loss with Revision Total Knee Arthroplasty: Defect Classification and Alternatives for Reconstruction," *Instr Course Lect,* Vol. 48, 1999, pp. 167–175.

[41] Engh G. A., Herzwurm P. J., and Parks N. L., "Treatment of Major Defects of Bone with Bulk Allografts and Stemmed Components During Total Knee Arthroplasty," *J Bone Joint Surg Am,* Vol. 79, 1997, pp. 1030–1039.

[42] Engh G. A. and Parks N. L., "The Management of Bone Defects in Revision Total Knee Arthroplasty," *Instr Course Lect,* Vol. 46, 1997, pp. 227–236.

[43] Enneking W. F. and Campanacci D. A., "Retrieved Human Allografts: a Clinicopathological Study," *J Bone Joint Surg Am,* Vol. 83, 2001, pp. 971–986.

[44] Enneking W. F. and Mindell E. R., "Observations on Massive Retrieved Human Allografts," *J Bone Joint Surg Am,* Vol. 73, 1991, pp. 1123–1142.

[45] Fernyhough J. C., Schimandle J. J., Weigel M. C., Edwards C. C., and Levine A. M., "Chronic Donor Site Pain Complicating Bone Graft Harvesting from the Posterior Iliac Crest for Spinal Fusion," *Spine,* Vol. 17, 1992, pp. 1474–1480.

[46] Finkelstein J. A., Chapman J. R., and Mirza S., "Anterior Cortical Allograft in Thoracolumbar Fractures," *J Spinal Disord,* Vol. 12, 1999, pp. 424–429.

[47] Floyd T. and Ohnmeiss, D., "A Meta-analysis of Autograft Versus Allograft in Anterior Cervical Fusion," *Eur Spine J,* Vol. 9, 2000, pp. 398–403.

[48] Fowler J. L., Gie G. A., Lee A. J., and Ling R. S., "Experience with the Exeter Total Hip Replacement Since 1970," *Orthop Clin North Am,* Vol. 19, 1988, pp. 477–489.

[49] Franzen H., Toksvig-Larsen S., Lidgren L., and Onnerfalt R., "Early Migration of Femoral Components Revised with Impacted Cancellous Allografts and Cement. A

Preliminary Report of Five Patients," *J Bone Joint Surg Br*, Vol. 77, 1995, pp. 862–864.

[50] Friedenberg Z. B., Brighton C. T., Michelson J. D., Bednar J., Schmidt R., and Brockmeyer T., "The Effects of Demineralized Bone Matrix and Direct Current on an "In Vivo" Culture of Bone Marrow Cells," *J Orthop Res*, Vol. 7, 1989, pp. 22–27.

[51] Fuchs M. D., Salvati E. A., Wilson P. D., Jr., Sculco T. P., and Pellicci P. M., "Results of Acetabular Revisions with Newer Cement Techniques," *Orthop Clin North Am*, Vol. 19, 1988, pp. 649–655.

[52] Galea G., Kopman D., and Graham B. J., "Supply and Demand of Bone Allograft for Revision Hip Surgery in Scotland," *J Bone Joint Surg Br*, Vol. 80, 1998, pp. 595–599.

[53] Garbuz D., Morsi E., and Gross A. E., "Revision of the Acetabular Component of a Total Hip Arthroplasty With a Massive Structural Allograft. Study with a Minimum Five-year Follow-up," *J Bone Joint Surg Am*, Vol. 78, 1996, pp. 693–697.

[54] Garbuz D., Morsi E., Mohamed N., and Gross A. E., "Classification and Reconstruction in Revision Acetabular Arthroplasty with Bone Stock Deficiency," *Clin Orthop Rel Res*, Vol. 324, 1996, pp. 98–107.

[55] Gazdag A. R., Lane J. M., Glaser D., and Forster R. A., "Alternatives to Autogenous Bone Graft: Efficacy and Indications," *J Am Acad Orthop Surg*, Vol. 3, 1995, pp. 1–8.

[56] Gebhardt M. C., Lord F. C., Rosenberg A. E., and Mankin H. J., "The Treatment of Adamantinoma of the Tibia by Wide Resection and Allograft Bone Transplantation," *J Bone Joint Surg Am*, Vol. 69, 1987, pp. 1177–1188.

[57] Ghazavi M. T., Stockley I., Yee G., Davis A., and Gross A. E., "Reconstruction of Massive Bone Defects with Allograft in Revision Rotal Knee Arthroplasty," *J Bone Joint Surg Am*, Vol. 79, 1997, pp. 17–25.

[58] Gie G. A., Linder L., Ling R. S., Simon J. P., Slooff T. J., and Timperley A. J., "Impacted Cancellous Allografts and Cement for Revision Total Hip Arthroplasty," *J Bone Joint Surg Br*, Vol. 75, 1993, pp. 14–21.

[59] Grogan D. P., Kalen V., Ross T. I., Guidera K. J., and Pugh L. I., "Use of Allograft Bone for Posterior Spinal Fusion in Idiopathic Scoliosis," *Clin Orthop Rel Res*, Vol. 369, 1999, pp. 273–278.

[60] Gross A. E., Agnidis Z., and Hutchison C. R., "Osteochondral Defects of the Talus Treated With Fresh Osteochondral Allograft Transplantation," *Foot Ankle Int*, Vol. 22, 2001, pp. 385–391.

[61] Gross A. E., Allan D. G., Lavoie G. J., and Oakeshott R. D., "Revision Arthroplasty of the Proximal Femur Using Allograft Bone," *Orthop Clin North Am*, Vol. 24, 1993, pp. 705–715.

[62] Grossman W., Peppelman W. C., Baum J. A., and Kraus D. R., "The Use of Freeze-Dried Fibular Allograft in Anterior Cervical Fusion," *Spine*, Vol. 17, 1992, pp. 565–569.

[63] Haddad F. S., Garbuz D. S., Masri B. A., Duncan C. P., Hutchison C. R., and Gross A. E., "Femoral Bone Loss in Patients Managed with Revision Hip Replacement: Results of Circumferential Allograft Replacement," *Instr Course Lect*, Vol. 49, 2000, pp. 147–162.

[64]   Harris A. I., Gitelis S., Sheinkop M. B., Rosenberg A. G., and Piasecki P., "Allograft Prosthetic Composite Reconstruction for Limb Salvage and Severe Deficiency of Bone at the Knee or Hip," *Sem Arthroplasty*, Vol. 5, 1994, pp. 85–94.

[65]   Harris A. I., Poddar S., Gitelis S., Sheinkop M. B., and Rosenberg A. G., "Arthroplasty with a Composite of an Allograft and a Prosthesis for Knees with Severe Deficiency of Bone," *J Bone Joint Surg Am*, Vol. 77, 1995, pp. 373–386.

[66]   Head W. C., Berklacich F. M., Malinin T. I., and Emerson R. H., Jr., "Proximal Femoral Allografts in Revision Total Hip Arthroplasty," *Clin Orthop Rel Res*, Vol. 225, 1987, pp. 22–36.

[67]   Head W. C., Emerson R. H., Jr., and Malinin T. I., "Structural Bone Grafting for Femoral Reconstruction," *Clin Orthop Rel Res*, Vol. 369, 1999, pp. 223–229.

[68]   Head W. C. and Malinin T. I., "Results of Onlay Allografts," *Clin Orthop Rel Res*, Vol. 371, 2000, pp. 108–112.

[69]   Head W. C., Malinin T. I., and Berklacich F., "Freeze-dried Proximal Femur Allografts in Revision Total Hip Arthroplasty. A Preliminary Report," *Clin Orthop Rel Res*, Vol. 215, 1987, pp. 109–121.

[70]   Head W. C., Malinin T. I., Emerson R. H., Jr. and Mallory T. H., "Restoration of Bone Stock in Revision Surgery of the Femur," *Int Orthop*, Vol. 24, 2000, pp. 9–14.

[71]   Head W. C., Malinin T. I., Mallory T. H., and Emerson R. H., Jr., "Onlay Cortical Allografting for the Femur," *Orthop Clin North Am*, Vol. 29, 1998, pp. 307–312.

[72]   Heekin R. D., Engh C. A., and Vinh T., "Morselized Allograft in Acetabular Reconstruction. A Postmortem Retrieval Analysis," *Clin Orthop Rel Res*, Vol. 319, 1995, pp. 184–190.

[73]   Hiki Y. and Mankin H. J., "Radical Resection and Allograft Replacement in the Treatment of Bone Tumors," *Nippon Seikeigeka Gakkai Zasshi*, Vol. 54, 1980, pp. 475–500.

[74]   Hornicek F. J., Gebhardt M. C., Tomford W. W., Sorger J. I., Zavatta M., Menzner J. P., and Mankin H. J., "Factors Affecting Nonunion of the Allograft-host Junction," *Clin Orthop Rel Res*, Vol. 382, 2001, pp. 87–98.

[75]   Hozack W. J., Bicalho P. S., and Eng K., "Treatment of Femoral Osteolysis with Cementless Total Hip Revision," *J Arthroplasty*, Vol. 11, 1996, pp. 668–672.

[76]   Iwata H., Hanamura H., Kaneko M., Yasuhara N., Terashima Y., et al., "Chemosterilized Autolyzed Antigen-extracted Allogeneic (AAA) Bone Matrix Gelatin for Repair of Defects from Excision of Benign Bone Tumors: a Preliminary Report," *Clin Orthop Rel Res*, Vol. 154, 1981, pp. 150–155.

[77]   Jasty M., "Jumbo Cups and Morselized Graft," *Orthop Clin North Am*, Vol. 29, 1998, pp. 249–254.

[78]   Jofe M. H., Gebhardt M. C., Tomford W. W., and Mankin H. J., "Reconstruction for Defects of the Proximal Part of the Femur Using Allograft Arthroplasty," *J Bone Joint Surg Am*, Vol. 70, 1988, pp. 507–516.

[79]   Jorgenson S. S., Lowe T. G., France J., and Sabin J., "A Prospective Analysis of Autograft Versus Allograft in Posterolateral Lumbar Fusion in the Same Patient. A Minimum of 1-year Follow-up in 144 Patients," *Spine*, 1994, Vol. 19, pp. 2048–2053.

[80] Kado K. E., Gambetta L. A., and Perlman M. D., "Uses of Grafton for Reconstructive Foot and Ankle Surgery," *J Foot Ankle Surg*, Vol. 35, 1996, pp. 59–66.

[81] Kakiuchi M., Hosoya T., Takaoka K., Amitani K., and Ono K., "Human Bone Matrix Gelatin as a Clinical Alloimplant. A Retrospective Review of 160 Cases," *Int Orthop*, Vol. 9, 1985, pp. 181–188.

[82] Karrholm J., Hultmark P., Carlsson L., and Malchau H., "Subsidence of a Non-Polished Stem in Revisions of the Hip Using Impaction Allograft. Evaluation with Radiostereometry and Dual-energy X-ray Absorptiometry," *J Bone Joint Surg Br*, Vol. 81, 1999, pp. 135–142.

[83] Kawabe N., Ehrlich M. G., and Mankin H. J., "Growth Plate Reconstruction Using Chondrocyte Allograft Transplants," *J Pediatr Orthop*, Vol. 7, 1987, pp. 381–388.

[84] Khan M. T., Stockley I., and Ibbotson C., "Allograft Bone Transplantation: a Sheffield Experience, " *Ann R Coll Surg Engl*, Vol. 80, 1998, pp. 150–153.

[85] Killian J. T., Wilkinson L., White S., and Brassard M., "Treatment of Unicameral Bone Cyst with Demineralized Bone Matrix," *J Pediatr Orthop*, Vol. 18, 1998, pp. 621–624.

[86] Knight J. L., Fujii K., Atwater R., and Grothaus L., "Bone-grafting for Acetabular Deficiency During Primary and Revision Total Hip Arthroplasty. A Radiographic and Clinical Analysis," *J Arthroplasty*, Vol. 8, 1993, pp. 371–382.

[87] Krishnamurthy A. B., MacDonald S. J., and Paprosky W. G., "5- to 13-year Follow-up Study on Cementless Femoral Components in Revision Surgery," *J Arthroplasty*, Vol. 12, 1997, pp. 839–847.

[88] Kwong L. M., Jasty M., and Harris W. H., "High Failure Rate of Bulk Femoral Head Allografts in Total Hip Acetabular Reconstructions at 10 Years," *J Arthroplasty*, Vol. 8, 1993, pp. 341–346.

[89] Lachiewicz P. F. and Hussamy O. D., "Revision of the Acetabulum Without Cement With Use of the Harris- Galante Porous-coated Implant. Two to Eight-year Results," *J Bone Joint Surg Am*, Vol. 76, 1994, pp. 1834–1839.

[90] Lachiewicz P. F. and Poon E. D., "Revision of a Total Hip Arthroplasty with a Harris-Galante Porous-coated Acetabular Component Inserted Without Cement. A Follow-up Note on the Results at Five to Twelve Years," *J Bone Joint Surg Am*, Vol. 80, 1998, pp. 980–984.

[91] Langlais F., Lambotte J. C., and Thomazeau H., "Long-term Results of Hemipelvis Reconstruction with Allografts," *Clin Orthop Rel Res*, Vol. 388, 2001, pp. 178–186.

[92] Lawrence J. M., Engh C. A., and Macalino G. E., "Revision Total Hip Arthroplasty. Long-term Results Without Cement," *Orthop Clin North Am*, Vol. 24, 1993, pp. 635–644.

[93] Lawrence J. M., Engh C. A., Macalino G. E., and Lauro,G. R., "Outcome of Revision Hip Arthroplasty Done Without Cement," *J Bone Joint Surg Am*, Vol. 76, 1994, pp. 965–973.

[94] Leopold S. S., Berger R. A., Rosenberg A. G., Jacobs J. J., Quigley L. R., and Galante J. O., "Impaction Allografting with Cement for Revision of the Femoral Component. A Minimum Four-year Follow-up Study with Use of a Precoated Femoral Stem," *J Bone Joint Surg Am*, Vol. 81, 1999, pp. 1080–1092.

[95] Leopold S. S., Rosenberg A. G., Bhatt R. D., Sheinkop M. B., Quigley L. R., and Galante J. O., "Cementless Acetabular Revision. Evaluation at an Average of 10.5 Years," *Clin Orthop Rel Res*, Vol. 369, 1999, pp. 179–186.

[96] Liljenqvist U., O'Brien J. P., and Renton P., "Simultaneous Combined Anterior and Posterior Lumbar Fusion with Femoral Cortical Allograft," *Eur Spine J*, Vol. 7, 1998, pp. 125–131.

[97] Ling R. S., "Femoral Component Revision Using Impacted Morselized Cancellous Graft," *J Bone Joint Surg Br*, Vol. 79, 1997, p. 874.

[98] Ling R. S., Timperley A. J., and Linder L., "Histology of Cancellous Impaction Grafting in the Femur. A Case Report," *J Bone Joint Surg Br*, Vol. 75, 1993, pp. 693–696.

[99] Lofgren H., Johannsson V., Olsson T., Ryd L., and Levander B., "Rigid Fusion after Cloward Operation for Cervical Disc Disease Using Autograft, Allograft, or Xenograft: a randomized study with radiostereometric and clinical follow-up assessment," *Spine*, Vol. 25, 2000, pp. 1908–1916.

[100] Lord C. F., Gebhardt M. C., Tomford W. W., and Mankin H. J., "Infection in Bone Allografts. Incidence, Nature, and Treatment," *J Bone Joint Surg Am*, Vol. 70, 1988, pp. 369–376.

[101] Macdonald S. J., Paprosky W. G., Jablonsky W. S., and Magnus R. G., "Periprosthetic Femoral Fractures Treated with a Long-stem Cementless Component," *J Arthroplasty*, Vol. 16, 2001, pp. 379–383.

[102] Macewen W., "Intrahuman Bone Grafting and Reimplantation of Bone, " *Ann Surg*, Vol. 50, 1909, pp. 959–968.

[103] Maloney W. J., Herzwurm P., Paprosky W., Rubash H. E., and Engh C. A., "Treatment of Pelvic Osteolysis Associated With a Stable Acetabular Component Inserted Without Cement as Part of a Total Hip Replacement," *J Bone Joint Surg Am*, Vol. 79, 1997, pp. 1628–1634.

[104] Maloney W. J., Peters P., Engh C. A., and Chandler H., "Severe Osteolysis of the Pelvic in Association with Acetabular Replacement Without Cement," *J Bone Joint Surg Am*, Vol. 75, 1993, pp. 1627–1635.

[105] Mankin H. J., Doppelt S., and Tomford W., "Clinical Experience with Allograft Implantation. The First Ten Years," *Clin Orthop Rel Res*, Vol. 174, 1983, pp. 69–86.

[106] Mankin H. J., Doppelt S. H., Sullivan T. R., and Tomford W. W., "Osteoarticular and Intercalary Allograft Transplantation in the Management of Malignant Tumors of Bone," *Cancer*, Vol. 50, 1982, pp. 613–630.

[107] Mankin H. J. and Fogelson F. S., Thrasher, A. Z., and Jaffer F., "Massive Resection and Allograft Transplantation in the Treatment of Malignant Bone Tumors," *N Engl J Med*, Vol. 294, 1976, pp. 1247–1255.

[108] Mankin H. J., Gebhardt M. C., Jennings L. C., Springfield D. S., and Tomford W. W., "Long-term Results of Allograft Replacement in the Management of Bone Tumors," *Clin Orthop Rel Res*, Vol. 324, 1996, pp. 86–97.

[109] Masterson E. L., Masri B. A., and Duncan C. P., "The Cement Mantle in the Exeter Impaction Allografting Technique. A Cause for Concern," *J Arthroplasty*, Vol. 12, 1997, pp. 759–764.

[110] Masterson E. L., Masri B. A., Duncan C. P., Rosenberg A., Cabanela M., and Gross M., "The Cement Mantle in Femoral Impaction Allografting. A Comparison of

Three Systems from Four Centres," *J Bone Joint Surg Br*, Vol. 79, 1997, pp. 908–913.

[111] McFarland E. G., Lewallen D. G., and Cabanela M. E., "Use of Bipolar Endoprosthesis and Bone Grafting for Acetabular Reconstruction," *Clin Orthop Rel Res*, Vol. 268, 1991, pp. 128–139.

[112] McGann W. A., Welch R. B., and Picetti G. D., III, "Acetabular Preparation in Cementless Revision Total Hip Arthroplasty," *Clin Orthop Rel Res*, Vol. 235, 1988, pp. 35–46.

[113] McGoveran B. M., Davis A. M., Gross A. E., and Bell R. S., "Evaluation of the Allograft-prosthesis Composite Technique for Proximal Femoral Reconstruction After Resection of a Primary Bone Tumour," *Can J Surg*, Vol. 42, 1999, pp. 37–45.

[114] Meding J. B., Ritter M. A., Keating E. M., and Faris P. M., "Impaction Bone-Grafting Before Insertion of a Femoral Stem with Cement in Revision Total Hip Arthroplasty. A Minimum Two-year Follow-up Study," *J Bone Joint Surg Am*, Vol. 79,1997, pp. 1834–1841.

[115] Michelson J. D. and Curl L. A., "Use of Demineralized Bone Matrix in Hindfoot Arthrodesis," *Clin Orthop Rel Res*, Vol. 325, 1996, pp. 203–208.

[116] Mizutani H. and Urist M. R., "The Nature of Bone Morphogenetic Protein (BMP) Fractions Derived from Bovine Bone Matrix Gelatin," *Clin Orthop Rel Res*, Vol. 171, 1982, pp. 213–223.

[117] Moreland J. R. and Bernstein M. L., "Femoral Revision Hip Arthroplasty with Uncemented, Porous-coated Stems," *Clin Orthop Rel Res*, Vol. 319, 1995, pp. 141–150.

[118] Muscolo D. L., Ayerza M. A., Calabrese M. E., and Gruenberg M., "The Use of a Bone Allograft for Reconstruction After Resection of Giant-cell Tumor Close to the Knee," *J Bone Joint Surg Am*, Vol. 75, 1993, pp. 1656–1662.

[119] Nather A., "Use of Allografts in Spinal Surgery," *Ann Transplant*, Vol. 4, 1999, pp. 19–22.

[120] Nelissen R. G., Bauer T. W., Weidenhielm L. R., LeGolvan D. P., and Mikhail W. E., "Revision Hip Arthroplasty with the Use of Cement and Impaction Grafting. Histological Analysis of Four Cases," *J Bone Joint Surg Am*, Vol. 77, 1995, pp. 412–422.

[121] Nivbrant B. and Karrholm J., "Migration and Wear of Hydroxyapatite-coated Press-fit Cups in Revision Hip Arthroplasty: a radiostereometric study," *J Arthroplasty*, Vol. 12, 1997, pp. 904–912.

[122] Padgett D. E., Kull L., Rosenberg A., Sumner D. R., and Galante J. O., "Revision of the Acetabular Component Without Cement After Total Hip Arthroplasty. Three to Six-year Follow-up," *J Bone Joint Surg Am*, Vol. 75, 1993, pp. 663–673.

[123] Pak J. H., Paprosky W. G., Jablonsky W. S., and Lawrence J. M., "Femoral Strut Allografts in Cementless Revision Total Hip Arthroplasty, " *Clin Orthop Rel Res*, Vol. 295, 1993, pp. 172–178.

[124] Paprosky W. G., "Distal Fixation with Fully Coated Stems in Femoral Revision: a 16-year follow-up," *Orthopedics*, Vol. 21, 1998, pp. 993–995.

[125] Paprosky W. G., Bradford M. S., and Younger T. I., "Acetabular Reconstruction with Massive Allograft and Cementless Prosthesis," *Chir Organi Mov*, Vol. 79, 1994, pp. 379–86.

[126] Paprosky W. G., Bradford M. S., and Younger T. I., "Classification of Bone Defects in Failed Prostheses," *Chir Organi Mov*, Vol. 79, 1994, pp. 285–291.

[127] Paprosky W. G., Bradford M. S., and Younger T. I., "Femoral Reconstruction with Massive Allograft and Cementless Prosthesis," *Chir Organi Mov*, Vol. 79, 1994, pp. 313–318.

[128] Paprosky W. G., Greidanus N. V., and Antoniou J., "Minimum 10-year Results of Extensively Porous-coated Stems in Revision Hip Arthroplasty," *Clin Orthop Rel Res*, Vol. 369, 1999, pp. 230–242.

[129] Paprosky W. G. and Sekundiak T. D., "Total Acetabular Allografts," *Instr Course Lect*, Vol. 48, 1999, pp. 67–76.

[130] Parks N. L. and Engh G. A., "The Ranawat Award. Histology of Nine Structural Bone Grafts Used in Total Knee Arthroplasty," *Clin Orthop Rel Res*, Vol. 345, 1997, pp. 17–23.

[131] Pekkarinen J., Alho A., Lepisto J., Ylikoski M., Ylinen P., and Paavilainen T., "Impaction Bone Grafting in Revision Hip Surgery. A High Incidence of Complications," *J Bone Joint Surg Br*, Vol. 82, 2000, pp. 103–107.

[132] Perry C. R., "Bone Repair Techniques, Bone Graft, and Bone Graft Substitutes," *Clin Orthop Rel Res*, Vol. 360, 1999, pp. 71–86.

[133] Peters C. L., Curtain M., and Samuelson K. M., "Acetabular Revision with the Burch-Schnieder Antiprotrusio Cage and Cancellous Allograft Bone," *J Arthroplasty*, Vol. 10, 1995, pp. 307–312.

[134] Ragni P. and Lindholm T. S., "Interaction of Allogeneic Demineralized Bone Matrix and Porous Hydroxyapatite Bioceramics in Lumbar Interbody Fusion in Rabbits," *Clin Orthop Rel Res*, Vol. 272, 1991, pp. 292–299.

[135] Razack N., Green B. A., and Levi A. D., "The Management of Traumatic Cervical Bilateral Facet Fracture-Dislocations with Unicortical Anterior Plates," *J Spinal Disord*, Vol. 13, 2000, pp. 374–381.

[136] Roffman M., Silbermann M., and Mendes D. G., "Viability and Osteogenicity of Bone Graft Coated with Methylmethacrylate Cement," *Acta Orthop Scand*, Vol. 53, 1982, pp. 513–519.

[137] Rosson J. and Schatzker J., "The Use of Reinforcement Rings to Reconstruct Deficient Acetabula," *J Bone Joint Surg Br*, Vol. 74, 1992, pp. 716–720.

[138] Russell J. L. and Block J. E., "Clinical Utility of Demineralized Bone Matrix for Osseous Defects, Arthrodesis, and Reconstruction: impact of processing techniques and study methodology," *Orthopedics*, Vol. 22, pp. 524–31; quiz 532–533, 1999.

[139] Saleh K. J., Jaroszynski G., Woodgate I., Saleh L., and Gross A. E., "Revision Total Hip Arthroplasty with the Use of Structural Acetabular Allograft and Reconstruction Ring: a Case Series with a 10-Year Average Follow-Up," *J Arthroplasty*, Vol. 15, 2000, pp. 951–958.

[140] Sandhu H. S., Grewal H. S., and Parvataneni H., "Bone Grafting for Spinal Fusion," *Orthop Clin North Am*, Vol. 30, 1999, pp. 685–698.

[141] Sarwat A. M., O'Brien J. P., Renton P., and Sutcliffe J. C., "The Use of Allograft (and avoidance of autograft) in Anterior Lumbar Interbody Fusion: a Critical Analysis," *Eur Spine J*, Vol. 10, 2001, pp. 237–241.

[142] Sassard W. R., Eidman D. K., Gray P. M., Block J. E., Russo R., Russell J., et al., "Augmenting Local Bone with Grafton Demineralized Bone Matrix for

Posterolateral Lumbar Spine Fusion: avoiding second site autologous bone harvest," *Orthopedics*, Vol. 23, 2000, pp.1059–1064; discussion, 1064–1105.

[143] Schmalzried T. P., Fowble V. A., and Amstutz H. C., "The Fate of Pelvic Osteolysis After Reoperation. No Recurrence with Lesional Treatment," *Clin Orthop Rel Res*, Vol. 350, 1998, pp. 128–37.

[144] Schmalzried T. P., Guttmann D., Grecula M., and Amstutz H. C., "The Relationship Between the Design, Position, and Articular Wear of Acetabular Components Inserted Without Cement and the Development of Pelvic Osteolysis," *J Bone Joint Surg Am*, Vol. 76, 1994, pp. 677–688.

[145] Schmalzried T. P., Kwong L. M., Jasty M., Sedlacek R. C., Haire T. C., O'Connor D. O., et al., "The Mechanism of Loosening of Cemented Acetabular Components in Total Hip Arthroplasty. Analysis of Specimens Retrieved at Autopsy," *Clin Orthop Rel Res*, Vol. 274, 1992, pp. 60–78.

[146] Schnee C. L., Freese A., Weil R. J., and Marcotte P. J., "Analysis of Harvest Morbidity and Radiographic Outcome Using Autograft for Anterior Cervical Fusion," *Spine*, Vol. 22, 1997, pp. 2222–2227.

[147] Schreurs B. W., Slooff T. J., Buma P., Gardeniers J. W., and Huiskes R., "Acetabular Reconstruction with Impacted Morselised Cancellous Bone Graft and Cement. A 10- to 15-Year Follow-up of 60 Revision Arthroplasties," *J Bone Joint Surg Br*, Vol. 80, 1998, pp. 391–395.

[148] Scott R. D., "Use of a Bipolar Prosthesis with Bone Grafting in Revision Surgery," *Tech Orthop*, Vol. 2, 1987, pp. 84–89.

[149] Shina, A. A. and Harris W. H., "Bulk Structural Autogenous Grafts and Allografts for Reconstruction of the Acetabulum in Total Hip Arthroplasty. Sixteen-year-Average Follow-up," *J Bone Joint Surg Am*, Vol. 79, 1997, pp. 59–68.

[150] Silverton C. D., Rosenberg A. G., Sheinkop M. B., Kull L. R., and Galante J. O., "Revision of the Acetabular Component Without Cement after Total Hip Arthroplasty. A Follow-up Note Regarding Results at Seven to Eleven Years," *J Bone Joint Surg Am*, Vol. 78, 1996, pp. 1366–1370.

[151] Simmonds R. J., Holmberg S. D., and Hurwitz R. L., "Transmission of Human Immunodeficiency Virus Type 1 from a Seronegative Organ and Tissue Donor," *N Engl J Med*, Vol. 326, 1992, pp. 726–732.

[152] Slooff T. J., Buma P., Schreurs B. W., Schimmel J. W., Huiskes R., and Gardeniers J., "Acetabular and Femoral Reconstruction with Impacted Graft and Cement," *Clin Orthop Rel Res*, Vol. 324, 1996, pp. 108–115.

[153] Slooff T. J., Huiskes R., van Horn J., and Lemmens A. J., "Bone Grafting in Total Hip Replacement for Acetabular Protrusion," *Acta Orthop Scand*, Vol. 55, 1984, pp. 593–596.

[154] Smith R. J. and Mankin H. J., "Allograft Replacement of Distal Radius for Giant Cell Tumor, " *J Hand Surg [Am]*, Vol. 2, 1977, pp. 299–308.

[155] Stockley I., McAuley J. P., and Gross A. E., "Allograft Reconstruction in Total Knee Arthroplasty," *J Bone Joint Surg Br*, Vol. 74, 1992, pp. 393–397.

[156] Sutherland C. J., "Treatment of Type III Acetabular Deficiencies in Revision Total Hip Arthroplasty Without Structural Bone-Graft," *J Arthroplasty*, Vol. 11, 1996, pp. 91–98.

[157] Swank M. L., Lowery, G. L., Bhat, A. L., and McDonough, R. F., "Anterior Cervical Allograft Arthrodesis and Instrumentation: Multilevel Interbody Grafting or Strut Graft Reconstruction," *Eur Spine J*, Vol. 6, 1997, pp. 138–143.

[158] Tiedeman J. J., Connolly J. F., Strates B. S., and Lippiello L., "Treatment of Nonunion by Percutaneous Injection of Bone Marrow and Demineralized Bone Matrix. An Experimental Study in Dogs," *Clin Orthop Rel Res*, Vol. 268, 1991, pp. 294–302.

[159] Tiedeman J. J., Garvin K. L., Kile T. A., and Connolly J. F., "The Role of a Composite, Demineralized Bone Matrix and Bone Marrow in the Treatment of Osseous Defects," *Orthopedics*, Vol. 18, 1995, pp. 153–158.

[160] Tiedeman J. J., Huurman W. W., Connolly, J. F. and Strates, B. S., "Healing of a Large Nonossifying Fibroma After Grafting with Bone Matrix and Marrow. A Case Report, " *Clin Orthop Rel Res*, Vol. 265, 1991, pp. 302–305.

[161] Tsahakis, P. J., Beaver, W. B., and Brick, G. W., "Technique and Results of Allograft Reconstruction in Revision Total Knee Arthroplasty," *Clin Orthop Rel Res*, Vol. 265, 1994, pp. 86–94.

[162] Upton J. and Glowacki J., "Hand Reconstruction with Allograft Demineralized Bone: twenty-six implants in twelve patients," *J Hand Surg Am*, Vol. 17, 1992, pp. 704–713.

[163] Urist M. R., "Bone: Formation by autoinduction," *Science*, Vol. 150, 1965, pp. 893–899.

[164] Van Limbeek J., Jacobs W. C., Anderson P. G., and Pavlov P. W., "A Systematic Literature Review to Identify the Best Method for a Single Level Anterior Cervical Interbody Fusion," *Eur Spine J*, Vol. 9, 2000, pp. 129–136.

[165] Voggenreiter G., Klaes W., Assenmacher S., and Schmit-Neuerburg K. P., "Massive Intercalary Bone Allografts in the Treatment of Primary and Secondary Bone Tumors. A Report on 21 Cases," *Arch Orthop Trauma Surg*, Vol. 114, 1995, pp. 308–318.

[166] Westrich G. H., Mollano A. V., Sculco T. P., Buly R. L., Laskin R. S., and Windsor R., "Rotating Hinge Total Knee Arthroplasty in Severly Affected Knees," *Clin Orthop Rel Res*, Vol. 379, 2000, pp. 195–208.

[167] Wetzel F. T., Hoffman M. A., and Arcieri R. R., "Freeze-dried Fibular Allograft in Anterior Spinal Surgery: Cervical and Lumbar Applications," *Yale J Biol Med*, Vol. 66, 1993, pp. 263–275.

[168] Whiteman D., Gropper P. T., Wirtz P., and Monk P., "Demineralized Bone Powder. Clinical Applications for Bone Defects of the Hand," *J Hand Surg Br*, Vol. 18, 1993, pp. 487–490.

[169] Wilkins R. M., Kelly C. M., and Giusti D. E., "Bioassayed Demineralized Bone Matrix and Calcium Sulfate: use in bone-grafting procedures," *Ann Chir Gynaecol*, Vol. 88, 1999, pp. 180–185.

[170] Wilson M. G., Nikpoor N., Aliabadi P., Poss R., and Weissman B. N., "The Fate of Acetabular Allografts after Bipolar Revision Arthroplasty of the Hip. A Radiographic Review," *J Bone Joint Surg Am*, Vol. 71, 1989, pp. 1469–1479.

[171] Wilson P. D., Jr., "A Clinical Study of the Biomechanical Behavior of Massive Bone Transplants used to Reconstruct Large Bone Defects," *Clin Orthop Rel Res*, Vol. 87, 1972, pp. 81–109.

[172] Wimmer C., Krismer M., Gluch H., Ogon M., and Stockl B., "Autogenic Versus Allogenic Bone Grafts in Anterior Lumbar Interbody Fusion," *Clin Orthop Rel Res*, Vol. 122, 1999, pp. 122–126.

[173] Wittenberg R. H., Moeller J., Shea M., White A. A., III, and Hayes W. C., "Compressive Strength of Autologous and Allogenous Bone Grafts for Thoracolumbar and Cervical Spine Fusion," *Spine*, Vol. 15, 1990, pp. 1073–1078.

[174] Woolson S. T. and Adamson G. J., "Acetabular Revision Using a Bone-ingrowth Total Hip Component in Patients Who Have Acetabular Bone Stock Deficiency," *J Arthroplasty*, Vol. 11, 1996, pp. 661–667.

[175] Yoshida Y., Osaka S., and Mankin H. J., "Hemipelvic Allograft Reconstruction after Periacetabular Bone Tumor Resection," *J Orthop Sci*, Vol. 5, 2000, pp. 198–204.

[176] Young W. F. and Rosenwasser R. H., "An Early Comparative Analysis of the Use of Fibular Allograft Versus Autologous Iliac Crest Graft for Interbody Fusion After Anterior Cervical Diskectomy," *Spine*, Vol. 18, 1993, pp. 1123–1124.

[177] Younger E. M. and Chapman M. W., "Morbidity at Bone Graft Donor Sites," *J Orthop Trauma*, Vol. 3, 1989, pp. 192–195.

[178] Zdeblick T. A. and Ducker T. B., "The Use of Freeze-dried Allograft Bone for Anterior Cervical Fusions," *Spine*, Vol. 16, 1991, pp. 726–729.

[179] Zehntner M. K. and Ganz R., "Midterm Results (5.5–10 years) of Acetabular Allograft Reconstruction with the Acetabular Reinforcement Ring During Total Hip Revision," *J Arthroplasty*, Vol. 9, 1994, pp. 469–479.

[180] Zehr R. J., Enneking W. F., and Scarborough M. T., "Allograft-prosthesis Composite Versus Megaprosthesis in Proximal Femoral Reconstruction," *Clin Orthop Rel Res*, Vol. 322, 1996, pp. 207–223.

[181] Zhang M., Powers R. M., Jr., and Wolfinbarger L., Jr., "Effect(s) of the Demineralization Process on the Osteoinductivity of Demineralized Bone Matrix," *J Periodontol*, Vol. 68, 1997, pp. 1085–1092.

[182] Zhang M., Powers R. M., Jr., and Wolfinbarger L., Jr., "A Quantitative Assessment of Osteoinductivity of Human Demineralized Bone Matrix," *J Periodontol*, Vol. 68, 1997, pp. 1076–1084.

[183] Zicat B., Engh C. A., and Gokcen E., "Patterns of Osteolysis Around Total Hip Components Inserted With and Without Cement," *J Bone Joint Surg Am*, Vol. 77, 1995, pp. 432–439.

The Development of Bone Graft Materials Using Various Formulations of Demineralized Bone Matrix

by Mark Borden, [1] *Ph.D.*

INTRODUCTION

THE DISCOVERY OF THE PROTEINS CAPABLE of inducing bone formation can be traced back to the work by Marshall Urist in the mid-1960s [1]. When Urist discovered that the implantation of various preparations of demineralized bovine bone into rat muscle resulted in the deposition of ectopic bone, he began to investigate the cause of this response. This led to the eventual isolation and characterization of bone morphogenetic proteins (BMPs). Although Urist's early studies are often referred to as the "discovery of BMPs," they also introduced the scientific community to the osteoconductive capabilities of demineralized bone matrix. Following Urist's initial work, a significant amount of research has shown the ability of demineralized matrix (DBM) to induce bone formation [2–8]. The success of DBM in the laboratory eventually translated into its use as a clinical bone graft material. Particulate DBM saw its first use in patients as a bone void filler in dental and periodontal surgeries [9]. The range of applications soon expanded to include the current areas of orthopedics [10–13] and oral and maxillofacial surgery [14–17].

Although DBM and DBM products are currently used to treat a variety of skeletal defects, the initial use of this graft material was limited due to the difficulty in handling the particulate form of the DBM. DBM powder worked well in a contained defect, but delivery and graft migration became issues when moving to more open bone defects. However, in the early 1990s, Osteotech, Inc. (Eatonton, NJ) solved this problem with the introduction of Grafton® Gel. It was the first commercially available product that greatly improved DBM handling and opened the door for its widespread use in bone repair. Using glycerol as a carrier, DBM in Grafton® Gel was effectively delivered to the graft site thereby improving surgical placement. Since its release, a variety of DBM putties, pastes, and sheets have also become available. Each of these products enlists a different approach to delivering and containing DBM at the graft site. The focus of this chapter is to discuss the methodology for developing a DBM product, to review DBM products

---

[1] Interpore Cross International, 181 Technology Dr., Irvine, CA 92618.

currently available, and to introduce some of the issues surrounding DBM based graft materials.

DEVELOPMENT OF A DBM BONE GRAFT

The idea behind designing a DBM bone graft involves the combination of DBM particles with an appropriate carrier to aid in graft delivery and containment. Conceptually, this sounds like an easy task; however, there are several important factors that need to be taken into consideration. The list of available biomaterials capable of effectively delivering the DBM to the graft site is significantly reduced by adding a few bone-specific requirements. The development of a DBM bone graft must incorporate specific design criteria related to bone regeneration in order to maximize the osteoinductive potential of the DBM. First and foremost, the carrier must be biocompatible with both surrounding soft tissue and bone. However, this does not immediately qualify a material for use as a bone graft carrier. Development of a fibrous capsule around a biocompatible carrier in a bone defect can interfere with proper bone healing and should be avoided. For bone grafting applications, the carrier must also be osteocompatible. Osteocompatibility is defined as the ability of a material to provide a suitable environment for bone regeneration without interfering with the bone healing mechanism. Such a carrier will allow for proper healing at the defect site and exposure of the DBM to the surrounding tissue.

In addition to being compatible with the defect site, the carrier should also be compatible with the DBM. The sole purpose of the DBM carrier is to effectively deliver the particles to the graft site and to maintain graft placement. However, this must be accomplished without compromising the biological activity of the DBM powder. The ability of DBM to induce bone formation has been associated with the diffusion of BMPs from the collagen matrix of the DBM particles to the surrounding regeneration site [18]. Work by Reddi showed that the presence of host enzymes during the initial inflammatory phase of healing may be responsible for the release of osteoinductive proteins by breaking down the highly cross-linked collagen matrix of DBM [19]. Therefore, the exposure of DBM to the local host environment is crucial to the success of DBM putty or gel. In order to accomplish this task, the carrier must be resorbable within a relatively short period of time or be porous enough to allow for diffusion of bone morphogenetic proteins (BMPs). If the carrier is impervious to local enzymes and cells, or the material degrades too slowly, diffusion of the proteins from the DBM may not occur or may be delayed reducing the ability of the graft to regenerate bone. With the exception of collagen and gelatin sponges embedded with DBM, most carriers are solid gels and pastes. Typically, these types of carriers are designed to resorb within the first few days of implantation. A carrier that resorbs at a slower pace during the initial healing phase could possibly interfere with the interaction of DBM with the surrounding tissue, and the eventual in-growth of bone and blood vessels.

In addition to the accessibility of the BMPs to the graft site, the long-term interaction between DBM and carrier is also of vital importance to the success of the graft. From the time of manufacture, DBM products may sit on the shelf for extended periods of time before implantation. Typically, manufacturing shelf-life validations assess only the sterility of the packaging over time, not the osteoinductivity of the DBM. It has been shown that freeze-dried DBM is stable for up to 9 months [20]; however, many manufacturers have expiration dates beyond one year. In addition, the 9-month time frame applies to dry DBM and not DBM in prolonged contact with a carrier. Therefore, it is important that the long-term effects of the carrier on the activity of the DBM product are evaluated.

Potential problems that may occur with extended contact include: 1) extraction of the BMPs from the DBM, 2) a reduction or complete loss of activity due to denaturation of the osteoinductive proteins by the carrier, and 3) a change to the handling properties of the DBM/carrier formulation. Regarding extractability of BMPs from DBM, this concept was first introduced by Urist. Using various ionic solutions, it was shown that the osteoinductive proteins of DBM could be extracted from the residual collagen matrix [21,22]. In this process, the activity of the proteins was maintained by partially purifying the extract and minimizing its contact with the extraction solution. This prevented degradation of the inductive proteins by the extraction solution. In DBM putties and gels where the carrier is capable of extracting BMPs, prolonged exposure of the DBM to the carrier could potentially lead to inactivation and a reduction in the osteoinductive potential of the graft material. The denaturation of the BMPs could also potentially occur through the absorption or swelling of the DBM by the carrier. As long as the carrier is in direct contact with the DBM particles, there could be a chance of inactivation.

In addition to the loss of osteoinductivity, a long shelf life may also change the physical properties of the putty or gel. Water-based carriers can dry out leaving the putty or gel crumbly or excessively sticky. Other carriers can be slowly absorbed by the DBM changing the consistency and handling of the product over time. Although the osteoinductivity may be maintained, if the graft is difficult to handle or does not maintain its placement, its effectiveness is reduced. Although these issues can result in decreased function of the DBM product, they are not insurmountable problems. With a comprehensive evaluation of the various DBM/carrier interactions of new putties and gels, these carrier problems can be avoided.

In addition to carrier properties, there are several characteristics related to developing an effective DBM putty or gel. The optimal properties of a DBM bone graft are shown in Table 1. The optimal product would consist of an easy to handle, osteoinductive putty/gel that effectively delivers DBM to the graft site. It would be stable on the shelf for extended periods of time, provide excellent graft handling and containment, and be resistant to irrigation at the implant site. The carrier would also be resorbable in a short period of time and would be compatible with the DBM so that long-term exposure would not reduce its osteoinductive potential. Additionally, the product would be compatible with minimally invasive delivery systems and capable of being mixed with other graft materials (e.g., autograft), growth factors, and/or marrow cells.

With the goal of providing an effective means of delivering DBM to a graft site, several manufacturers have released DBM products to the bone grafting market. Table 2 shows a listing of DBM products currently available. As seen from the list, manufacturers have used a variety of carriers to produce a range of DBM products. The specific formulation of each product is shown in Table 3. A brief description of several commercially available DBM products follows.

TABLE 1— Characteristics of an optimal DBM-based putty or gel.

DBM Maintains Its Osteoinductivity for the Life of the Product	Excellent Handling/Moldability
Long Term Stability of the Handling Properties	Excellent Graft Containment
Quick Resorption of the Carrier	Resistant to Irrigation
Biocompatible and Osteocompatible	Mixable with Other Graft Materials, Growth Factors and/or Marrow Cells
No Mixing Required	Compatible with Minimally Invasive Delivery Systems
No Refrigeration, Heating or Special Processing Required	History of Clinical Use (Carrier)

TABLE 2— Summary of the various DBM-based products.

Company	Product Line	Carrier	DBM Source	Sterilization Method	Product Form
GenSci Orthobiologics Irvine, CA	DynaGraft®, OrthoBlast®, CollaPro™	Poloxamer 407 Water Human Collagen (Matrix only)	Various Tissue Banks	Electron Beam Sterilization	Gel, Putty, Sheet
Interpore Cross Irvine, CA	InterGro™	Lecithin	Various Tissue Banks	Aseptic Processing	Putty
Musculoskeletal Transplant Foundation Edison, NJ	DBX™	Hyaluronic Acid Water	MTF	Aseptic Processing	Gel
Osteotech Eatontown, NJ	Grafton®	Glycerol	Various Tissue Banks	Aseptic Processing	Gel, Putty, Sheet
Regeneration Technologies Alachua, FL	Osteofil®	Porcine Gelatin Water	Various Tissue Banks	Aseptic Processing	Paste, Strips, Disc
Wright Medical Technologies Memphis, TN	Allomatrix®	Calcium Sulfate Carboxymethyl-Cellulose, Water	AlloSource, DCI	E-beam sterilization	Putty

TABLE 3—Composition of the various DBM formulations used for bone grafting applications.

Product	Company	DBM	Carrier	Other Tissue	Other Components
CollaPro™ Matrix	GenSci	Particles	Human collagen		
DynaGraft® Gel	GenSci	Particles	Poloxamer 407 in water		
DynaGraft® Putty	GenSci	Particles	Poloxamer 407 in water		
OrthoBlast™	GenSci	Particles	Poloxamer 407 in water	Cancellous Chips	
InterGro™	Interpore-Cross	Particles	Lecithin		
DBX™	MTF	Particles	Hyaluronic acid in water		
Grafton® Crunch	Osteotech	Fibers	Glycerol	Demineralized cortical cubes	
Grafton® Flex	Osteotech	Fibers	Glycerol		
Grafton® Gel	Osteotech	Particles	Glycerol		
Grafton® Putty	Osteotech	Fibers	Glycerol		
OPTEFORM®	RTI	Particles	Porcine gelatin in water (disc)	Cancellous Chips	
OSTEOFIL®	RTI	Particles	Porcine gelatin in water		
OSTEOFIL® IC	RTI	Particles	Porcine gelatin in water (paste)	Cancellous Chips	
OSTEOFIL® ICM	RTI	Particles	Porcine gelatin in water (strip)	Cancellous Chips	
OSTEOFIL® RT	RTI	Particles	Porcine gelatin (freeze dried)		
ALLOMATRIX®	Wright Medical	Particles	Calcium sulfate		Carboxymethyl-cellulose, water
ALLOMATRIX® C	Wright Medical	Particles	Calcium sulfate	Cancellous Chips (in powder)	Carboxymethyl-cellulose, water
ALLOMATRIX® Custom	Wright Medical	Particles	Calcium sulfate	Cancellous Chips (in powder and additional vial)	Carboxymethyl-cellulose, water
ALLOMATRIX® DR	Wright Medical	Particles	Calcium sulfate	Cancellous Chips (in powder)	Carboxymethyl-cellulose, water

Grafton®

With its release in 1991, Grafton® Gel became the first DBM product available to surgeons. The initial formulation used a mixture of glycerol and DBM particles to create an extrudable bone graft "gel." Since the release of Grafton® Gel, Osteotech has developed several other DBM-based bone graft materials (Fig. 1). Grafton® Putty is a modified version of Gel that uses DBM fibers instead of particles to impart more of a doughy feel to the graft (Fig. 2). In this product, glycerol is used to swell the DBM fibers and to aid in the cohesion of the putty. Grafton® Flex also uses elongated DBM fibers and glycerol; however, in the Flex form, the fibers are pressed into a non-woven sheet (Fig. 1). A newer addition to the Grafton® family is Grafton® Crunch which is a version of the Putty that additionally contains demineralized cortical cubes (Fig. 1).The bone used in the

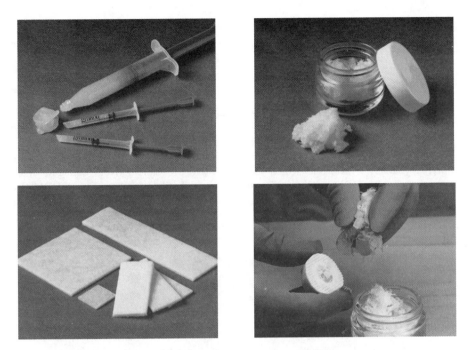

FIG. 1—Grafton® family of DBM products (manufactured by Osteotech, Inc.) includes Grafton® Gel (upper left), Grafton® Putty (upper right), Grafton® Flex (lower left), and Grafton® Crunch (lower right).

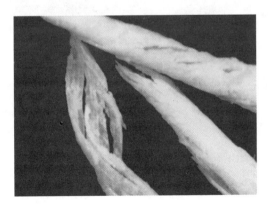

FIG. 2—DBM fibers unique to Osteotech are found in Grafton® Putty, Flex, and Crunch.

Grafton® product line is obtained from a variety of Tissue Banks accredited by the American Association of Tissue Banks (AATB). Osteotech aseptically processes the bone into DBM and aseptically manufactures its Grafton® DBM products.

DynaGraft®

The DynaGraft® Line of DBM products are produced by GenSci Orthobiologics, Inc. (Irvine, CA) and include DynaGraft® Gel, DynaGraft® Putty, OrthoBlast™, and CollaPro™ Matrix (Fig. 3). GenSci's products use two types of carriers to deliver DBM to the graft site. The first product that GenSci released was CollaPro™ Matrix (originally called DynaGraft® Matrix), which consists of a human derived collagen foam impregnated with DBM particles. In this product, both the collagen and DBM are obtained from the same donor to avoid any cross-donor issues. During implantation, the foam is designed to absorb local blood, provide an osteoconductive scaffold for bone regeneration, and deliver DBM to the site.

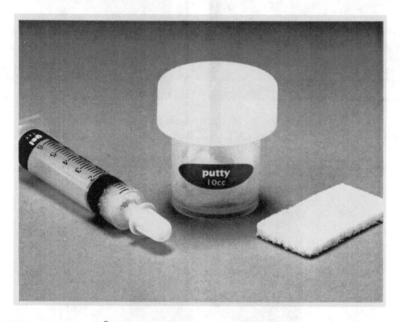

FIG. 3—DynaGraft® line of products manufactured by GenSci Orthobiologics. (From left to right: DynaGraft® Gel, DynaGraft® Putty, and CollaPro™ Matrix.) Dynagraft® Gel and Putty use a copolymer carrier while CollaPro™ Matrix uses a human collagen carrier.

The putty/gel line of products uses a different approach to deliver the DBM particles to the site (Fig. 3). The carrier in these products is a copolymer called poloxamer 407 that exhibits unique thermal properties. Poloxamer 407 is a reverse phase tri-block copolymer (polyethylene oxide–polypropylene oxide–polyethylene oxide) that is liquid at low temperatures (<20°C) and gels at room temperature [23]. Depending on the concentration of DBM in the carrier, a moldable putty or extrudable gel can be formed. GenSci has also added additional osteoconductivity to its putty with the inclusion of cancellous chips in OrthoBlast™ [DBM + cancellous chips + poloxamer 407]. The porous architecture of the chips increases the surface area available for bone growth. Similar to DynaGraft® matrix, the tissue in OrthoBlast™ is also from the same donor. In the manufacture of its products, GenSci uses DBM, cancellous chips, and soft tissue from a variety of AATB Tissue Banks. All products manufactured by GenSci are terminally sterilized using electron beam radiation.

OSTEOFIL®

Similar to GenSci's collagen-based CollaPro™ Matrix, Regeneration Technologies, Inc. (RTI) has also developed a naturally derived DBM product called OSTEOFIL® Paste (Fig. 4). OSTEOFIL® Allograft Paste uses porcine (pig) gelatin mixed with human DBM

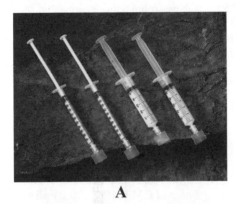

A

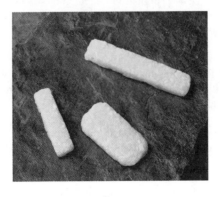

B

FIG. 4—DBM products available from RTI. OSTEOFIL® Allograft Paste (top) is a mix of DBM in a gelatin carrier whereas OSTEOFIL® ICM Allograft Strips (bottom) have cortical cancellous bone chips added to the DBM/gelatin mix. Both formulations are rigid gels at room temperature that soften into moldable pastes at 43–49°C.

to create a thermoplastic DBM composition that is provided in a syringe. OSTEOFIL® Paste is provided to the surgeons in a variety of formulations. RTI has released a version with cortical cancellous chips (CCC) added to the DBM/gelatin mix called OSTEOFIL® IC Moldable Paste. In additional to extrudable pastes, the OSTEOFIL® Paste/CCC formulation is also provided as moldable strips (OSTEOFIL® ICM Allograft Strips) and as a custom shape designed specifically for acetabular cup reconstruction (OPTEFORM® Allograft Paste, Disc).

In order to maintain the biological (osteoinductive) property and structural integrity of the natural components of OSTEOFIL®, RTI ships its products frozen. At the time of surgery, OSTEOFIL® is thawed and heated to 43–49°C to soften the graft material into an extrudable paste (syringe form) or moldable putty (strip form). RTI also manufactures a freeze-dried version of OSTEOFIL® Paste called OSTEOFIL® RT Allograft Paste (DBM + gelatin) that is rehydrated with any available sterile fluid at the time of surgery. This freeze-dried product is stable at room temperature and does not require refrigeration. As in all OSTEOFIL® formulations, once it is delivered to the implant site, the product firms back into a gel as it cools to body temperature. In this form, the graft is resistant to irrigation and maintains graft placement. RTI uses a variety of Tissue Recovery Agencies to procure allograft bone, which it uses to process and prepare DBM. RTI products are produced aseptically and do not require terminal sterilization.

ALLOMATRIX®

Wright Medical Technologies entered the DBM market with its first DBM product, ALLOMATRIX® (Fig. 5). Using a carrier composed of calcium sulfate and carboxy-methylcellulose (CMC), ALLOMATRIX® is provided in a kit form that requires mixing at the time of implantation. The ALLOMATRIX® kit consists of a vial of sterile water and a dry powder mix of DBM, surgical grade calcium sulfate hemihydrate, and CMC. The kit is terminally sterilized by electron beam radiation. The unique formulation of ALLOMATRIX® is based on Wright's core calcium sulfate bone graft technology. Typically, the reaction of calcium sulfate hemihydrate and water results in a paste that thickens into a dough, and then hardens into rigid calcium sulfate dihydrate. The presence of CMC in ALLOMATRIX® prevents the calcium sulfate dihydrate from completely hardening, which results in a moldable putty that can be extruded from a syringe or placed directly at the graft site.

Wright has also developed a newer version of ALLOMATRIX® (called ALLOMATRIX® C) which contains cancellous chips mixed into the DBM/calcium sulfate/CMC powder. Additional versatility is added with the ALLOMATRIX® Custom Kit. Similar in composition to ALLOMATRIX® C, the Custom Kit contains an additional vial of larger sized cancellous chips. ALLOMATRIX® Custom allows the surgeon to customize the consistency of the graft by adjusting the cancellous chip content based on the specific application. Wright's DBM and cancellous chips are provided by AlloSource and DCI Donor Services, Inc. (both accredited by the AATB).

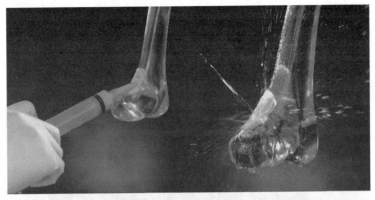

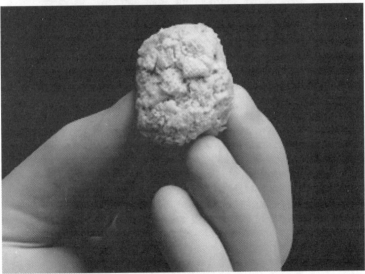

FIG. 5—Top: ALLOMATRIX® putty from Wright Medical is an extrudable putty that maintains graft placement and is resistant to irrigation. Bottom: ALLOMATRIX® Custom adds cancellous chips to the original ALLOMATRIX® formulation.

New DBM Putties

The newer additions to the DBM market include *DBX*™, manufactured by MTF and distributed by Synthes, and *InterGro*™, manufactured and distributed by Interpore Cross Intl. DBX™ Putty consists of DBM particles mixed with a sodium hyaluronate/water gel. Hyaluronic acid is a commonly used biomaterial that gives DBX™ an extrudable putty consistency. DBX™ is aseptically manufactured from DBM processed by MTF. Interpore's new DBM putty, InterGro™, consists of DBM mixed with a lecithin derived phospholipid carrier (Fig. 6). This naturally derived carrier is a common substance found

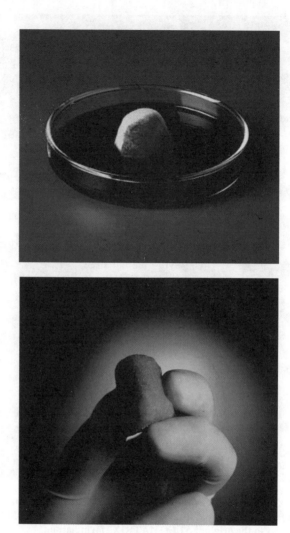

FIG. 6—Interpore Cross's new DBM putty based on a lecithin phospholipid carrier. In addition to effectively delivering DBM to the site, the InterGro™ Putty is resistant to irrigation and exposure to body fluids such as blood.

in the body and has been shown to provide an effective vehicle for DBM delivery. Additionally, due to the lipid nature of lecithin, InterGro is resistant to irrigation. Interpore sources its DBM from various AATB Tissue Banks and aseptically manufactures its putty.

THE OSTEOINDUCTIVITY ISSUE

As seen from the previous products, manufacturers have enlisted a variety of techniques to formulate DBM pastes, putties, and gels for bone grafting applications. However, with different carriers, DBM sources, methods of sterilization, and manufacturing techniques, the question arises as to whether the products are equally effective. Clinical effectiveness has typically been linked to the osteoinductive potential of the DBM in the various products. Methods of assessing the osteoinductivity of particulate DBM have ranged from in vitro tissue culture assays [24–30] to in vivo subcutaneous and intra-muscular implantations in rodents [5,31–35]. However, testing of the final product form of DBM putties and gels (consisting of both carrier and DBM) is not as straightforward. Culturing cells in the presence of a DBM carrier can often interfere with obtaining an accurate assessment of osteoinductivity. Therefore, evaluations of the off-the-shelf form of DBM putties and gels has been limited to in vivo models.

In recent years, the standard model used to assess osteoinductivity has been the athymic rodent assay. The use of an athymic animal allows for the implantation of human DBM without a xenogenic immune response. This model has been shown to be both reproducible and sensitive to varying levels of inductivity [32]. However, recent controversy regarding the athymic model has arisen from reports showing large variability in the inductive response of commercially available DBM putties [36–38]. The data indicated that some DBM materials were highly osteoinductive, whereas others did not show any osteoinductive properties at all. Although the products seemed to have variable levels of inductivity, the issue is not as straightforward as these data indicate. Table 2 shows that DBM products not only differ in the type of carrier, but also the source of DBM, and the method of sterilization. The complexity of the osteoinductivity issue lies in the fact that multiple factors have been shown to effect osteoinductivity. Variables such as donor [39–41], method of demineralization [42], and method of sterilization [43–45] all have been shown to effect the osteoinductivity of particulate DBM. To reduce some of the variability associated with the DBM component, some manufacturers have relied on testing the DBM powder before mixing with the carrier. Although these assays may help eliminate donor and tissue bank variability, it does not take into account the interaction of the DBM with the carrier. As discussed previously, this interaction can have a significant effect on the osteoinductivity of the final DBM product.

The solution seems to be the establishment of an accurate assay capable of measuring the osteoinductivity of the final DBM product (DBM + carrier). However, the broad range of products makes it difficult to choose a specific, all-purpose assay that accounts for the individual chemical and physical properties of each carrier. In past studies, the athymic rat assay has been used to compare some of the various commercial DBM formulations. Although the results have shown prominent differences in the osteoinductivity of the different products, variations in the experimental parameters such as implantation time, implant amount, and implant site can have significant effects on the resulting data. For example, one DBM putty was shown to be highly osteoinductive in one study [38], whereas separate studies showed that it was highly toxic with 100% mortality [46,47]. The main difference between these two models was an increased dose.

Other work [unpublished data] has shown that putties implanted at 28 days in the abdominal region showed little to no induction while the same putty implanted for 35 days in the biceps femoris showed excellent induction. By slightly modifying the experimental parameters of the athymic rat assay, completely different results can be obtained. Although the assay seems highly variable, if it is optimized for each individual product, athymic implantation can serve as an effective method of pre-qualifying a lot of DBM for manufacture. In a proposed scenario, the manufacturer could take a small amount of DBM, prepare a few milliliters of the final putty or gel product (DBM + carrier), and implant those samples into their optimized assay. This would eliminate any DBM lots with a low osteoinductivity while testing the material in the final, sterile form. Although there is an investment of time and money into such testing, it would improve the overall quality of DBM products entering the marketplace and ultimately being used by surgeons.

CONCLUSION

It is clear that the osteoinductivity of DBM putties and gels is dependent on a multitude of factors relating to both the DBM and the carrier in which it is delivered. It is also clear that newer methods for assessing the osteoinductivity of the final, sterile product need to be established. Current techniques utilizing athymic implantations offer a method of evaluating DBM products in an "off-the-shelf" scenario. This takes into account final processing, sterilization of the product, and interactions between DBM and the carrier. However, experimental parameters in the assay need to be optimized for individual products. This will encompass the range in properties of the carriers and provide a product-specific assessment of osteoinductivity. Although it would be difficult to compare various products in the same assay, it would provide manufacturers with a method of quality control ensuring that the most osteoinductive bone graft possible is reaching the surgeon's hands.

REFERENCES

[1]   Urist M. R., "Bone: Formation by Autoinduction," *Science,* Vol. 150, 1965, pp. 893–899.

[2]   Urist M. R., Silverman B. F., Buring K., Dubuc F. L., and Rosenberg J. M., "The Bone Induction Principle," *Clin Orthop Rel Res,* Vol. 53, 1967, pp. 243–283.

[3]   Urist M. R. and Strates B. S., "Bone Formation in Implants of Partially and Wholly Demineralized Bone Matrix. Including Observations on Acetone-fixed Intra and Extracellular Proteins," *Clin Orthop Rel Res,* Vol. 71, 1970, pp. 271–278.

[4]   Bauer F. C., Nilsson O. S., and Tornkvist H., "Formation and Resorption of Bone Induced by Demineralized Bone Matrix Implants in Rats," *Clin Orthop Rel Res,* Vol. 191, 1984, pp. 139–143.

[5]   Harakas N. K., "Demineralized Bone-matrix-induced Osteogenesis," *Clin Orthop Rel Res,* Vol. 188, 1984, pp. 239–251.

[6]   Reddi A. H., Wientroub S., and Muthukumaran N., "Biologic Principles of Bone Induction," *Orthop Clin North Am,* Vol. 18, 1987, pp. 207–212.

[7]   Ripamonti U., "Bone Induction in Nonhuman Primates. An Experimental Study on the Baboon," *Clin Orthop Rel Res,* Vol. 269, 1991, pp. 284–294.

[8]   Tuli S. M. and Singh A. D., "The Osteoinductive Property of Decalcified Bone Matrix. An Experimental Study," *J Bone Joint Surg Br,* Vol. 60, 1978, pp. 116–123.

[9]   Libin B. M., Ward H. L., and Fishman L., "Decalcified, Lyophilized Bone Allografts for Use in Human Periodontal Defects," *J Periodontol,* Vol. 46, 1975, pp. 51–56.

[10]   Iwata H., Sakano S., Itoh T., and Bauer T. W., "Demineralized Bone Matrix and Native Bone Morphogenetic Protein in Orthopedic Surgery," *Clin Orthop Rel Res,* Vol. 395, 2002, pp. 99–109.

[11]   Shapiro S., Connolly P., Donaldson J., and Abel T., "Cadaveric Fibula, Locking Plate, and Allogeneic Bone Matrix for Anterior Cervical Fusions after Cervical Discectomy for Radiculopathy or Myelopathy," *J Neurosurg,* Vol. 95, Suppl, 2001, pp. 43–50.

[12]   Ladd A. L. and Pliam N. B., "Use of Bone-graft Substitutes in Distal Radius Fractures," *J Am Acad Orthop Surg,* Vol. 7, 1999, pp. 279–290.

[13]   Sandhu H. S., "Anterior Lumbar Interbody Fusion with Osteoinductive Growth Factors," *Clin Orthop Rel Res,* Vol. 371, 2000, pp. 56–60.

[14]   Ferretti C. and Ripamonti U., "Human Segmental Mandibular Defects Treated With Naturally Derived Bone Morphogenetic Proteins," *J Craniofac Surg,* Vol. 13, 2002, pp. 434–444.

[15]   Landi L., Pretel R. W., Jr., Hakimi N. M., and Setayesh R., "Maxillary Sinus Floor Elevation Using a Combination of DFDBA and Bovine-derived Porous Hydroxyapatite: a Preliminary Histologic and Histomorphometric Report," *Int J Periodon, Restorat Dent,* Vol. 20, 2000, pp. 574–583.

[16]   Groeneveld E. H., van den Bergh J. P., Holzmann P., ten Bruggenkate C. M., Tuinzing D. B., and Burger E. H., "Histomorphometrical Analysis of Bone

Formed in Human Maxillary Sinus Floor Elevations Grafted with OP-1 Device, Demineralized Bone Matrix or Autogenous Bone. Comparison with Non-grafted Sites in a Series of Case Reports," *Clin Oral Implants Res,* Vol. 10, 1999, pp. 499–509.

[17]   Groeneveld E. H., van den Bergh J. P., Holzmann P., ten Bruggenkate C. M., Tuinzing D. B., and Burger E. H., "Mineralization Processes in Demineralized Bone Matrix Grafts in Human Maxillary Sinus Floor Elevations," *J Biomed Mater Res,* Vol. 48, 1999, pp. 393–402.

[18]   Lohmann C. H., Andreacchio D., Koster G., Carnes D. L., Jr., Cochran D. L., Dean D. D., et al., "Tissue Response and Osteoinduction of Human Bone Grafts in Vivo," *Arch Orthop Trauma Surg,* Vol. 121, 2001, pp. 583–590.

[19]   Landesman R. and Reddi A. H., "In Vivo Analysis of the Half-life of the Osteoinductive Potential of Demineralized Bone Matrix Using Diffusion Chambers," *Calcif Tissue Int,* Vol. 45, 1989, pp. 348–353.

[20]   Pinholt E. M. and Solheim E., "Effect of Storage on Osteoinductive Properties of Demineralized Bone in Rats," *Ann Plast Surg,* Vol. 33, 1994, pp. 531–535.

[21]   Urist M. R., Sato K., Brownell A. G., Malinin T. I., Lietze A., Huo Y. K., et al., "Human Bone Morphogenetic Protein (hBMP)," *Proc Soc Exp Biol Med,* Vol. 173, 1983, pp. 194–199.

[22]   Hanamura H., Higuchi Y., Nakagawa M., Iwata H., Nogami H., and Urist M. R., "Solubilized Bone Morphogenetic Protein (BMP) from Mouse Osteosarcoma and Rat Demineralized Bone Matrix," *Clin Orthop Rel Res,* Vol. 148, 1980, pp. 281–290.

[23]   Cabana A., Ait-Kadi A., and Juhasz J., "Study of the Gelation Process of Polyethylene Oxide-Polypropylene Oxide-Polyethylene Oxide Copolymer (Poloxamer 407) Aqueous Solutions," *J Colloid Interface Sci,* Vol. 190, 1997, pp. 307–312.

[24]   Glowacki J., "Cellular Reactions to Bone-derived Material," *Clin Orthop Rel Res,* Vol. 324, 1996, pp. 47–54.

[25]   Shteyer A., Kaban L. B., and Kao R. T., "Effect of Demineralized Bone Powder on Osteoblast-like Cells in Culture. A Potential Rapid Quality Control Assay," *Int J Oral Maxillofac Surg,* Vol. 19, 1990, pp. 370–373.

[26]   Friedenberg Z. B., Brighton C. T., Michelson J. D., Bednar J., Schmidt R., and Brockmeyer T., "The Effects of Demineralized Bone Matrix and Direct Current on an "In Vivo" Culture of Bone Marrow Cells," *J Orthop Res,* Vol. 7, 1989, pp. 22–27.

[27]   Torricelli P., Fini M., Giavaresi G., and Giardino R., "In Vitro Osteoinduction of Demineralized Bone," *Artif Cells Blood Substit Immobil Biotechnol,* Vol. 26, 1998, pp. 309–315.

[28]   Becerra J., Andrades J. A., Ertl D. C., Sorgente N., and Nimni M. E., "Demineralized Bone Matrix Mediates Differentiation of Bone Marrow Stromal Cells in Vitro: Effect of Age of Cell Donor," *J Bone Miner Res,* Vol. 11, 1996, pp. 1703–1714.

[29]   Wolfinbarger L., Jr. and Zheng Y., "An in Vitro Bioassay to Assess Biological Activity in Demineralized Bone," *In Vitro Cell Dev Biol Anim,* Vol. 29A, 1993, pp. 914–916.

[30] Wilkins R. M., Kelly C. M., and Giusti D. E., "Bioassayed Demineralized Bone Matrix and Calcium Sulfate: Use in Bone-grafting Procedures," *Ann Chir Gynaecol,* Vol. 88, 1999, pp. 180–185.

[31] Munting E., Wilmart J. F., Wijne A., Hennebert P., and Delloye C., "Effect of Sterilization on Osteoinduction. Comparison of Five Methods in Demineralized Rat Bone," *Acta Orthop Scand,* Vol. 59, 1988, pp. 34–38.

[32] Edwards J. T., Diegmann M. H., and Scarborough N. L., "Osteoinduction of Human Demineralized Bone: Characterization in a Rat Model," *Clin Orthop Rel Res,* Vol. 357, 1998, pp. 219–228.

[33] Aspenberg P. and Andolf E., "Bone Induction by Fetal and Adult Human Bone Matrix in Athymic Rats," *Acta Orthop Scand,* Vol. 60, 1989, pp. 195–199.

[34] Lindholm T. S. and Urist M. R., "A Quantitative Analysis of New Bone Formation by Induction in Composite Grafts of Bone Marrow and Bone Matrix," *Clin Orthop Rel Res,* Vol. 150, 1980, pp. 288–300.

[35] Ripamonti U., Magan A., Ma S., van den Heever B., Moehl T., and Reddi A. H., "Xenogeneic Osteogenin, a Bone Morphogenetic Protein, and Demineralized Bone Matrices, Including Human, Induce Bone Differentiation in Athymic Rats and Baboons," *Matrix,* Vol. 11, 1991, pp. 404–411.

[36] Wang J. C., Davies M. C., and Kanim L. E., "Prospective Comparison of Commercially Available Demineralized Bone Matrix for Spinal Fusion," *Proc N Am Spine Soc,* Vol. 15, 2000, pp. 35–37.

[37] Takikawa S., Bauer T. W., and Konbic H., "A Comparative Evaluation of the Osteoinductivity of Two Formulations of Human Demineralized Bone Matrix," *Tran Soc Biomaterials,* Vol. 24, 2001, pp. 302.

[38] Fox W. C., Aufdemorte T. B., and Sandhu H., "Comparative Histologic and Calcium Content Evaluation of Osteofil, Grafton, and Dynagraft Putty Bone Inductive Materials in the Nude Rat at 28 Days," *Proc N Am Spine Soc,* Vol. 15, 2000, pp. 38–39.

[39] Schwartz Z., Somers A., Mellonig J. T., Carnes D. L., Jr., Dean D. D., Cochran D. L., and Boyan B. D., "Ability of Commercial Demineralized Freeze-dried Bone Allograft to Induce New Bone Formation is Dependent on Donor Age but not Gender," *J Periodontol,* Vol. 69, 1998, pp. 470–478.

[40] Schwartz Z., Mellonig J. T., Carnes D. L., Jr., de la Fontaine J., Cochran D. L., Dean D. D., et al., "Ability of Commercial Demineralized Freeze-dried Bone Allograft to Induce New Bone Formation," *J Periodontol,* Vol. 67, 1996, pp. 918–926.

[41] Maddox E., Zhan M., Mundy G. R., Drohan W. N., and Burgess W. H., "Optimizing Human Demineralized Bone Matrix for Clinical Application," *Tissue Eng,* Vol. 6, 2000, pp. 441–448.

[42] Zhang M., Powers R. M., Jr., and Wolfinbarger L., Jr., "Effect(s) of the Demineralization Process on the Osteoinductivity of Demineralized Bone Matrix," *J Periodontol,* Vol. 68, 1997, pp. 1085–1092.

[43] Wientroub S. and Reddi A. H., "Influence of Irradiation on the Osteoinductive Potential of Demineralized Bone Matrix," *Calcif Tissue Int,* Vol. 42, 1988, pp. 255–260.

[44] Buring K. and Urist M. R., "Effects of Ionizing Radiation on the Bone Induction Principle in the Matrix of Bone Implants," *Clin Orthop Rel Res,* Vol. 55, 1967, pp. 225–234.

[45] Aspenberg P., Johnsson E., and Thorngren K. G., "Dose-dependent Reduction of Bone Inductive Properties by Ethylene Oxide," *J Bone Joint Surg Br,* Vol. 72, 1990, pp. 1036–1037.

[46] Bostrom M. P., Yang X., Kennan M., Sandhu H., Dicarlo E., and Lane J. M., "An Unexpected Outcome During Testing of Commercially Available Demineralized Bone Graft Materials: How Safe Are the Non-allograft Components?" *Spine,* Vol. 26, 2001, pp. 1425–1428.

[47] Wang J. C., Kanim L. E., Nagakawa I. S., Yamane B. H., Vinters H. V., and Dawson E. G., "Dose-dependent Toxicity of a Commercially Available Demineralized Bone Matrix Material," *Spine,* Vol. 26, 2001, pp. 1429–1435.

Standards Development Perspectives on the Use of Bone Graft Substitutes Based Upon Allografts

by John S. Kirkpatrick, [1] *M. D.*

THE DEVELOPMENT OF BONE GRAFT substitutes has had explosive growth recently. Bone graft substitutes include collagen or mineral void fillers, processed bone allografts, extracted allograft products such as demineralized bone matrix, and combination products of implants and bone morphogenetic proteins [1,2]. Bone morphogenetic protein products are in need of standardization for a number of issues including dose, concentration of product, carrier factors, and threshold of bone induction [2]. One example of the complex nature of evaluating bone graft substitutes is the recently Food and Drug Administration (FDA) approved "InFUSE"™ Bone Graft/"LT-CAGE"™ Lumbar fusion device. This product includes three components: a metallic device, a collagen sponge, and recombinant human bone morphogenetic protein-2 (rhBMP-2) [3]. The manufacturer provided basic science and clinical data from a several year, multi-center investigation in order to obtain approval for the product. Only one component of the product was subject to a standardized evaluation, and that was the cage component. The remaining components (the collagen sponge and rhBMP-2) had no standardized testing or specifications. This resulted in data that may not be comparable for future products, nor does it allow clinicians to know what key components are needed for specific clinical problems. These problems result in significant added cost to the consumer and health care system, and delays in implementing treatments that are beneficial to patients.

Many questions have been raised regarding the relative efficacy of bone graft substitute products, the relative safety from biologic contaminants, the safety of possible residual processing chemicals, the safety of additives and their safety profiles, and the appropriate dose and form of the various products. How can these questions be answered for all products? When the products are combined, the complexity of the evaluations increases. Should product improvements involving one component of combination

[1] Division of Orthopaedic Surgery, University of Alabama at Birmingham and division of Orthopaedic Surgery, Birmingham Veterans Administration Medical Center, 1813 Sixth Avenue South, MEB 601, Birmingham, AL 35294.

products require re-evaluation of the entire product or can one component be evaluated? These questions need to be addressed quickly through standardized evaluations and possibly standardized processing of the products to ensure the safety and efficacy of each product.

Regulatory agencies in general, and the Food and Drug Administration (FDA) in particular, use consensus standards in the approval process. Section 514(c) of the Food, Drug, and Cosmetic act addresses recognition of consensus standards to satisfy certain regulatory requirements. The use of consensus standards is an integral part of the FDA's implementation of the least burdensome approach in medical device regulation [4]. Standards for describing, testing, and efficacy of products are therefore an integral component of getting such products into clinical use. Consensus standards are developed for specific areas by an interactive process involving the input from producers, users, regulatory bodies, and general interest participants. Consensus standards generally require unanimous agreement on the scientific content of the standard.

Autograft-based bone graft substitutes may involve one or more of the following: synthetic products, the use of human cells, tissue, and cellular and tissue-based products (HCT/Ps), or allograft products. HCT/Ps are the most complex and have three potential pathways for market approval through the Food and Drug Administration. Description of these three pathways serves as an overview for the alternatives for all potential graft products. One pathway applies if the material is considered banked human tissue, it must then conform to appropriate transplant guidelines and regulations issued by the Public Health Service. The second pathway is through the FDA Center for Biologics Evaluation and Research (CBER), which offers a biologic licensing application (BLA) or a new drug application. The Center for Devices and Radiological Health (CDRH) offers the third pathway, which is pre-market approval application (PMA). Some confusion may occur since the products may be considered devices by some and biological products by others. This results in uncertainty in whether the evaluation should occur through the biological regulatory pathway or the devices regulatory pathway. Some considerations exist to aid the determination of whether a product may be a "device" or "biologic" product. The FDA has formed the "tissue reference group" (TRG), made up of representatives from both the Center for Biologics Evaluation and Research (CBER) and the Center for Devices and Radiological Health (CDRH). This group reviews products based on guidelines of what makes a product a "device" versus a "biologic" and which center would be most appropriate for regulatory review. HCT/Ps are considered as "articles containing or consisting of human cells or tissues that are intended for implantation, transplantation, infusion, or transfer. Articles NOT considered as HCT/Ps are: organs, blood or blood components, secreted or extracted products, bone marrow, ancillary products, animal cells, tissues, organs, IVDs." Next is the determination of whether the HCT/P is regulated as a device or as a biologic product. The conditions for being regulated as a device or biologic product include:

(1)   The HCT/P is minimally manipulated, and
(2)   The HCT/P is intended for homologous use only, as reflected by labeling, advertising, or other indications of manufacturer's objective intent, and
(3)   The manufacture of the HCT/P does not involve the combination of the cell or tissue component with a drug or device, except for a sterilizing, preserving, or

storage agent, if the addition of the agent does not raise new clinical safety concerns with respect to the HCT/P, and

(4)   The HCT/P does not have a systemic effect or is not dependent upon the metabolic activity of living cells for its primary function (exception if autologous use, allogeneic use in a first-degree or second-degree relative, or reproductive use).

(5)   Is the HCT/P a biological product, drug, medical device, or combination product?

Homologous vs. non-homologous use refers to the use of an allograft tissue similar to its tissue type. Products for homologous use are potentially devices if they meet additional criteria. Allografts designated as devices must show that they have been "minimally manipulated." To date, allograft bone, which has been cut, shaped, or demineralized is considered minimally manipulated. The intended use or labeling is considered, as is the marketing intent. These factors aid the FDA in the appropriate center for review of each product. Additional information on the tissue reference group can be obtained from the FDA website [5].

Legislation signed in October 2002 establishes an "office of combination products" within the FDA. The responsibilities of this office and how it will function are unavailable at this time but are expected to be detailed by early 2003.

Consensus standards are important to producers and surgeons regardless of the center evaluating a product. The center for devices operates under amendments passed in 1997 that provide for the recognition of voluntary consensus standards. The center for biologics operates with the development of independent FDA standards, but is moving toward the use of consensus standards. Both sections of the FDA require the submission of data based upon testing accomplished according to standards, either consensus or internal. Surgeons seeking the most safe and effective product for their patients would be well served by efficacy data from standardized evaluations, and rely upon procurement and processing standards to ensure their patient's safety from contamination.

Many standards relevant to allograft tissues already exist through the American Association of Tissue Banks [6]. These standards cover critical issues of safe procurement, storage of tissues, and appropriate delivery of tissues to the surgeon. The existence of these recognized standards results in the use of existing standards for allografts and requires less administrative and regulatory cost to the company bringing that product to market. The use of allograft tissues as raw material for products is not well standardized and is the potential source of ethical controversy as well. Those allograft products that receive more than "minimal manipulation" are subject to a much higher level of regulatory scrutiny leading to higher premarket costs and product cost. Part of this higher cost is the demonstration of safety and efficacy of the product in the absence of existing standards. Ethical controversy resulting from the use of allograft-based systems for bone graft substitutes stems from the original source of such allografts as anatomical gifts. The motivation for the donation of these gifts made by families in traumatic situations is altruistic. Such a major "gift of life" should not be a source of profit for medical product companies charging more for a product than the costs of processing. If such a profit occurs, the public trust is broken and the source of such anatomical gifts, and ultimately the bone graft substitute, is likely to be limited. Caution needs to be used in allocating processing costs when pricing allograft-based products.

ASTM International is active in device standards and has taken steps to provide a variety of standards in the area of tissue engineering. Medical and surgical device standards have been developed since 1962 in Committee F 04 on Medical and Surgical Materials and Devices. The standards process within ASTM is a consensus process. There must be agreement on the scientific principles and appropriate application of terms, classifications, specifications, and test methods. It is important for all interested parties to be represented in the development process and not just those with products to be marketed. Producers have an incentive to participate because they want to get their products to market in an efficient manner. Users of the products (surgeons) also are required to make sure that standards are clinically relevant and result in clear indications for use. The users also are needed to ensure safety and efficacy of the products and represent the interests of the patients. General interest participants and regulatory agencies are needed to represent the public health, provide additional representation for the patients, and ensure enforceable standards.

The standards development process generally begins with the concept for a draft standard that is reviewed by a subcommittee and a task group is assigned. The task group writes a draft standard that is then circulated among the subcommittee members with a ballot. The ballot requires specific suggestions for revision if it is not for approval of the standard. At the next subcommittee meeting, the objections are considered and determined to be persuasive, leading to a change in the standard, non-persuasive, or withdrawal by the objector if explanation by the task group clarifies the source of the objection. After a standard is approved by the subcommittee, it then is subject to a main committee ballot where the process is repeated. The ballot process ensures that all members of the subcommittee and committee review the standard for approval, including those who could not be present for meetings. Following main committee approval, the standard is then published and used as needed.

Four types of standards can be applied to issues related to bone graft substitutes. These include Terminology standards, Classifications, Specifications, and Test Methods. Terminology standards provide definitions of technical terms related to a particular area. Terminology important to define includes terms related to bone graft incorporation and evaluation. Specific terms raised by workshop participants are listed in Table 1. The importance of uniform definitions is critical to surgeons using the product and to producers. If the definition of bone includes only the microscopic description of osteoid and mineral and not the presence of cells, then a surgeon may select a bone graft substitute that does not lead to a viable bone replacement. Similarly, if one producer considers a critical size defect smaller than another producer, then the surgeon would not be able to fairly compare the two products.

Classification standards guide the sorting of products in a variety of ways. Suggestions for possible classification standards include classification by process, by chemical composition, by structure, or by biological activity. Structural considerations include morphology, organization of the tissue, powder, solid, porous, or fiber, demineralized vs. nondemineralized, and cell and matrix composition. Biological activity would include descriptive and quantitative measures of osteoconduction, osteoinduction, and/or facilitating bone formation.

Specification standards potentially needed relevant to bone graft substitutes may include existing standards from other organizations or the development of new standards.

The American Association of Tissue Banks (AATB) has standards related to procurement, processing, and sterilization of allograft tissues.

TABLE 1 —Terminology.

Terminology
Bone graft incorporation terms
Bone
Bone induction
Bone conduction
Union/nonunion
Resorption
Resorbable
New bone
Evaluation terms
Minimal manipulation
Critical size defect
Homologous use
Safety
Viral inactivation

Fresh frozen processing, freeze-dried processing, and any additional treatments would be determined by standard specifications. Bone graft substitutes, which are not allograft transplants but instead are products based upon allografts, require additional standards. Specifications for possible development of graft substitutes include concentration/dose, carrier, molecular structure, and physical characteristics. For load bearing graft substitutes, specifications of mechanical strength would need to be standardized and would also need an accompanying test method standard.

Test method standards are needed to clarify the relevance and efficacy of a particular product to its intended use. Standards needed in this area are bioactivity, safety (viral, biocompatibility, etc.), and animal models. A bioactivity standard should address the problem of a volume of one product possibly having a different effect than the same amount of another product. This standard may be developed as a cell culture model, animal model in muscle, critical size defect in long bone, or spine fusion model. Some safety standards may already exist for viral and other infectious agents in processing, but additional standards specific to bone grafts may also need development. Animal models are controversial as to the specific site of the model (muscle pouch, spine, or long bone) as well as species and relevance to human biology. Agreement on relevant models is essential to the safe and appropriate pre-clinical evaluation of bone graft substitutes.

The majority of standards relative to bone graft substitutes other than allograft are most appropriately developed in the Tissue Engineered Medical Products (TEMPs) group (ASTM Committee F04.40- Division IV on TEMPs). This group is the pioneer standards body internationally regarding TEMPs, and includes international participation in developing standards. This division currently has subcommittee activity in Classification and Terminology (F04.41), Biomaterials and Biomolecules (F04.42), Cells and Tissue Engineered Constructs (F04.43), Assessment (F04.44), and Safety (F04.45). Meetings of the TEMPs division are held twice a year and include teleconference participation for international regulatory agencies, manufacturers, users (physicians), and general interest participants.

The standards development process related to bone graft substitutes or TEMPs is in its infancy. There is only one standard published that is specific to bone, F1581-99 Standard Specification for Composition of Anorganic Bone for Surgical Implants. Some TEMP standards, which are nonspecific to bone, include F2149-01 related to automated analyses of cells, F2027-00e01 related to the characterization of substrates for TEMPs, F2150-02e1 on characterization of biomaterial scaffolds, F2103-01 on Chitosan salts as starting materials, and F2064-00 on characterization of alginates. There is one standard under development of a test method for in vitro activity of recombinant human Bone Morphogenetic Protein-2. Additional areas of concern which have little or no activity include: normal biology of bone, assessment of critical size defects, mechanical testing of bone of bone functional replacements, guide for fabricated biomaterials used for bone replacement, and a guide for assessment of bone TEMPs.

One other standards body may become involved in developing standards related to tissue engineered medical products. The International Standards Organization (ISO) Technical Committee 150 (TC150) has recently begun Working Group 11 (WG 11) to explore standards for Tissue Engineered Implants (TEI). They currently have no standards in development but are expected to begin some activity in the area. A formal liaison between ASTM F04 and ISO TC 150 WG11 exists in the form of the US Technical Advisory Group to ISO TC 150 (US-TAG ISO TC 150.)

As bone graft substitutes are developed, appropriate standards are needed for the characterization, marketing, and clinical applications of these products. Such standards will allow clear definition of the expectations of the product (efficacy) and allow the surgeon to choose products that meet specific needs. Standards relevant to safety concerns will ensure protection of the patient from risks disproportionate to the benefit of a product. Standards will allow manufacturers to provide regulatory agencies with appropriate data for the marketing approval of their products. Standards will hopefully allow all parties a clear understanding of terms, classifications, specifications, and test methods relevant to bone graft substitutes and help ensure their appropriate use, safety, and efficacy.

CONCLUSION

Bone graft substitute products based on allograft tissues are being developed and marketed in increasing numbers. Those products that are not significantly modified and are simply transplanted tissue currently have standards, predominantly produced by the AATB. Those products, which are combination products or are manipulated before marketing, have few existing regulatory standards. The development of standards for allograft that is manipulated, combination products, and tissue-engineered products is underway at ASTM International. These standards will facilitate regulatory approval and enable surgeons to make appropriate decisions regarding the safety and efficacy of products for their patients.

REFERENCES

[1]   Finkmeier C., "Bone-Grafting and Bone-Graft Substitutes," *J Bone Joint Surg Am,* Vol. 84, 2002, pp. 454–464.
[2]   Boden S. D., Andersson G. J., Anderson D. G., Damien S., Ebara S., Helm G., et al., "Summary Statement: Overview of Bone Morphogenetic Proteins for Spine Fusion," *Spine*, Vol. 27, 2002, p. S1.
[3]   New Device Approvals: InFuse[TM] Bone Graft /LT Cage[TM] Lumbar Tapereed Fusion Device-P000058. Available at: www.fda.gov/cdrh/pdf/p000058.html.
[4]   "Frequently Asked Questions on the Recognition of Consensus Standards," Guidance for Industry and for FDA Staff, July 22, 2002. Available at: www.fda.gov/cdrh/ost/guidance/109.pdf.
[5]   Manual of Standard Operating Procedures and Policies, Regulatory-General Information, Tissue Reference Group. Available at: www.fda.gov/cber/regsopp/8004.html.
[6]   Standards for Tissue Banking. Available at: www.aatb.org.

Section II: Cellular Systems and Growth Factor-Based Systems for Use as Bone Graft Substitutes

OVERVIEW

Parallel developments in both cell biology and molecular biology have ushered in a new era in the generation of bone graft substitutes. In the past, bone grafting was generally limited to the use of autologous bone or allografts. Native bone products have been extended to include various forms of demineralized bone matrix as an adjunctive material for use in bone grafting. There have been exciting developments in the field of mesenchymal stem cell (MSC) biology. The experimental work detailing the existence of MSCs and the methods of manipulating these cells for use in bone healing or regeneration is detailed in the comprehensive chapters by Bruder and coworkers and by Lieberman and coworkers. Techniques for isolating stem cells from bone marrow, periosteum, muscle, and fat have been developed. These cells can be maintained in tissue culture and manipulated by specific cytokines and growth factors to differentiate along tissue-specific pathways, including fat, connective tissue, muscle, bone, and cartilage. Stem cells are known to be an important component of normal bone healing, as in fracture repair. Cells from the marrow and periosteum differentiate into cartilage and bone, yielding the ossifying fracture callus tissue, which results in mechanical stability of the fracture and ultimately, reconstitution of the bone structure and function. Because of the plastic phenotypic nature of MSCs during differentiation, they are able to provide both the cartilage and bone formation essential to fracture healing. MSCs can be expanded in culture before inducing differentiation or implantation, allowing for larger populations of effective bone healing cells to be obtained. MSCs have been used in a wide variety of models to enhance healing of fractures or bone defects. In vivo, the cells have the ability to spontaneously respond to the microenvironment and locally produced factors and cytokines and differentiate into bone forming cells. The microenvironment is extremely important in MSC differentiation, and matrix component contact, scaffolding materials, and mechanical forces all influence the differentiation process of the cells.

MSCs isolated from bone marrow and injected into fracture or nonunion sites with or without partial purification to concentrate the stem cells have been used successfully both in animal models and in several clinical trials. Enhancement of bone healing by transduction of MSCs with osteoinductive genes such as BMPs has also shown efficacy in healing bone defects in animal models. Thus the use of cell-based and growth factor approaches to bone graft substitutes are complementary. This has led to tremendous growth in research on bone tissue engineering, combining appropriate cells, scaffolds or matrices, and protein growth factors or cytokines to create tissue with potential utility and improved handling characteristics as bone graft substitutes. Both organic and inorganic mineral materials have been used individually and in combination to produce scaffolding materials, which will support osteogenic differentiation and growth with appropriate cellular elements. An advantage of the use of MSCs is the ability to produce an autogenous, patient-specific material from the individual's own cells, obviating immunologic issues associated with allograft transplantation. The possibility also exists of producing embryonic or genetically modified stem cell lines, which have low antigenicity and could be used allogeneically in the clinical setting. Some scaffolding materials may include variously processed forms of allograft bone or demineralized bone matrix.

The dramatic progress in molecular biology in the past decade has resulted in the cloning and subsequent production of recombinant human bone morphogenetic proteins (BMPs) has opened entirely new frontiers. Experimental and clinical studies have validated the use of these single osteogenic proteins as effective agents in causing bone induction to a degree that is clinically useful in bone repair and regeneration. Other growth factors such as transforming growth factor-beta's (TGF-βs), fibroblast growth factors (FGFs), and insulin-like growth factors (IGFs) may stimulate bone formation in some circumstances. The current state of growth factor osteoinduction, comparing the scientific data with these various growth factors, is well summarized in the chapter by Cheung et al.

A large number of promising applications not only in bone regeneration, but also in the control of stem cell differentiation and cartilage formation, are emerging as the knowledge of the BMPs and related factors accumulates. The ability of these molecules to induce an entire cascade of cellular proliferation, differentiation, and matrix formation is one of the most intriguing and exciting discoveries in musculoskeletal science. Their use both as single factor osteoinductive agents and as components of tissue engineering are reviewed. A wonderful chapter by the pioneering scientists in the field, Drs. Sampath and Reddi describes the latest developments and challenges in the use of BMPs. Clinical trials demonstrating efficacy and safety have been conducted, and two of the BMPs, BMP-2 and OP-1 (BMP-7) have recently been approved by the Food and Drug Administration for selective and specific indications in patients (spinal arthrodesis for BMP-2, and refractory tibial nonunions for OP-1). These agents are used in conjunction with a delivery device consisting of a collagen sponge, and the device containing BMP-2 is used in conjunction with a metal cage implant for spine arthrodesis.

The translation of the basic research on BMPs into the clinical arena is a major milestone in orthopedics, although much research remains to be done. The BMPs need to be used at much higher than physiologic dosages to induce bone in higher animals and humans, and the reasons are not clear. Also, the optimum clinical indications, timing of administration, delivery devices and dosages of molecules, and potential complications all need much investigation for these new tools to find their appropriate applications in treatment of bone healing in patients. The role of BMP inhibitor molecules such as chordin and noggin, which can offset effects of exogenous BMPs has not been thoroughly studied. Also, the potential effects of antibodies, which may form in the host in response to use of BMPs, remain incompletely understood, although initial clinical trials have not demonstrated adverse systemic effects.

Other new and exciting approaches for delivery of osteoinductive molecules to specific sites to enhance bone healing include use of gene therapies, in which the gene encoding the BMP or other protein is introduced into cells, which then produce and secrete the protein locally. Also, intracellular regulatory molecules such as LMP1 have been identified, which can stimulate cells to produce high levels of BMPs, and this has been successfully used in stimulation of bone healing. Thus an array of new approaches using molecular biologic tools to enable clinical applications of osteoinduction with protein growth factors is emerging, and holds tremendous promise.

The development of combination products as bone graft substitutes, which may contain scaffolding materials or matrices, cellular components, and potentially protein growth factors such as BMPs or their genes, presents a set of complex challenges not only at the experimental level, but in the regulatory arena. An excellent review of the current status of the regulation of bone graft substitutes follows in the chapters by Gadaleta and Arinzeh, which also provide insights into the inherent complexities of regulation of these types of biologic products. Whether a bioengineered tissue product is classified as a medical device, a biologic product, a drug, or a combination of these determines which agency within the Food and Drug Administration (FDA) oversees its review and regulation. Obviously, many of these new products may cross traditional regulatory boundaries. New guidelines for regulation of human cellular and tissue-based produces have been introduced, and also cover minimally manipulated tissues such as allograft products, and use of tissues for homologous or non-homologous clinical uses. In addition, the FDA is working with researchers, industry, and ASTM International to produce standards for various types of bone graft substitutes.

The new developments in use of cell- and growth factor-based approaches to bone graft substitutes have ushered in an exciting new era in the translation of basic research to clinical applications in the musculoskeletal field. Although many challenges remain, evidence suggests tremendous promise for the future. The following chapters provide excellent reviews of the state of the art in cell- and factor-based growth factor approaches to bone graft substitutes, and the regulatory processes that are evolving to deal with these new types of medical products.

Mohammed Attawia, M.B.B.Ch.

Section Leader

Randy Rosier, M.D., Ph.D.

Section Leader

Cell-Based Approaches for Bone Graft Substitutes

by Mohamed Attawia, [1,2] *M.B.B.Ch., Sudha Kadiyala,* [1] *Ph.D.,*
Kim Fitzgerald, [1] *B.S., Karl Kraus,* [3] *D.V.M., and*
Scott P. Bruder, [1,4] *M.D., Ph.D.*

INTRODUCTION

THE PROCESS OF BONE HEALING is an exquisite and complex phenomenon that requires the interaction of three key ingredients: 1) competent bone-forming cells, 2) a suitable framework or scaffold, and 3) the presence of biological stimulants. The principal actors in the process of bone formation are the bone-forming cells, the osteoblasts, and their precursors, the mesenchymal stem cells (MSC). Bone formation is the direct result of the self-assembly and mineralization of the extracellular matrix (ECM) produced by the osteoblasts. The osteoblast arises from the MSC and progresses through a series of maturation steps, eventually becoming an osteoblast. In this process, the cell stages of the maturation sequence are known by distinct names. The term osteoprogenitor is commonly used to refer to all the cell stages preceding the osteoblast, including the MSC.

To function properly, and synthesize ECM, the cells, referred to above, require attachment to a scaffold. In addition to providing the framework for cells to synthesize the bone, the scaffold also serves to present (or transduce) stimulatory signals, which is the third important ingredient involved in the bone formation process. Biological stimulants, or "signals," direct the synthetic activity of the osteoblasts and regulate the formation and remodeling of bone. The stimulatory signals can take a variety of forms such as chemical (growth factors), mechanical loading (Wolff's law), electromagnetic stimuli, or even nutritional cues such as partial pressure of oxygen.

In summary, one needs an adequate supply of osteoblasts on an appropriate scaffold in the presence of appropriate stimuli to successfully form new bone. Although the specific process and rate of bone healing is dependent on the complex interaction of multiple factors both temporally and spatially, the general process can be simplified to a series of steps as described below.

Stages of New Bone Formation

The injury to bone causes release of specific growth factors into the surrounding environment, and activation of the platelet-mediated wound healing response. The

[1] DePuy AcroMed, Inc., a Johnson & Johnson Company, Raynham, MA 02767.
[2] Department of Chemical Engineering, Drexel University, Philadelphia, PA 19104.
[3] Orthopedic Research Laboratory, Tufts University, School of Veterinary Medicine, North Grafton, MA 01536.
[4] Department of Orthopaedics, Skeletal Research Center, Case Western Reserve University, Cleveland, OH 44106.

released factors, at a given concentration gradient, act as "attracting agents" causing white blood cells and osteoprogenitor cells, such as the MSCs, to migrate to the wound site. This stage is commonly termed chemotaxis, during which white blood cells such as macrophages migrate to the site, clear the wound of damaged and necrotic tissue, and also release additional chemotactic factors to attract even more MSCs.

After the MSCs and other osteoprogenitor cells arrive at the site, they begin to multiply to reach a critical mass that is required for the bone healing process. This stage is termed proliferation. Following proliferation, these cells undergo maturation into osteoblasts or chondrocytes and start the phenomenon of bone formation through a process of membranous or endochondral bone formation. The differentiated function of the osteoblast is to synthesize the bone matrix (osteoid) that eventually mineralizes into mature bone. The above process can be summed as a sequence of steps starting with chemotaxis followed by proliferation and differentiation, and ending with optimal differentiated function (Fig. 1).

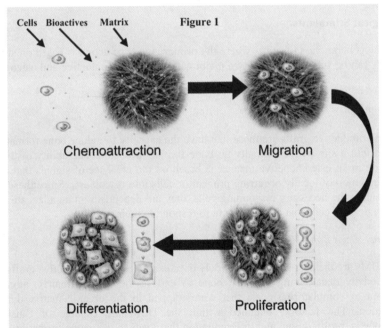

FIG. 1— **Graphical representation of the cellular events (Chemotaxis, Proliferation, and Differentiation) that lead to bone regeneration. Reproduced with permission from DePuy AcroMed.**

Due to the complex nature of the bone healing process, it is possible to manipulate the process at various stages of the healing cascade. Thus, various types of graft materials have been developed, or are under investigation, for use in the clinical setting. These materials can be grouped according to various different classification schemes. One convenient method to classify these graft materials is on the basis of their principal mode of action: osteoconductive, stimulatory, or osteogenic.

TYPES OF GRAFT MATERIALS

Osteoconductive Grafts

Osteoconductive materials refer to scaffolds that provide the appropriate framework for bone to grow in sites where bone naturally occurs. They function as substrates on which locally residing osteoblasts can attach. These materials rely on the presence of sufficient cues in the local environment to direct the bone formation process, and depend on direct physical contact with exposed surfaces of viable bone.

Examples of osteoconductive scaffolds include naturally occurring materials such as mineralized cancellous chips (allograft), as well as synthetic substrates such as tricalcium phosphates (TCP) or hydroxyapatite (HA). Due to their relatively passive role, these materials have limited utility on their own. However, they can be mixed with autograft and adequately serve as autograft extenders. Also, they are essential for the delivery of cells and/or stimulatory signals.

Biological Stimulants

The general class of grafts where the primary mode of action is based on stimulatory signals can be sub-divided into two major categories: osteoinductive and osteopromotive grafts.

Osteoinductive Grafts

Osteoinductive grafts are those that have the capacity to induce bone formation when placed into a site where normally no bone formation occurs. The ability of the graft to function in an osteoinductive manner is based on the presence of signals that can cause differentiation of locally occurring progenitor cells into osteoblasts. Since these grafts do not contain the necessary responding cells, they are dependent on an adequate supply of locally derived cells that are competent to respond to their stimuli.

Demineralized Bone Matrix (DBM)

DBMs are the best-known and widely used example of osteoinductive grafts. DBM is prepared by decalcifying allograft bone to expose the organic matrix, along with a plethora of stimulatory signals that were trapped in the organic matrix during bone formation. The factors contained within the DBM are capable of causing MSC chemotaxis, proliferation, and differentiation that leads to new bone formation. Also, the underlying matrix provides a suitable scaffold for cell attachment.

The majority of DBM use is in the form of particulates (powders or fibers) requiring the use of a carrier to impart desirable handling properties to the graft. A variety of inert carriers have been used including glycerol and gelatin. These carriers are largely considered non-contributory to the biological events but work solely to improve handling characteristics. DBM is typically considered to be an autograft extender rather than a replacement. This is due to the limited bioactivity of DBM. However, when combined with the appropriate supplement such as platelet rich plasma (PRP), the biological potency is raised to a level that may impart function as an optimal bone graft.

Bone Morphogenetic Protein (BMP)

Urist postulated that the inductivity of DBM was due to the presence of specific proteins trapped inside [1]. He coined the term "bone morphogenetic protein" to describe them [2]. A large family of BMPs were purified from the DBM and eventually cloned [3–6]. During this process, it was determined that rather than a single protein, there are a series of BMP molecules, as well as related molecules, that may also be isolated from non-bony tissue including cartilage. The BMPs are members of the TGF-β superfamily of growth factors [7–9] that includes the TGF-βs, Cartilage-derived growth factors (CDGF) and other proteins termed Growth and Differentiation Factors (GDF).

Osteopromotive Grafts

Osteopromotive grafts have the ability to enhance the natural bone formation process by providing stimulatory signals at various stages of the bone healing process. However, they differ from osteoinductive grafts in that they do not have the capacity, by themselves, to induce new bone formation at non-skeletal sites. Thus, osteopromotive grafts are best used where there are: 1) natural differentiation cues sufficient to initiate bone formation in the local environment, 2) osteoinductive graft materials such as DBM, or 3) osteogenic graft materials, such as autograft bone and marrow. The best example of an osteopromotive graft material is platelet rich plasma (PRP), which can be used in all the aforementioned settings.

Platelet Rich Plasma (PRP)

Platelet rich plasma is prepared by collecting and concentrating platelets from whole blood obtained from the patient immediately before or during surgery. Platelets are a rich source of multiple growth factors, and thus by concentrating platelets from blood, the surgeon has a ready and ample source of autologous growth factors. Various methods can be used to concentrate platelets from whole blood with the resulting suspension containing growth factor levels increased proportionally to the increased platelet count [10].

Some of the growth factors that have been shown to be concentrated in platelets are Transforming Growth Factor–Beta (TGF-β), Platelet Derived Growth Factor (PDGF) and Vascular Endothelial Growth Factor (VEGF). TGF-β is one of the most potent chemotactic agents for osteoprogenitor cells and also has a very important role in supporting differentiated function of the osteoblasts [11]. PDGF is a potent mitogenic agent and posseses chemotactic properties. VEGF is the best-known inducer of angiogenesis, or blood vessel formation. Thus, by providing a variety of concentrated growth factors, PRP can play an important role in enhancing the bone healing process and, when used with the appropriate bone graft such as DBM or autograft, contributes to an optimal bone healing environment. In addition, since platelet concentrates readily form a fibrin-based clot, this attribute may be used as an adjuvant to impart desirable handling characteristics to bone grafts used in surgery. Furthermore, the fibrin mesh that is formed during the clotting process also provides scaffolding needed for bone repair.

The benefit of adding PRP to various bone grafts in preclinical studies has been published previously [12]. In the clinical arena, there is extensive data available in the context of bone reconstruction in oral and maxillofacial surgery [13]. For instance, Marx et al. [14] demonstrated a significant benefit in the healing rate and bone density due to the addition of PRP to autograft. In the setting of spine, studies showing the benefits of PRP have just recently appeared in the literature [15].

PRP has also enjoyed widespread use outside of bone grafting serving as a wound healing accelerant in a variety of areas including plastic surgery and general surgery. The growth factors within the PRP work in conjunction with the local tissue specific signals in order to promote tissue healing. Thus in the setting of the bone, PRP is typically used in conjunction with a bone graft such as DBM or autograft, and works by enhancing the healing response and providing a useful handling system for the graft itself.

Osteogenic Grafts

Osteogenic material refers to a mixture that contains all the necessary elements required for direct bone formation. Upon implantation into the body, such grafts can form bone without any additional elements from the surrounding environment other than nutritional and metabolic support. The basis of such powerful bone-forming potential lies in the fact that these grafts contain the necessary synthetic machinery namely, living cells. Not only must these grafts contain the cells, but they must include a scaffold that orients the cells and provides access to the stimulatory signals, which may be synthesized by the cells themselves.

Cortico-cancellous Bone Autograft

Today's "gold-standard" in bone grafting continues to be autologous bone harvested from the iliac crest. Autograft is clearly the best example of an osteogenic graft. When harvested from the iliac crest, autograft provides a mixture of cells from fully differentiated osteoblasts lining the cancellous bone to undifferentiated stem cells in the marrow compartment. The cells, combined with the matrix and signals provided by the bone morsels, yield a mixture that leads to reproducible bone formation when placed into the surgical site.

There are, however, many drawbacks associated with the harvesting and use of iliac crest autograft. One such drawback is the potential morbidity and a resulting post-operative pain that can last for several years [16]. Some studies show the incidence of such complications, including, infection to be as high as 20% [17]. Limited supply and quality of autograft is sometimes problematic for patients undergoing procedures that require large graft volumes. Due to these considerations, some surgeons have reverted to using autograft from the local site. However, it is well documented that local bone (especially from the spine) does not possess the same level of biologic activity as iliac crest autograft due to the poor cellularity. Furthermore, the amount of local bone available is usually so small that it is insufficient to use alone, and requires combination with DBM or another scaffold type material.

Another limitation with the use of autograft is its poor handling characteristics. Autograft is typically morselized during harvest and is not easily placed or retained at the surgical site. More recently, however, PRP has been used effectively to impart desirable handling characteristics to autograft, as well as to provide a source of concentrated growth factors that may further enhance the bone healing process.

Bone Marrow-based Grafts

Another class of potent osteogenic graft materials is based on cells and stimulatory signals from bone marrow. Though not widely used in patients at present, the biologic potential of marrow has been appreciated by surgeons for nearly 100 years [18]. Unlike autograft, bone marrow can be obtained from the iliac crest using a simple needle aspiration, which does not cause morbidity. These grafts have typically been prepared by mixing small amounts of aspirated marrow with an osteoconductive graft such as TCP granules or osteoinductive grafts such as DBM. The bone marrow provides a rich source of cells ranging from the MSCs, which are the undifferentiated stem cells, to cells that have already committed down the osteogenic lineage and are destined to become osteoblasts.

Despite the favorable bone forming capacity of bone marrow-based grafts, they have not enjoyed widespread use as a replacement for iliac crest cancellous autograft for three reasons: 1) The variability resulting from inconsistent and substandard aspiration technique, 2) the very low osteoprogenitor content of these small aspirates, and 3) the combination of marrow cells with sub-optimal scaffold materials. Because the osteoprogenitors constitute a very small fraction of the cells in the marrow, and may occur as infrequently as one in 100 000 cells [19], optimizing the aspiration, cell selection, and delivery system is critical to graft success. Despite the relative scarcity of these progenitors, it is important to remember that the bone marrow and periosteum provide a richer source of these cells than any other tissue.

Culture-Expanded Cell Technology

Because it is impractical to obtain large quantities of mature osteoblasts for tissue repair and regeneration, strategies aimed at collecting their progenitors have gained popularity. One such approach is to isolate bone marrow, which can be used as a source of MSCs that can be culture expanded in the laboratory for several weeks. These progenitor cells may then be directed into the osteoblastic lineage prior to their combination with a delivery vehicle. In an attempt to accelerate bone formation, several investigators have explored the use of differentiated osteoblasts in tissue engineering of bone. Culturing MSCs with dexamethasone, ascorbic acid and B-glycerophosphate directs the cells into the osteogenic lineage [20–23]. Theoretically, these predifferentiated osteoblasts then can be used to treat various bone defects.

Okumura et al. [24] and Yoshikawa et al. [25] cultured bone marrow derived rat MSCs with dexamethasone on porous hydroxyapatite to allow cell attachment to the matrix and promote lineage progression while still in vitro. Implantation of the differentiated cell and matrix combination into an ectopic subcutaneous site supports an accelerated bone formation compared with samples implanted with undifferentiated marrow cells. Bone formation occurred on the surface of the hydroxyapatite and moved toward the center of the pore, suggesting that a stable bone-matrix interface was forming. Implants seeded with osteoblasts had a 10-fold higher level of bone gamma carboxylated glutamic acid (Gla) protein at 4 weeks than did the implants seeded with fresh marrow. These data indicate that the use of predifferentiated osteoblasts enhanced the rate and extent of bone regeneration.

Breitbart et al. [26] also used predifferentiated osteoblasts to achieve tissue engineered bone repair. For these studies, a polyglycolic acid nonwoven resorbable fiber was used as a scaffold for cell delivery. The fibers were seeded with cells derived from rabbit periosteal tissue, and cultured with dexamethasone in vitro to promote osteoblastic differentiation. The osteoblast-seeded fibers were used to treat full thickness calvarial defects in rabbits. Twelve weeks after implantation, the cell seeded fibers produced significant bone, whereas little repair was seen in defects that had been left untreated or were implanted with fibers not containing cells. Together, these studies suggest that committed osteoblasts could form the basis for rapid and effective repair of bone defects.

To show clinical applicability of tissue regeneration therapies using such MSCs, a series of preclinical studies was performed. These investigations, all aimed at achieving osseous regeneration in a critical sized defect of the femur, were designed to compare the efficacy and effective dosing when the cellular source was escalated from rodents to large animals, and eventually to humans. In the first study, culture expanded, marrow-derived MSCs were used to repair a segmental defect in the femur of rats [27]. Syngeneic MSCs at a density of 7.5×10^6 cells/mL were loaded onto a porous HA/TCP cylinder and implanted in an 8 mm long diaphyseal defect. By 8 weeks, nearly every pore of the implants contained considerable new bone (Fig. 2a). In contrast, cell-free implants were well vascularized, but displayed little if any bone formation within the pores (Fig. 2b). In the defects treated with MSC-loaded implants, substantial new bone formation occurred at the interface between the host and the implant, leading to a continuous span of bone across the defect. Furthermore, a periosteal callus of bone also was present in samples loaded with MSCs but not with cell-free implants. These studies established the proof of principle for MSC-based tissue regeneration therapy in bone.

The ability of MSC-loaded implants to repair defects in larger animals was examined in a critical-sized canine femoral gap defect model [28,29]. The healing of a 21 mm osteoperiosteal defect was studied using ceramic implants made from porous hydroxyapatite/ß-tricalcium phosphate that had been loaded with autologous culture expanded MSCs at a density of 7.5×10^6 cells/mL. At 16 weeks, atrophic nonunion occurred in all of the femurs that had untreated defects, and only a small amount of trabecular bone formed at the cut ends of the cortex of the host bone in this group (Fig. 2c). In contrast, radiographic union was established rapidly at the interface between the host bone and the implants in samples that had been loaded with MSCs. Numerous fractures, which became more pronounced with time, developed in the implants that had not been loaded with cells. Significantly more bone was found in the pores of the implants loaded with MSCs than in the cell-free implants. In addition, a large collar of bone formed around the implants that had been loaded with cells; this collar became integrated and contiguous with callus that formed in the region of the periosteum of the host bone. The collar of bone remodeled during the study, ultimately resulting in a size and shape that was comparable with the segment of bone that had been resected. Osseous callus did not develop around the cortex of the host bone or around the implant in any of the specimens in the control groups.

Culture expanded *human* MSCs also have been shown to effect bone repair in a segmental gap defect model [30]. Human MSCs were loaded onto ceramic cylinders similar to those described above, and used to repair an identical femoral defect created in athymic rats. Because these rats lack T-lymphocytes, transplantation of xenogeneic material does not lead to graft rejection. Like the studies using syngeneic rat MSCs, substantially more bone was found in defects that received cylinders loaded with human MSCs than in those that received cell-free implants. With the MSC-loaded implants, complete union between bone and implant was achieved at 12 weeks. Before that time, there was an increasing amount of bone formed between the 4- and 8-week evaluation points. Biomechanical testing, at 12 weeks, confirmed that femurs implanted with MSC-loaded ceramics were significantly stronger than those that received cell-free ceramics (Fig. 2*d*). Measurement of stiffness and torque showed increases of 245% and 212%, respectively, in the MSC-loaded samples compared with the cell-free carrier samples. These studies show that human and rat MSCs are capable of healing a clinically significant bone defect in a well established model of bone repair.

The three studies described above show the success of using mesenchymal stem cells to regenerate bone in segmental defects. Using rat, canine, or human mesenchymal stem cells, bone fill ranged from 40–47% of available space, a value not likely to be exceeded given the nature of the scaffold and the requirement for vasculature and associated soft tissue [27,28,30]. The cellular doses required to effect bone repair were constant across species, and the process of bone repair remained the same. The ability of the therapeutic approach to scale up in a predictable manner increases one's confidence that cell-based therapies for bone repair will be effective in the treatment of human disease.

These studies indicate that culture-expanded MSCs can be presented in sufficient numbers in a supportive delivery vehicle to provide bony regeneration of a large, osteoperiosteal femoral defect in both small and large animals. Figure 3 depicts how this experience may potentially be used to construct an *autologous* cell-matrix composite for excision-repair of femoral gaps and other osseous defects in humans. In the case pictured, we suggest that the use of an external fixator could allow load-bearing by the patient shortly after implantation. If the fixator could be constructed to incrementally transfer partial load to the implant, the fixator could be sequentially off-loaded so that more and more load can be gradually transferred to the implant. As the MSCs differentiate into osteoblasts and fabricate bone onto the walls of the porous implant, the incremental loading would serve to orient the new bone and stimulate its acquisition of mechanical integrity. Eventually, the implant would carry 100% of the load and the external fixator could be removed so that no metal devices would remain. The delivery vehicle would be naturally replaced as osteoclasts resorb its matrix and osteoblasts replace it with new, host-derived bone as governed by the natural turnover sequence. The selection of appropriate biomaterials and configurations for each formulation will depend on the anatomic site for regeneration, the mechanical loads present at the site, and the desired rate of incorporation. It may also be possible to use allogeneic MSCs for these massive osseous repairs. In this case, the immunoreactive groups on the MSCs would need to be muted or inactive. The availability of allogeneic cell therapy, or universal donor cells, would provide easy access for trauma-related skeletal reconstruction or for gene therapy applications. In addition, such allogeneic cells may be incubated in osteoinductive media prior to implantation to cause them all to enter the osteogenic pathway. These osteogenic, or jump-started, cells could be loaded into the delivery vehicle thereby accelerating the bone formation. In addition, the allo-MSCs would become either osteocytes or would expire as osteoblasts. This accelerated bone formation conceivably would attract host-

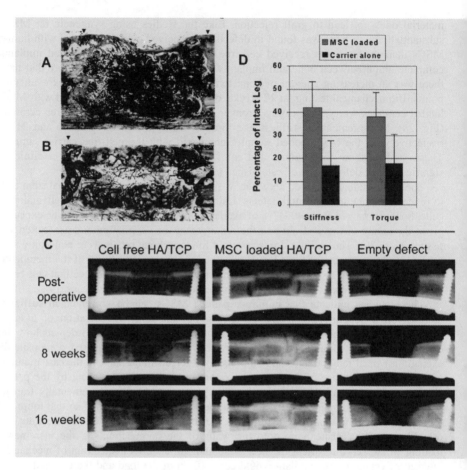

FIG. 2—MSC-mediated bone regeneration in preclinical animal studies of segmental defect repair. (A) Rat segmental defects fitted with a HA/TCP carrier loaded with syngeneic rat mesenchymal stem cells form a solid osseous union with the host, and contain substantial new bone throughout the pores by 8 weeks. (B) Defects fitted with a cell free HA/TCP carrier do not contain bone within the pores of the implant, nor is there significant union at the interfaces, indicated by the arrowheads. (Stain, Toluidine blue-O, original magnification x16.) (C) Radiographic appearances of bone healing in a 21 mm canine femoral gap defect 16 weeks after surgery. Animals that did not receive an implant had a fibrous nonunion. Animals that received a mesenchymal stem cell loaded HA/TCP cylinder had a substantial amount of bone regeneration at the defect site, including a peri-implant callus that remodeled to the size of the original bone by 16 weeks. Those animals receiving cell free implants did not achieve healing of their defects, as is evident by the lack of new bone and the multiple fractures throughout the body of the implant material. (D) Results of biomechanical torsion testing performed on athymic rat femurs 12 weeks after implantation with human mesenchymal stem cell loaded ceramics. Load to failure and overall stiffness was more than twice that of controls at the same time. Reproduced with permisson from DePuy AcroMed.

derived osteogenic cells to the repair site and the bulk of the repair bone would then become of host origin. Eventually, when the repair bone turned-over, the allogeneic osteocyte-containing bone would be replaced by host bone and immunosuppression therapy, if used, could be discontinued.

Although these culture-expanded techniques have the potential to yield a large number of repair-competent cells, the logistics of the process pose considerable challenges for use in a hospital or private practice setting. Combined with our own observations that minor manipulations of autologous marrow in appropriate carriers creates sufficient osteogenic potential to heal critical sized defects [31], we believe that intra-operative manipulation of bone marrow has the potential to revolutionize treatment options for patients requiring augmentation of bone formation. Figure 3 suggests a paradigm under which fresh marrow, as well as culture-expanded MSCs, can be the basis of the bone graft material.

Selective Cell Retention Technology

Recently, techniques to aspirate bone marrow have identified an optimal way to minimize its dilution with peripheral blood, resulting in samples with reproducibly high cellularity and osteogenic potential [32]. An automated and simple methodology for the active intra-operative concentration of cells participating in the bone healing process is currently in the late stages of development. This technique relies on the selective retention of the osteoprogenitor cells from bone marrow onto substrates that are directly implantable.

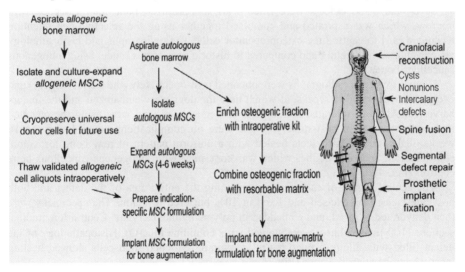

FIG. 3—Diagram of clinical strategies for allogeneic MSC-, autologous MSC-, and bone marrow-based bone regeneration. (MSC = mesenchymal stem cell.) Reproduced with permission from DePuy AcroMed.

The technique is based on controlled flow of marrow through matrices of specific geometry, chemistry and biocompatibility. By properly designing the substrate or mixture of substrates, very potent osteogenic bone grafts can be easily prepared in a matter of minutes intra-operatively.

For instance, Takigami et al. [33] used the selective cell retention technique to capture the osteoprogenitor cells on a bed of DBM powder. Using this cell-enhanced mixture of allograft, they were able to reproducibly obtain spine fusion in a canine model. The results were comparable to those achieved with autograft, and significantly better than that observed when whole bone marrow or the allograft mixture alone was implanted [33].

Initial clinical results in interbody spine fusion and long bone defect repair using this technique at the Cleveland Clinic Foundation have yielded encouraging results. While the selective cell retention method has great promise, the widespread use of this technique will require the development of kits that allow easy integration into the flow and timing of the surgical procedure. Moreover, identification of substrate mixtures that provide optimal cell capture, orientation and presentation to the stimulatory signals could tranform the way we think about, and practice, the art of bone grafting.

In our recent efforts, we have evaluated a mixture of demineralized bone fibers and cancellous bone chips enriched with bone marrow to repair critical sized femoral defects in dogs. As described above, we employed the unilateral 21 mm osteoperiosteal defect in the femoral diaphysis of dogs, and stabilized it with a stainless steel fixation plate [29]. These critical sized defects were filled with an optimized bone matrix seeded with marrow, which was aspirated and combined together using the selective cell retention technique [33] to capture the osteoprogenitor cells. The radiographs and histopathology were evaluated for healing and compared to historic data of this model using autogenous cancellous bone.

Cranial to caudal radiographs were obtained post-operatively (the day of surgery) and every four weeks for 16 weeks, at which time the dogs were euthanized and the femurs harvested. All dogs tolerated the surgical procedure well, and were using the operated limb within two days post-surgery. There were no complications noted during the 16 weeks of the study. All defects healed with a uniform pattern of new bone formation, consolidation, and remodeling, which was consistent with autogenous cancellous bone controls (Fig. 4).

The central region of each femur, containing the entire area of the defect and both host interfaces, was excised and fixed in 10% buffered formalin. The specimens were then dehydrated, cleared, and embedded in polymethylmethacrylate. Central longitudinal sections (100 μm thickness were stained with Toluidine blue-O). Histopathology of the defect filled with allograft bone matrix containing enriched stem cells showed healing mostly by trabecular-like bone (Fig. 5).

In conclusion, this study showed that the use of allograft demineralized bone fibers and mineralized cancellous chips enriched in bone marrow derived cells (using selective cell retention technique) results in regeneration of a critically sized segmental bone defect in dogs. In addition, it appears that this regeneration of bone is radiographically comparable to regeneration of similar defects filled with autogenous cancellous bone.

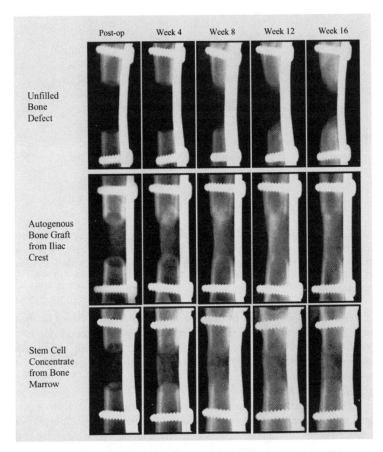

FIG. 4—Radiographs of the canine segmental defect treated with autogenous cancellous bone, optimized allograft bone matrix enriched in stem cell concentrate from bone marrow and a controlled defect left unfilled. Autogenous cancellous bone and optimized allograft bone enriched in bone marrow derived cells healed in a consistent pattern of calcification and early remodeling, but the empty defect did not unite. Reproduced with permission from DePuy AcroMed.

Summary

There are a wide variety of bone graft substitutes available to the surgeon for the repair or augmentation of bone. Although the specific mode of action may be different for each of the graft materials, the underlying physiological process that leads to bone formation is the same. The process of bone formation relies on the recruitment of osteoprogenitor cells to the site, followed by their differentiation into osteoblasts. These differentiated osteoblasts are responsible for the synthesis of the new bone. This new bone is then remodeled under the influence of the mechanical environment. Different graft materials function by specifically

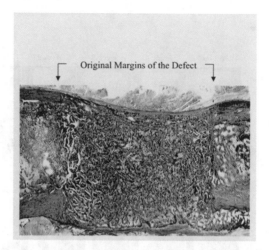

Original Margins of the Defect

FIG. 5—**Low power photomicrograph of a central longitudinal section from the femoral defect harvested 16 weeks after implantation. (100 μm thick section of nondecalcified material embedded in methylmethacrylate, stained with Toluidine blue-O). The defect zone shows a new trabecular-like bone growth. Reproduced with permission from DePuy AcroMed.**

enhancing one or more of the steps in the bone formation process. Based on their mode of action, these grafts can be classified into four categories: 1) osteoconductive materials that provide a scaffold; 2) osteoinductive material that can cause osteoblastic differentiation of progenitor cells; 3) osteopromotive materials that can enhance the bone formation process; and, 4) osteogenic grafts that contain repair-competent osteoprogenitor cells (Table 1).

It is important for the surgeon to understand the efficacy of each type of graft relative to other grafts. In general, we feel osteoconductive grafts may have limited potency and may be restricted to small voids or defects when used alone. Osteoinductive grafts have a wide array of efficacy ranging from moderate, when combined with DBM, to high, when associated with purified or recombinant BMPs. With a highly osteoinductive growth factor, such as BMP, the identification of an appropriate carrier for the delivery and presentation of the growth factor is critical. Osteopromotive grafts, such as PRP, are not used by themselves, but are typically added to the surgeon's graft of choice to enhance the bone formation rate. Thus, the efficacy of the combination graft containing osteopromotive material is driven in part by the performance characteristics of the underlying graft material. Osteogenic grafts rely on the presence of competent osteoprogenitor cells for their ability to form bone and their efficiency is governed in part by the concentration of these cells.

In choosing the appropriate graft for the application, the surgeon has to consider a variety of factors in addition to the efficacy of the graft. These factors include morbidity to the patient and the economic burden on both the patient and society. The majority of the bone grafts available today rely on a single feature for their action, which limits their use to narrow indications. In humans, although some grafts have been shown to be equivalent to autograft in a very narrow indication, none have proven to be superior to autograft or as versatile as autograft. However, as our understanding of the complex phenomena of bone formation increases, potent combination grafts that are based on osteoprogenitor cells delivered on the appropriate scaffold in the presence of the appropriate stimulatory signals will become more widely available, and, could potentially become the superior alternative.

TABLE 1—Different graft materials enhancing one or more steps in the bone formation process.

	Physiologic Principle	Examples
Osteoconduction	Ingrowth of bone from margins of defect with gradual resorption of scaffold	Cortical segments, banked allogeneic bone, resorbable biomaterials
Osteopromotion	Enhancement or acceleration of the natural cascade of bone repair	Platelet rich plasma, electromagnetic stimulation, certain bioactive factors (FGF)
Osteoinduction	Promotes phenotypic conversion of undifferentiated cells into osteoblasts	Demineralized bone matrix, bone extracts, peptides, recombinant morphogenetic proteins
Osteogenesis	Transplantation of viable osteoblasts and precursors	Autogenous cancellous bone, marrow and periosteum

REFERENCES

[1] Urist M. R., "Bone Formation by Autoinduction," *Science*, Vol. 150, 1965, pp. 893–899.

[2] Urist M. R., DeLange R. J., and Finerman G. A. M., "Bone Cell Differentiation and Growth Factors," *Science*, Vol. 220, 1983, pp. 680–686.

[3] Bentz H., Nathan R. M., Rosen D. M., Armstrong R. M., Thompson A.Y., Segarini P. R., et al., "Purification and Characterization of a Unique Osteoinductive Factor from Bovine Bone," *J Biol Chem*, Vol. 264, 1989, pp. 20805–20810.

[4] Luyten F. P., Cunningham N. S., Ma S., Muthukumaran N., Hammonds R. G., Nevins W. B., et al., "Purification and Partial Amino Acid Sequence of Osteogenin, a Protein Initiating Bone Differentiation," *J Biol Chem*, Vol. 264, 1989, pp. 13377–13380.

[5] Wang E. A., Rosen V., D'Alessandro J. S., Bauduy M., Cordes P., Harada T., et al., "Recombinant Human Bone Morphogenetic Protein Induces Bone Formation," *Proc Natl Acad Sci USA*, Vol. 87, 1990, pp. 2220–2224.

[6]   Wozney J. M., Rosen V., Celeste A. J., Mitsock L. M., Whitters M. J., Kriz R. W., et al., "Novel Regulators of Bone Formation: Molecular Clones and Activity," *Science*, Vol. 242, 1988, pp. 1528–1534.

[7]   Lyons K., Graycar J. L., Lee A., Hashmi S., Lindquist P. B., Chen E. Y., et al., "Vgr-1, A Mammalian Gene Related Xenopus Vg-1 is a Member of the Transforming Growth Factor-β Gene Superfamily," *Proc Natl Acad Sci USA*, Vol. 86, 1989, pp. 4554–4558.

[8]   Ozkaynak E., Rueger D. C., Drier E. A., Corbett C., Ridge R. J., Sampath T. K., et al., "OP-1 cDNA Encodes and Osteogenic Protein in the TGF-β Family," *Eur Mol Biol Organ J*, Vol. 9, 1990, pp. 2085–2093.

[9]   Wozney J. M., "Bone Morphogenetic Proteins," *Prog Growth Factor Res*, Vol. 1, 1989, pp. 267–280.

[10]   Kevy S. V., Jacobson M. S., Blasetti L., and Fagnant A., "Preparation of Growth Factor Enriched Autologous Platelet Gel," Harvard Medical School, Center for Blood Research Laboratory, *Tran Soc Biomater*, Vol. XXIV, 2001, p. 262.

[11]   Wergedal J. E., Mohan S., Lundy M., and Baylink D. J., "Skeletal Growth Factor and Growth Factors Known to be Present in Bone Matrix Stimulate Proliferation and Protein Synthesis in Human Bone Cells," *J Bone Miner Res*, Vol. 5, 1990, pp. 179–186.

[12]   Walsh W., Nicklin S., Loefler A., Yu Y., and Arm D., "Autologous Growth Factor Gel (AGF) and Spinal Fusion," *Orthop Research Society, 47th Annual Meeting*, Vol. 26, 2001, p. 951.

[13]   Whitman D. H., Berry R. L., and Green D. M., "Platelet Gel: An Autologous Alternative to Fibrin Glue with Applications in Oral and Maxillofacial Surgery," *J Oral Maxillofacial Surg*, Vol. 55, 1997, pp. 1294–1299.

[14]   Marx R. E., Carlson E. R., Eichstaedt R. M., Schimmele S. R., Strauss J. E., and Georgeff K. R., "Platelet-Rich Plasma, Growth Factor Enhancement for Bone Grafts," *Oral Surg Oral Med Oral Pathol Oral Radiol Endod*, Vol. 85, 1998, pp. 638–646.

[15]   Sethi P., Miranda J., Grauer J., Friedlaender S., Kadiyala S., and Patel T., "The Use of Platelet Concentrate in Posterolateral Fusion: Biomechanical and Histologic Analysis," *Int Soc Study Lumbar Spine*, 2001, p. 27.

[16]   Gupta A. R., Shah N. R., Patel T. C., and Grauer J. N., "Perioperative and Long-Term Complications of Iliac Crest Bone Graft Harvesting for Spinal Surgery: A Quantitative Review of Literature," *Int Med J*, Vol. 8, 2001, pp. 163–166.

[17]   Chapman M. W. and Younger E. M., "Morbidity at Bone Graft Donor Sites," *J Orthop Trauma*, Vol. 3, 1989, pp. 192–195.

[18]   Goujon E., "Recherches Experimentales sur les Proprietes Physiologiques de la Moelle Desos," *Journal de l'Anatomie et de Physiologic Normales et Patholgiques de l'Homme et des Animaux*, Vol. 6, 1869, p. 399.

[19]   Bruder S. P., Jaiswal N., and Haynesworth S. E., "Growth Kinetics, Self-Renewal and the Osteogenic Potential of Purified Human Mesenchymal Stem Cells During Extensive Subcultivation and Following Cryopreservation," *J Cell Biochem*, Vol. 64, 1997, pp. 278–294.

[20] Kadiyala S., Young R. G., Thiede M. A., and Bruder S. P., "Culture-Expanded Canine Mesenchymal Stem Cells Possess Osteochondrogenic Potential In Vivo and In Vitro," *Cell Transplant*, Vol. 6, 1997, pp. 125–134.

[21] Lennon D. P., Haynesworth S. E., Bruder S. P., Jaiswal N., and Caplan A. I., "Development of a Serum Screen for Mesenchymal Progenitor Cells from Bone Marrow," *In Vitro Cell Dev Biol*, Vol. 32, 1996, pp. 602–611.

[22] Maniatopoulos C., Sodek J., and Melcher A. H., "Bone Formation In Vitro by Stromal Cells Obtained from Marrow of Young Adult Rats," *Cell Tissue Res*, Vol. 254, 1988, pp. 317–330.

[23] Owen M., "Lineage of Osteogenic Cells and Their Relationship to the Stromal System," *Bone Min*, 3rd ed., W. J. Peck, Ed., Elsevier, Amsterdam, 1985, pp. 1–25.

[24] Okumura M., Ohgushi H., and Dohi Y., "Osteoblastic Phenotype Expression on the Surface of Hydroxyapatite Ceramics," *J Biomed Mater Res*, Vol. 37, 1997, pp. 122–129.

[25] Yoshikawa T., Ohgushi H., and Tamai S., "Immediate Bone Formation Capability of Prefabricated Osteogenic Hydroxyapatite," *J Biomed Mater Res*, Vol. 32, 1996, pp. 481–492.

[26] Breitbart A. S., Grande D. A., and Kessler R., "Tissue Engineered Bone Repair of Calvarial Defect Using Cultured Periosteal Cells," *Plast Reconstr Surg*, Vol. 101, 1998, pp. 567–574.

[27] Kadiyala S., Jaiswal N., and Bruder S. P., "Culture-Expanded, Bone Marrow-Derived Mesenchymal Stem Cells Can Regenerate a Critical-Sized Segmental Bone Defect," *Tissue Eng*, Vol. 3, 1997, pp. 173–185.

[28] Bruder S. P., Kraus K. H., Goldberg V. M., and Kadiyala S., "The Effect of Implants Loaded with Autologous Mesenchymal Stem Cells on the Healing of Canine Segmental Bone Defects," *J Bone Joint Surg Am*, Vol. 80, 1998, pp. 985–99.

[29] Kraus K., Kadiyala S., Wotton H. M., Kurth A., Shea M., Hannan M., et al., "Critically Sized Osteo-Periosteal Femoral Defects: A Dog Model," *J Invest Surg*, Vol. 12, 1999, pp. 115–124.

[30] Bruder S. P., Kurth A. A., Shea M., Hayes W. C., Jaiswal N., and Kadiyala S., "Bone Regeneration by Implantation of Purified, Culture-expanded Human Mesenchymal Stem Cells," *J Orthop Res*, Vol. 16, 1998, pp. 155–162.

[31] Bruder S. P., "Bone Regeneration: From Embryonic Chicks to Human Clinical Therapy," *52nd Annual Meeting of the Association of Bone and Joint Surgeons*, San Antonio, TX, Vol. 52, 2000, p. 26.

[32] Muschler G. F., Boehm C., and Easley K., "Aspiration to Obtain Osteoblast Progenitor Cells from Human Bone Marrow: The Influence of Aspiration Volume," *J Bone Joint Surg Am*, Vol. 79, 1997, pp. 1699–1709.

[33] Takigami H., Muschler G., Matsukura Y., Boehm C., Valdevit A., Kambic H., et al., "Spine Fusion Using Allograft Bone Matrix Enriched in Bone Marrow Cells and Connective Tissue Progenitors," *Trans Orthop Res Soc*, Vol. 27, 2002, p. 807.

Clinical Issues in the Development of Cellular Systems for Use as Bone Graft Substitutes

by Peter G. Whang,[1] M.D. and Jay R. Lieberman,[1] M.D.

INTRODUCTION

THE SUCCESSFUL REPAIR of skeletal defects is essential to the treatment of numerous orthopedic conditions such as fracture nonunion, spinal fusion, revision total joint arthroplasty, and segmental bone loss secondary to trauma or tumor resection. Various approaches to augment bone formation are presently available, but all of these treatment options are associated with significant limitations to their use. Autologous bone graft is still considered to be the gold standard and remains the most widely used therapy to stimulate bone repair. Unfortunately, only limited quantities of autograft may be harvested from the skeleton, and this invasive process often gives rise to considerable donor site morbidity, including persistent pain, paresthesia, infection, fracture or gait disturbance [1–4]. Cadaveric allograft bone has poor osteoinductive potential, and there continues to be concerns about graft resorption, inadequate revascularization, and possible transmission of pathogens [5–7]. Demineralized bone matrices are prepared by the acid extraction of allograft bone, resulting in the loss of the mineralized component while retaining collagen and noncollagenous proteins, including growth factors. However, demineralized bone matrices contain only minimal quantities of these growth factors. Because of differences in their processing, these substances possess variable osteoinductive activity and should generally be used as osteoconductive agents [8,9]. Clearly, alternative approaches for enhancing bone formation need to be developed.

Bone regeneration is a complex process consisting of a tightly regulated cascade of cellular interactions. As part of the acute inflammatory response, bioactive molecules are released, which promote the influx of pluripotential mesenchymal progenitor cells into the site of bony injury. In response to other bone-specific growth factors, these stem cells proliferate and differentiate into osteoblasts capable of secreting osteoid, which is subsequently mineralized to form new bone [10–18]. Thus, successful bone repair requires the following components: growth and differentiation factors that generate an osteoinductive signal, responsive osteoprogenitor cells, an osteoconductive matrix to support cell adhesion and migration, and adequate vascularity to facilitate the entry of oxygen, osteogenic cytokines, and other nutrients into the defect.

Tissue engineering is an innovative science whose objective is the fabrication of complex, functional tissues using cells, signaling molecules, and biologic matrices [19].

---

[1] UCLA Department of Orthopedic Surgery, Center for Health Sciences 76-134, 10833 LeConte Avenue, Los Angeles, CA 90095.

An increased understanding of the molecular and cellular interactions underlying bone formation and fracture healing has led to the development of novel tissue engineering strategies to address challenging bone repair problems. By providing an alternative to traditional bone grafting techniques, tissue engineering methods may transform the ways in which bone defects are treated.

Growth factors such as the bone morphogenetic proteins (BMPs) are thought to play an indispensable role in the process of bone formation by inducing uncommitted pluripotential cells to undergo osteogenic differentiation, and the introduction of recombinant BMPs has been shown to promote osseous repair of segmental defects in several different animal models [20–26]. Other growth factors such as transforming growth factor-β and fibroblast growth factor enhance bone healing by activating cellular proliferation [27–29]. In humans, the doses of recombinant proteins necessary to obtain healing are considerably higher than the levels observed during normal bone regeneration, possibly because these purified agents undergo rapid degradation in vivo or the carrier systems currently being used do not deliver the growth factors in a physiologic manner [30,31].

Autologous growth factor concentrate prepared from platelets represents another factor-based strategy that may be applied in conjunction with a source of osteogenic cells. This platelet-rich plasma is believed to contain multiple growth factors that collectively may function to enhance bone healing. Although platelet-derived growth factors have already been shown to stimulate bone formation in an animal model and have also been used to augment lumbar spinal fusion in humans [32,33], further studies are necessary to identify the specific growth factors present in platelet concentrate and to determine their efficacy in various clinical situations.

Even though treatment with growth factors provides a direct osteoinductive stimulus, this strategy is still dependent upon the presence of osteoprogenitor cells able to respond to this signal. Thus, implantation of these exogenous bioactive factors may have limited efficacy in clinical scenarios with reduced osteogenic potential, such as those involving significant bone loss, poor vascularity, and inadequate soft tissue coverage. In addition, the carrier systems used to deliver these proteins need to be optimized. Therapies combining the administration of growth factors with cellular systems for use as bone graft substitutes may prove to have a synergistic effect by delivering both osteoinductive proteins and cells that may undergo subsequent osteoblastic differentiation.

There are three major strategies for bone regeneration, based on the essential elements involved in the repair process: matrix scaffolds, growth factors, and cells. Osteoprogenitor cells play an integral role in all of these treatments because they function as the bioreactors responsible for synthesizing new tissue. Whereas osteoconductive matrices and growth factor systems are dependent on the presence of local endogenous cells capable of undergoing osteogenic differentiation, cellular approaches to tissue engineering of bone involve the direct transfer of exogenous precursor cells to the site of repair, thereby increasing the number of cells available to participate in bone formation.

Several cell-based therapies are currently being developed for use as bone graft substitutes, including unfractionated bone marrow [34–50], pluripotential stem cells isolated from various mesenchymal tissues [10–15, 51–55], and gene therapy [56–62]. However, before replacing any of the standard treatment options for the repair of bone defects, these osteogenic techniques will need to show improved healing rates with minimal complications. Although the results of preclinical studies have been promising, the widespread acceptance of these cellular approaches will ultimately be dependent on the validation of three fundamental clinical objectives—efficacy, safety, and cost-effectiveness.

EFFICACY AND SAFETY OF CELLULAR SYSTEMS

The vast majority of orthopedic conditions are not fatal, and in many cases patients with impaired bone healing are relatively young and healthy with skeletal defects limited to a single extremity. As a result, when developing cellular systems for use as bone graft substitutes, the issue of safety takes on considerable importance and any significant morbidity related to these treatment strategies is unacceptable.

Bone marrow, mesenchymal stem cells, and gene therapy methods have already been shown to stimulate osteogenesis in vitro and promote healing of skeletal defects in multiple animal models [10–15,35–38,40–42,44–45,47,50–62,74]. Although these preclinical studies are required for the initial evaluation of cellular systems, due to certain inherent limitations the results obtained from in vitro and animal experiments may not necessarily be applicable to humans. In vitro osteogenesis occurs under ideal conditions in cell culture, and in most animal models of bone repair the healing tissue defect is supplied with adequate perfusion and soft tissue coverage. Consequently, these studies do not accurately simulate the inhospitable biological environment often observed in fracture nonunion, pseudarthrosis of the spine, and other clinical situations in which regeneration is complicated by substantial bone loss, poor vascularity, and exuberant scar tissue formation. Preclinical investigations also do not take into account other systemic risk factors for impaired bone repair that will influence the success of cell-based therapies, such as increased age, use of tobacco or other drugs, irradiation of the local tissue bed, metabolic disease (e.g., diabetes), and osteoporosis [63,64]. Before unfractionated bone marrow, mesenchymal stem cells, and gene therapy techniques are considered viable options for the treatment of bone defects, they should be evaluated by randomized, controlled clinical trials to confirm their efficacy and to establish appropriate indications for their use as bone graft substitutes.

Bone Marrow Cell Systems

Human bone marrow cells have been successfully applied to a variety of clinical settings, including the regeneration of bone. This osteogenic potential of bone marrow is mediated by the activity of osteoprogenitor cells as well as endogenous growth factors [65]. Numerous in vitro and in vivo studies have previously shown its capacity to stimulate bone formation [35–38,40–42,44–45,47,50]. Bone marrow aspirates have also been shown to be effective for the treatment of bone defects in humans. In conjunction with adequate mechanical stabilization, percutaneous injection of autologous marrow has been used to promote healing of fracture nonunions [39,43,46,48–49]. This procedure involves the extraction of bone marrow cells from the iliac crest, which may either be directly introduced into the osseous defect or first combined with demineralized bone matrix to form a composite graft with improved handling characteristics.

In the largest reported series consisting of 100 patients treated with autologous marrow injections to enhance osteogenesis, only 80% experienced significant regeneration of their skeletal defects, with the remaining 20% exhibiting minimal bone formation at the site, requiring repair [48]. The relatively low rate of healing associated with the use of unfractionated bone marrow may reflect the paucity of osteoprogenitor cells present in mature bone marrow. Even in healthy adults, only 36–55 of every million nucleated bone marrow cells will undergo osteogenic differentiation [66,67]. Furthermore, conditions such as advanced age and osteoporosis are accompanied by a further decline in the quantity of undifferentiated stem cells present in bone marrow, especially in women [66,68–70]. Because osseous regeneration is dependent on the number of cells available to participate in bone synthesis, patients with fewer local osteogenic precursors will typically generate an attenuated healing response, increasing the risk of nonunion and other complications related to deficient bone repair. As greater volumes of bone marrow are harvested from the iliac crest, the concentration of osteoprogenitor cells decreases because the sample undergoes considerable dilution with peripheral blood. Therefore, no more than 1–2 cc of bone marrow should be aspirated from any one site in order to maximize the number of osteoblast progenitors available to participate in bone formation [67]. Bone formation may be enhanced even further by loading the bone marrow onto an osteoconductive matrix before implantation.

Injection of unfractionated bone marrow maintains the best safety profile of all the cell-based therapies. Because bone marrow may be introduced percutaneously without surgical exposure of the site in need of repair, this approach represents a minimally invasive method for enhancing bone formation. Compared to the harvesting of iliac crest bone graft, aspiration of bone marrow is a less aggressive procedure associated with a reasonably low risk of complications such as pain, paresthesias, and infection. There were no instances of any donor site morbidity reported in the various clinical studies employing percutaneous bone marrow injection for the treatment of fracture nonunion [39,43,46,48,49]. Similar to iliac crest bone grafting, the transplantation of fresh bone marrow simply involves the transfer of autologous tissue to another anatomic location, so this technique is not subject to FDA regulation.

Mesenchymal Stem Cells

Bone marrow is known to contain a population of mesenchymal stem cells (MSCs) capable of differentiating into several different mesodermal tissues, including bone, cartilage, muscle, tendon, ligament, and fat. Because of their multilineage potential, MSCs are thought to facilitate the regeneration of various tissues and may prove to be a powerful treatment for the healing of musculoskeletal defects. Techniques have been developed for the isolation of MSCs from human bone marrow and their subsequent expansion in cell culture [11,16,71,72]. Even after extensive growth in vitro and after cryopreservation, MSCs retain their undifferentiated state without any loss of their developmental capacity [71]. Progression of MSCs within a particular lineage is an intricate, multistage process that occurs under specific conditions dictated by regulatory molecules, i.e., growth factors and cytokines (see Fig. 1). By providing the appropriate osteoinductive signals in vitro, MSCs may be directed to undergo differentiation into osteoblasts [10–14,16,17]. Similar to in vivo studies in which rat and canine MSCs were used to regenerate bone [10,11,13–15], implantation of culture-expanded human MSCs placed in a ceramic carrier has been shown to heal segmental defects in an athymic rat model [51]. These findings suggest that MSCs may be a viable alternative to autogenous bone graft for the repair of skeletal lesions in humans.

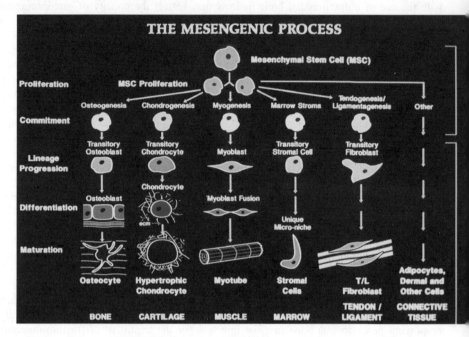

FIG. 1—The differentiation of mesenchymal stem cells into various tissues. Undifferentiated mesenchymal stem cells have the potential to develop into various different mesenchymal tissues, including bone, cartilage, skeletal muscle, bone marrow, tendon, ligament, adipose, and dermis. The progression of these stem cells within a lineage is regulated by specific growth factors and cytokines. Once these cells commit to a particular lineage, they lose their pluripotentiality. (Reprinted with permission from Caplan A. I., "The Mesengenic Process," *Clin Plastic Surg*, Vol. 21, 1994, p. 430.)

The use of autologous marrow-derived MSCs for the treatment for bone defects involves the direct transplantation of pluripotential cells into the area in need of augmentation, thereby ensuring that the healing response is not limited by an inadequate number of endogenous osteoprogenitor cells. As with all cell-based approaches, the combination of these cells with an osteoconductive carrier provides an even greater stimulus for the regeneration of bone. Clinical implementation of MSC therapy would also require ex vivo expansion of these stem cells to quantities sufficient for therapeutic purposes. In this process, MSCs are isolated from bone marrow aspirates and expanded in culture before being transferred into the osseous defect in conjunction with some type of biologic scaffold. Preclinical studies have suggested that the substantial increase in osteogenic cells provided by the expansion of MSCs in vitro generates greater bone formation than the use of unfractionated bone marrow, which generally yields only modest amounts of these cell types [66–70]. In an animal model, the addition of MSCs resulted in superior healing of critical-sized skeletal defects compared to that obtained with fresh bone marrow [13]. Because bone synthesis is dependent on the activity of osteogenic cells present at the site of injury, introduction of culture-expanded MSCs is a particularly attractive strategy for patients with diminished osteoprogenitor stores. Although the elderly and others with compromised tissues may have fewer cells available for bone repair, there is no loss in the in vitro developmental potential of their MSCs [11,16]. In these clinically challenging scenarios, autologous MSC therapy may be preferable to other bone grafting techniques that do not amplify the number of osteogenic precursor cells.

It is conceivable that more rapid and consistent bone formation may be achieved by initiating osteogenic differentiation of MSCs in vitro before delivery into defects. Culturing MSCs in the presence of dexamethasone, ascorbic acid, and other biologic factors induces these cells to undergo commitment to an osteogenic phenotype and promotes earlier biosynthetic activity by the mature osteoblasts [13,71,73]. Although there are currently no clinical trials using this approach, several animal studies have shown that treatment with predifferentiated osteoprogenitor cells may expedite healing of bony defects [74–76].

Multilineage stem cell populations with osteogenic potential have recently been identified in other mesenchymal tissues besides bone marrow. Both skeletal muscle [53,54,77] and fat [55] have been found to contain pluripotential cells that are readily expanded in culture and undergo osteogenic commitment following stimulation with specific osteoinductive factors, suggesting that these tissues may serve as alternative sources of autologous precursor cells capable of enhancing bone regeneration. Moreover, these undifferentiated stem cells are able be obtained conveniently from muscle biopsy specimens and liposuction procedures with less morbidity than traditional bone marrow harvesting. Unlike MSCs of bone marrow origin, however, pluripotential cells isolated from other mesodermal tissues have not been reported to effect healing of skeletal defects in animals.

Because only a limited number of pluripotential cells are present in bone marrow, skeletal muscle, and other mesenchymal tissues, the insertion of autologous MSCs into osseous defects necessitates the in vitro expansion of these cells to more clinically relevant levels sufficient to elicit bone regeneration. Consequently, unlike autograft or unfractionated bone marrow, treatment with culture-expanded MSCs is a two-step process that exposes patients to the attendant surgical and anesthetic hazards of a second operation. However, these risks are likely to be lower with the use of skeletal muscle or adipose, which may yield stem cells with reduced morbidity and minimal discomfort compared to bone marrow [53–55]. In addition, the potential for contamination of cell preparations is inherent to ex vivo approaches such as autologous MSC therapy.

GENE THERAPY

Gene therapy consists of the transfer of genetic material to cells for the purpose of generating therapeutic proteins. At this time, a large number of human clinical trials employing gene therapy methods are already in progress [78]. Although originally conceived for the treatment of genetic diseases such as cystic fibrosis and phenylketonuria, gene therapy systems are now being developed for other disorders that would benefit from the ongoing expression of specific bioactive factors. Gene transfer techniques have recently been applied to the science of tissue engineering. By increasing the local production of osteoinductive growth factors and cytokines, gene therapy has the potential to promote bone regeneration and facilitate the repair of osseous defects. Gene therapy may prove to be more efficacious than other approaches for enhancing bone regeneration such as the administration of recombinant proteins. Whereas a single dose of an exogenous growth factor may not be sufficient to elicit an adequate healing response in some clinical scenarios, the sustained local release of osteogenic factors provided by gene therapy strategies may serve as a more potent osteoinductive signal [58].

The successful application of gene therapy to the treatment of a certain disorder is dependent on the requisite duration of protein production. Because expression of the desired gene is only needed during the time of tissue formation, the majority of bone repair problems do not typically require the prolonged synthesis of osteogenic proteins. For this reason, bone regeneration seems to be well suited for gene therapy because the loss of protein expression over time that often limits its use for chronic diseases such as cystic fibrosis is actually preferable for the management of skeletal defects where long-term exposure to osteoinductive factors is not as essential. However, it is likely that the duration of protein delivery necessary for skeletal healing will vary from one clinical condition to another; for instance, the treatment of segmental bone defects may call for more extensive osteoinductive stimulation than spinal fusions or nonunions [63,64]. Other factors that will also certainly influence the potential success of gene therapy for the regeneration of bone include the anatomic location of the defect, the status of the surrounding soft tissue envelope, and the specific gene or combination of genes used to achieve tissue repair.

Gene therapy involves three fundamental elements: a sequence of DNA encoding a protein of interest, a vector that facilitates the entry of genetic material into cells, and target cells into which the gene will be inserted (see Fig. 2). The process by which DNA is transferred to target cells is known as transduction if viral vectors are employed or transfection if nonviral vectors are used. The advantages of nonviral vectors are that they are typically easier to generate and are more stable than viruses; moreover, since no infectious agents are introduced into the patient, these vectors are less antigenic and are associated with fewer safety concerns. Examples of nonviral vectors used to deliver genetic material into target cells include plasmids (circular DNA constructs) [79], gene-activated matrices or GAM (osteoconductive scaffolds implanted with plasmid DNA) [80,81], liposomes (plasmid-containing lipid vesicles able to fuse with cell membranes) [82,83], "gene guns" (gold particles loaded with DNA that are injected into cells at high velocities) [84,85], and DNA-ligand complexes (DNA bound to ligands that interact with specific cell-surface receptors) [86,87]. However, the use of these nonviral vectors is limited by relatively poor rates of gene transfer.

In general, transduction with viral vectors is more efficient than nonviral transfection strategies because the successful uptake and expression of genetic material by infected cells are obligatory for the survival and propagation of all normal viruses. For protein expression to occur, the DNA sequence of interest must gain access to the nucleus where transcription is initiated. The location of the therapeutic gene within the nucleus will have a significant effect upon the duration of its expression. Depending on the type of viral vector used, a particular gene may be incorporated into the target cell's chromosomes or remain episomal, i.e., outside the host genome. A gene that undergoes chromosomal integration will be passed on during cell replication, resulting in more prolonged protein

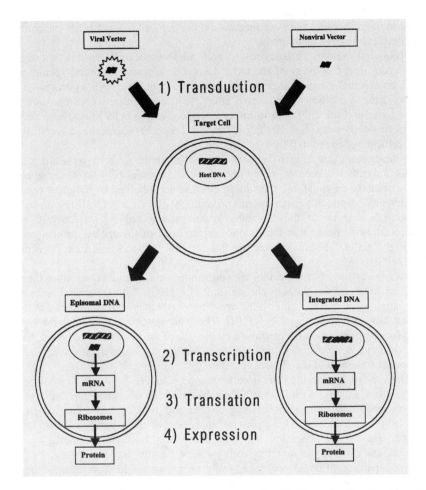

FIG. 2—The process of gene delivery to target cells. (1) Transduction involves the transfer of genetic material into the target cell using a viral vector (this process is referred to as transfection if nonviral vectors are employed). The DNA sequence of interest may be incorporated into the host genome or remain episomal (i.e., extrachromosomal). (2) Transcription is the process by which the DNA template is used to generate messenger RNA. (3) Translation is the process by which the messenger RNA is used to synthesize proteins. (4) Expression involves the production of the desired protein. An integrated gene will be transmitted to progeny cells and will likely result in more prolonged protein production, whereas the expression of episomal DNA is more transient because the gene is not passed on to daughter cells. (Reprinted with permission from Oakes D. A. and Lieberman J. R., "Osteoinductive Applications of Regional Gene Therapy: Ex Vivo Gene Transfer," *Clin Orthop Rel Res*, Vol. 379S, 2000, p. S103.)

production that is appropriate for long-term therapy. The expression of episomal DNA is more transient because the gene remains extra-chromosomal and is not transmitted from the transduced cell to its progeny.

Retroviral vectors, adenoviruses, and adeno-associated viruses show essential differences in the delivery of the target host cell. Whereas retroviral vectors are small RNA viruses that integrate their genetic material into the host cell's genome, giving rise to the stable and efficient transfer of DNA [88], they can only accommodate genes of limited size and are only able to infect actively dividing cells [89]. These vectors also insert randomly into cellular DNA, raising concerns about the theoretical risk of neoplastic transformation [90].

Adenoviruses are able to effectively deliver genes to both replicating and non-replicating cells without integrating into host chromosomes [91–94]. Because adenoviral vectors remain episomal, the transduced DNA is not inherited by daughter cells and the ensuing gene expression may diminish accordingly over time [95,96]. The presentation of adenoviral antigens to the immune system by infected cells frequently elicits an inflammatory response that also attenuates the level of therapeutic protein production, although "gutless" adenoviral vectors that are less immunogenic have been developed [97–99].

Adeno-associated viral vectors are nonpathogenic viruses that introduce their genetic material at a single site on chromosome 19 [100]. Like retroviral vectors, these integrating recombinant viruses bring about long-term gene expression but can only carry modest amounts of foreign DNA [101]. The most suitable viral vector for a particular gene therapy application is determined by the size of the gene to be delivered, the type of target cell to be transduced, and the duration of protein production required for the successful treatment of the clinical condition.

Delivery of a gene into target cells may be achieved by either in vivo or ex vivo methods (see Fig. 3). With in vivo techniques, insertion of a gene into the target cells is accomplished by directly administering the gene and its associated vector into the patient. This in vivo approach is less complex and more convenient to perform but is complicated by poor transduction efficiency, induction of a host inflammatory response against viral proteins, and difficulty in targeting cells for gene transfer. Ex vivo strategies call for the culture-expansion of target cells taken from the patient and in vitro transduction of these cells with a particular gene before autologous reimplantation into the desired anatomic site. Ex vivo gene therapy allows for the selection of a specific target cell type and is associated with higher transduction efficiencies. This method of gene delivery is also safer than in vivo techniques because no viruses or foreign DNA are injected systemically and the genetically modified cells can be screened for tumorigenicity before they are returned to the patient. However, because it necessitates an extra surgical procedure, ex vivo gene transfer is more complex, time-consuming, and expensive. Ex vivo gene therapy offers theoretical advantages over other cellular strategies for the tissue engineering of bone because this approach may supply both osteogenic cells and osteoinductive proteins to the site in need of osseous repair. Introduction of the appropriate DNA sequence into osteoprogenitor cells results in the sustained local release of osteoinductive factors that may act in both a paracrine as well as an autocrine fashion. In addition to inducing surrounding pluripotential cells to undergo differentiation into

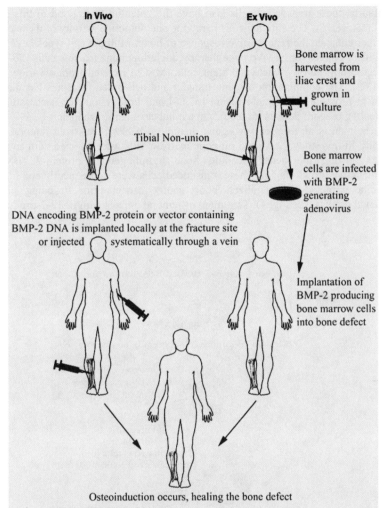

In Vivo Ex Vivo

Bone marrow is harvested from iliac crest and grown in culture

Tibial Non-union

Bone marrow cells are infected with BMP-2 generating adenovirus

DNA encoding BMP-2 protein or vector containing BMP-2 DNA is implanted locally at the fracture site or injected systematically through a vein

Implantation of BMP-2 producing bone marrow cells into bone defect

Osteoinduction occurs, healing the bone defect

FIG. 3—Comparison of in vivo and ex vivo gene therapy strategies to heal a tibial nonunion. In vivo gene therapy involves the direct administration of the gene and its associated vector into the patient. This method is easier to perform but is complicated by relatively poor transduction efficiencies and potential inflammatory responses against viral proteins. Ex vivo gene therapy required the removal and culture-expansion of autologous cells that are subsequently transduced in vitro prior to reimplantation into the site in need of repair. This approach is associated with higher transduction efficiencies and is safer because no foreign material is directly injected into the patient. However, ex vivo gene transfer is more complex and expensive because it requires an additional surgical procedure. (Reprinted with permission from Scaduto A. A. and Lieberman J. R., "Gene Therapy for Osteoinduction," *Orthop Clin North Am*, Vol. 30, 1999, p. 627.)

osteoblasts, these transduced cells also have the potential to respond to this osteogenic signal themselves. The simultaneous paracrine and autocrine activity of these cells serves to further enhance the regenerative response of bone. Multiple cell types have been used as cellular vehicles for ex vivo gene therapy, including bone marrow cells [56–58], buffy coat cells [60], and mesenchymal stem cells (MSCs) isolated from a variety of tissues [59,61,62]. The combination of gene transfer and cell-based therapies has already been shown to promote solid spinal fusion [57,60] and bring about the successful repair of non-healing osseous defects [56,58,62] in a number of animal models.

Lieberman et al. used ex vivo gene therapy to heal critical-sized femoral defects in rats [58]. In this study, harvested rat bone marrow cells were infected with an adenoviral vector carrying the gene encoding bone morphogenetic protein-2 (BMP-2), an osteoinductive growth factor. These transduced cells were subsequently combined with a guanidine-extracted demineralized bone matrix carrier prior to being placed into segmental defects (see Fig. 4). Treatment of femoral defects with BMP-2-producing bone

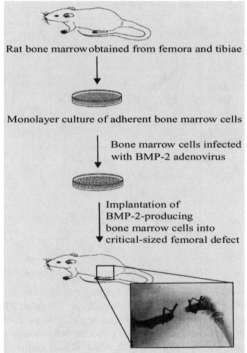

FIG. 4—Transduction of rat bone marrow cells with a recombinant human BMP-2-containing adenovirus and implantation into a femoral defect. Bone marrow cells were harvested from rats and expanded in cell culture. These cells were then infected with an adenovirus vector containing the gene encoding recombinant human BMP-2. These transduced cells were subsequently implanted into a critical-sized femoral defect. (Reprinted with permission from Lieberman J. R., Daluiski A., Stevenson S., et al., "The Effect of Regional Gene Therapy with Bone Morphogenetic Protein-2-Producing Bone-Marrow Cells on the Repair of Segmental Femoral Defects in Rats," *J Bone Joint Surg Am*, Vol. 81, 1999, p. 907.)

marrow cells resulted in the healing comparable to that observed with implantation of recombinant human BMP-2 protein (rhBMP-2) (see Fig. 5). Histologic and histomorphometric analyses of the specimens revealed that defects filled with the transduced bone marrow cells generated significantly greater amounts of dense trabecular bone than those administered rhBMP-2 protein, which demonstrated thin, lace-like patterns of bone formation; however, no differences in the biomechanical characteristics of these two groups were noted.

In another experiment, Viggeswarapu et al. used a similar gene transfer strategy in an attempt to induce single-level spinal fusion in rabbits [60]. A recombinant adenovirus containing the gene for LIM mineralization protein-1 (LMP-1), a signaling molecule involved in osteoblast differentiation, was delivered to buffy-coat cells derived from either bone marrow or peripheral blood. The infected cells were loaded into an osteoconductive matrix and implanted in the posterolateral spine of rabbits. Successful fusion of the spine was achieved in all animals receiving these transduced buffy-coat cells, further validating ex vivo gene therapy as a valuable technique for promoting bone formation.

Targeting autologous MSCs for ex vivo gene therapy would be particularly advantageous since these pluripotential cells may be culture-expanded before transduction, ensuring that there are more target cells available for gene transfer, and they may undergo subsequent osteogenic commitment in response to the growth factors they produce. Genetic material may be introduced into MSCs with relatively high efficiency, and these transduced cells are able to express the desired therapeutic protein without any compromise in their capacity to differentiate [102,103]. In preclinical studies, ex vivo gene therapy using bone marrow-derived MSCs as biologic carriers for the osteoinductive growth factor BMP-2 stimulated the repair of critical-sized bone defects in rats [56–58]. Despite these preliminary results that support ex vivo gene transfer as an effective technique for the tissue engineering of bone in humans, further research is required before gene therapy methods may be applied to clinical practice.

Although stem cells obtained from mesenchymal tissues other than bone marrow have not been shown to stimulate healing when directly implanted into skeletal defects, undifferentiated cells isolated from skeletal muscle and fat have been used successfully as effective vehicles for gene delivery. Ex vivo gene therapy using muscle-derived MSCs transduced with the recombinant human BMP-2 gene significantly augmented repair of critical-sized skull defects in mice [62]. Similarly, human fat cells genetically engineered to express BMP-2 protein have been shown to stimulate in vivo bone production in a murine model [104]. Nevertheless, additional preclinical studies are needed to validate the efficacy of autologous muscle and fat cells for inducing bone regeneration before ex vivo gene delivery and other cell-mediated strategies employing these types of MSCs may be applied to humans.

Since the gene therapy-related death of a patient in 1999, clinical trials applying gene transfer technology to humans have come under much closer scrutiny. Of particular concern is the safety of recombinant viruses, whose systemic effects have not been elucidated. Even though viral vectors are unable to replicate because portions of their genome are deleted and replaced with a particular therapeutic gene, it is possible that a

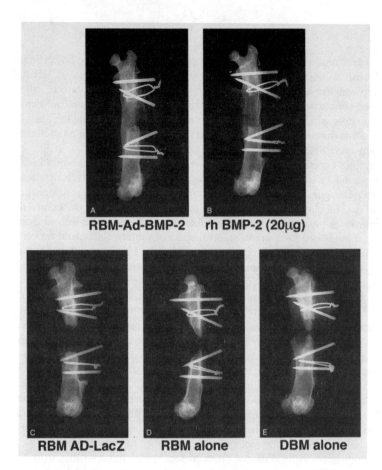

FIG. 5— Healing of femoral defects using BMP-2-producing bone marrow cells. (A) Defects treated with marrow cells transduced with the BMP-2 gene and demineralized bone matrix (DBM); (B) Defects treated with recombinant human BMP-2 protein and DBM (positive control); (C) Defects treated with marrow cells transduced with the LacZ gene and DBM (negative control); (D) Defects treated with nontransduced marrow cells with DBM (negative control); (E) Defects treated with DBM alone (negative control). Treatment with BMP-2-producing cells and DBM elicited healing comparable to that observed with implantation of recombinant human BMP-2 protein and DBM. (Reprinted with permission from Oakes, D. A. and Lieberman, J. R., "Osteoinductive Applications of Regional Gene Therapy: Ex Vivo Gene Transfer," *Clin Orthop Rel Res*, Vol. 379S, 2000, p. S108.)

defective virus could recombine with host cell DNA sequences and become replication-competent, resulting in uncontrolled viral propagation and ultimately cell death. Because retroviral vectors incorporate randomly into the host genome, it is conceivable that integration of the virus within a tumor suppressor gene or proto-oncogene could bring about malignant transformation of the cell. The use of adenoviral vectors is also limited by the potential host inflammatory response that may be induced by viral proteins. Ex vivo gene therapy approaches circumvent these problems because all of the genetic engineering occurs outside the patient and the transduced cells can undergo rigorous in vitro testing before being implanted. Although a technique that allows for the rapid infection of autologous peripheral blood cells immediately before implantation has recently been described [60], ex vivo gene delivery typically entails an additional surgery with all of its associated risks as well as the possibility of cell contamination. At this time the duration and level of protein expression cannot be regulated with any consistency, and the consequences of such unpredictable production of bioactive factors has not yet been determined. Gene therapy ultimately may prove to be effective for the treatment of skeletal defects, but further animal studies and Phase I clinical trials are needed to confirm the safety of this strategy prior to its widespread use in humans.

CARRIERS

Achieving successful bone healing with any of these cell-based therapies requires an acceptable matrix scaffold in which the cells may be carried. Certain carriers do not possess any inherent osteoinductive potential, so when used alone they rely solely on the migration of endogenous osteoprogenitors to generate new tissue. When combined with a source of osteogenic cells, osteoconductive scaffolds enhance bone repair even more by facilitating the delivery of these cells and restricting their movement away from the area of implantation. Besides providing a matrix that promotes cellular attachment, a carrier must also support bony ingrowth and neovascularization, resorb over time without inciting an inflammatory response, and possess desirable handling properties so that it is easy to use in the operating room. Several different carriers made up of a number of biologic or synthetic materials are presently available, including demineralized bone matrices, collagen sponges, ceramics, and various polymers. The most appropriate scaffold for a given clinical application is dependent upon the specific condition being treated, the type of cellular therapy to be implemented, the anatomic location of the defect and the biomechanical stresses the construct will be subjected to at that site.

COST OF CELLULAR SYSTEMS

Fractures and other bone defects are responsible for billions of dollars of direct and indirect costs annually, with millions more spent on bone grafts and fusion adjuncts [61]. The development of these new cellular systems has proven to be expensive, yet their widespread implementation as bone graft substitutes could result in considerable long-term financial benefits secondary to improved healing rates and reduced morbidity. Regardless of their relative efficacy and safety, in this era of increasingly limited health care resources the issue of cost may greatly influence which of these approaches are accepted as viable alternatives to conventional bone grafting techniques.

Bone marrow aspiration is less invasive than the procurement of iliac crest bone graft, and these cells may be introduced percutaneously into the area requiring augmentation without the need for another procedure. For these reasons, the injection of unfractionated bone marrow is the most inexpensive method of augmenting osseous repair. Autologous MSC therapy entails a minimum of two surgeries as well as the expansion of these undifferentiated cells in tissue culture. Although there are concerns about the cost of ex vivo strategies, a similar approach is already being used routinely for the treatment of articular cartilage defects. Autologous chondrocyte transplantation involves the harvesting and in vitro expansion of cartilage cells prior to their implantation into the defect [106,107]. Ex vivo gene therapy also requires the isolation of autologous tissue, but techniques that do not necessitate the culture expansion of target cells are being developed in order to reduce costs and make the process more convenient for the surgeon [60]. The successful implementation of any of these cellular approaches will also call for the selection of an appropriate carrier, which is determined by the specific biologic environment and mechanical requirements of the skeletal defect. If these cell-based therapies can be used to effectively treat difficult bone repair problems for which there are presently no satisfactory therapeutic options, then they will likely prove to be cost-effective as well.

All of the existing cellular systems are dependent upon the acquisition of tissue from each individual with or without subsequent in vitro expansion before its reimplantation. Allogeneic cell preparations could be administered to multiple patients and would represent a more economical method of stimulating bone healing than therapeutic strategies employing autologous cells. However, because of the potential for adverse immunologic reactions, at this time the treatment of skeletal defects with allogeneic cells is not feasible.

CONCLUSION

Cell-based approaches such as unfractionated bone marrow, culture-expanded mesenchymal stem cells, and ex vivo gene therapy are currently being developed to enhance the regeneration of bone. Recent findings suggest that these new tissue engineering strategies may be more efficacious than standard iliac crest bone grafting and may ultimately change the way in which patients with bone healing problems are treated. However, extensive preclinical studies and well-designed clinical trials are necessary to identify the optimal conditions for the application of each of these techniques and determine their specific clinical indications. In addition, before these cellular systems are available to orthopedic surgeons, their safety and cost-effectiveness must also be clearly established. As the mechanisms underlying the biology of bone formation and the role osteogenic cells play in fracture repair are better characterized, further advances in the field of cell-based therapies will likely continue in the future.

Acknowledgments

This work was supported by a grant from the National Institutes of Health (J. R. L. R01 AR46789-01A1).

REFERENCES

[1]   Younger E. M. and Chapman M. W., "Morbidity at Bone Graft Donor Sites," *J Orthop Trauma*, Vol. 3, 1989, pp. 192–195.

[2]   Summers B. N. and Eisenstein S. M., "Donor Site Pain from the Ilium: A Complication of Lumbar Spine Fusion," *J Bone Joint Surg Br*, Vol. 71, 1989, pp. 677–680.

[3]   Vail T. P. and Urbaniak J. R., "Donor Site Morbidity with Use of Vascularized Autogenous Fibular Grafts," *J Bone Joint Surg Am*, Vol. 78, 1996, pp. 204–211.

[4]   Goulet J. A., Senunas L. E., DeSilva G. L., and Greenfield M. L., "Autogenous Iliac Crest Bone Graft: Complications and Functional Assessment," *Clin Orthop Rel Res*, Vol. 339, 1997, pp. 76–81.

[5]   Goldberg V., Stevenson S., and Shaffer J., "Biology of Autografts and Allografts," *Bone and Cartilage Allografts: Biology and Clinical Applications*, G. E. Friedlaender and V. M. Goldberg, Eds., American Academy of Orthopedic Surgeons, Park Ridge, IL, 1991.

[6]   Muschler G. F. and Lane J. M., "Clinical Applications of Bone Grafting in Orthopedic Surgery," *Bone Grafting: From Basic Science to Clinical Applications*, M. Habel and A. H. Reddi, Eds., Saunders, New York, NY, 1992, pp. 375–407.

[7]   Buck B., Malinin T., and Brown M., "Bone Transplantation and Human Immunodeficiency Virus: An Estimate of Risk of Acquired Immunodeficiency Syndrome (AIDS)," *Clin Orthop Rel Res*, Vol. 240, 1989, pp. 129–134.

[8]   Khan S. N., Tomin E., and Lane, J. M., "Clinical Applications of Bone Graft Substitutes," *Orthop Clin North Am*, Vol. 31, 2000, pp. 389–398.

[9]   Yoon S. T. and Boden S. D., "Osteoinductive Molecules in Orthopedics: Basic Science and Preclinical Studies," *Clin Orthop Rel Res*, Vol. 395, 2002, pp. 33–43.

[10]   Dennis J. E., Haynesworth S. E., Young R. G., and Caplan A. I., "Osteogenesis in Marrow-Derived Mesenchymal Cell Porous Ceramic Composites Transplanted Subcutaneously: Effect of Fibronectin and Laminin on Cell Retention and Rate of Osteogenic Expression," *Cell Transplant*, Vol. 1, 1992, pp. 23–32.

[11]   Haynesworth S. E., Goshima J., Goldberg V. M., and Caplan A. I., "Characterization of Cells with Osteogenic Potential from Human Marrow," *Bone*, Vol. 13, 1992, pp. 81–88.

[12]   Cassiede P., Dennis J. E., Ma F., and Caplan A. I., "Osteochondrogenic Potential of Marrow Mesenchymal Progenitor Cells Exposed to TGF-β1 or PDGF-BB as Assayed In Vivo and In Vitro," *J Bone Mineral Res*, Vol. 11, 1996, pp. 264–1273.

[13]   Kadiyala S., Jaiswal N., and Bruder S. P., "Culture-Expanded Bone Marrow-Derived Mesenchymal Stem Cells Can Regenerate a Critical-Sized Segmental Bone Defect," *Tissue Eng*, Vol. 3, 1997, pp. 173–185.

[14]   Kadiyala S., Young R. G., Thiede M. A., and Bruder S. P., "Culture Expanded Canine Mesenchymal Stem Cells Possess Osteochondrogenic Potential In Vivo and In Vitro," *Cell Transplant*, Vol. 6, 1997, pp. 125–134.

[15]   Bruder S. P., Kraus K. H., Goldberg V. M., and Kadiyala S., "The Effect of Implants Loaded with Autologous Mesenchymal Stem Cells on the Healing of Canine Segmental Bone Defects," *J Bone Joint Surg Am*, Vol. 80, 1998, pp. 985–996.

[16]   Jaiswal N., Haynesworth S. E., Caplan A. I., and Bruder S. P., "Osteogenic Differentiation of Purified, Culture-Expanded Human Mesenchymal Cells In Vitro," *J Cell Biochem*, Vol. 64, 1997, pp. 295–312.

[17]   Grigoradis A., Heersche J. N. M., and Aubin J., "Differentiation of Muscle, Fat, Cartilage, and Bone from Progenitor Cells Present in a Bone-Derived Clonal Cell Population: Effect of Dexamethasone," *J Cell Biol*, Vol. 106, 1988, pp. 2139–2151.

[18]   Bruder S. P., Fink D. J., and Caplan A. I., "Mesenchymal Stem Cells in Bone Formation, Bone Repair, and Skeletal Regeneration Therapy," *J Cell Biochem*, Vol. 56, 1994, pp. 283–294.

[19] Vacanti C. A. and Vacanti J. P., "The Science of Tissue Engineering," *Orthop Clin North Am*, Vol. 31, 2000, pp. 351–355.

[20] Yasko A., Lane J. M., Fellinger E. J., Rosen V., Wozney J. M., and Wang E. A., "The Healing of Segmental Bone Defects, Induced by Recombinant Human Bone Morphogenetic Protein (rhBMP-2). A Radiographic, Histological, and Biomechanical Study in Rats," *J Bone Joint Surg Am*, Vol. 74, 1992, pp. 659–670.

[21] Gerhart T. N., Kirker-Head C. A., Kriz M. J., Holtrop M. E., Hennig G. E., Hipp J., et al., "Healing Segmental Femoral Defects in Sheep Using Recombinant Human Bone Morphogenetic Protein," *Clin Orthop Rel Res*, Vol. 293, 1993, pp. 317–326.

[22] Cook S. D., Baffes G. C., Wolfe M. W., Sampath T. K., and Rueger D. C., "Recombinant Human Bone Morphogenetic Protein-7 Induces Healing in a Canine Long-Bone Segmental Defect Model," *Clin Orthop Rel Res*, Vol. 301, 1994, pp. 302–312.

[23] Cook S. D., Baffes G. C., Wolfe M. W., Sampath T. K., Rueger D. C., and Whitecloud T. S., III, "The Effect of Recombinant Human Osteogenic Protein-1 on Healing of Large Segmental Bone Defects," *J Bone Joint Surg Am*, Vol. 76, 1994, pp. 827–838.

[24] Stevenson S., Cunningham N., Toth J., Davy D., and Reddi A. H., "The Effect of Osteogenin (A Bone Morphogenetic Protein) on the Formation of Bone in Orthotopic Segemental Defects in Rats," *J Bone J Surg Am*, Vol. 76, 1994, pp. 1676–1687.

[25] Cook S. D., Wolfe M. W., Salkeld S. L., and Rueger D. C., "Effect of Recombinant Human Osteogenic Protein-1 on Healing of Segmental Defects in Non-Human Primates," *J Bone Joint Surg Am*, Vol. 77, 1995, pp. 734–750.

[26] Riley E. H., Lane J. M., Urist M. R., Lyons K. M., and Lieberman J. R., "Bone Morphogenetic Protein-2. Biology and Applications," *Clin Orthop Rel Res*, Vol. 324, 1996, pp. 39–46.

[27] Centrella M., McCarthy T. L., and Canalis E., "Transforming Growth Factor-Beta and Remodeling of Bone," *J Bone Joint Surg Am*, Vol. 73, 1991, pp. 1418–1428.

[28] Aspenberg P. and Lohmander L. S., "Fibroblast Growth Factor Stimulates Bone Formation: Bone Induction Studied in Rats," *Acta Orthop Scand*, Vol. 60, 1989, pp. 473–476.

[29] Wang J. S. and Aspenberg P., "Basic Fibroblast Growth Factor Enhances Bone-Graft Incorporation: Dose and Time Dependence in Rats," *J Orthop Res*, Vol. 14, 1996, pp. 316–323.

[30] Friedlaender G. E., Perry C. R., Cole J. D., Cook S. D., Cierny G., Muschler G. F., et al., "Osteogenic Protein-1 (Bone Morphogenetic Protein-7) in the Treatment of Tibial Nonunions," *J Bone Joint Surg Am*, Vol. 83, 2001, pp. S151-S158.

[31] Boden S. D., Zdeblick T. A., Sandhu H. S., and Heim S. E., "The Use of rhBMP-2 in Interbody Fusion Cages," *Spine*, Vol. 25, 2000, pp. 376–381.

[32] Siebrecht M. A. N, De Rooij P. P., Arm D. A., Olsson M. L., and Aspenberg P., "Platelet Concentrate Increases Bone Ingrowth into Porous Hydroxyapatite," *Orthopedics*, Vol. 25, 2002, pp. 169–172.

[33] Lowery G. L., Kulkarni S., and Pennisi A. E., "Use of Autologous Growth Factors in Lumbar Spinal Fusion," *Bone*, Vol. 25, 1999, pp. 47S–50S.

[34] Takagi K. and Urist M. R., "The Role of Bone Marrow in Bone Morphogenetic Protein-Induced Repair of Femoral Massive Diaphyseal Defects," *Clin Orthop Rel Res*, Vol. 171, 1982, pp. 224–231.

[35] Nade S., Armstrong L., McCartney E., and Baggaley B., "Osteogenesis after Bone Marrow Transplantation: The Ability of Ceramic Materials to Sustain Osteogenesis

from Transplanted Bone Marrow Cells: Preliminary Studies," *Clin Orthop Rel Res*, Vol. 181, 1983, pp. 255–263.

[36] Paley D., Young M. C., Wiley A. M., Fornasier V. L., and Jackson R. W., "Percutaneous Bone Marrow Grafting of Fractures and Bone Defects: An Experimental Study in Rabbits," *Clin Orthop Rel Res*, Vol. 208, 1986, pp. 300–311.

[37] Connolly J., Guse R., Lippiello L., and Dehne R., "Development of an Osteogenic Bone Marrow Preparation," *J Bone Joint Surg Am*, Vol. 71, 1989, pp. 684–691.

[38] Ohgushi H., Goldberg V. M., and Caplan A. I., "Repair of Bone Defects with Marrow Cells and Porous Ceramic: Experiments in Rats," *Acta Orthop Scand*, Vol. 60, 1989, pp. 334–339.

[39] Healey J. H., Zimmerman P. A., McDonnell J. M., and Lane J. M., "Percutaneous Bone Marrow Grafting of Delayed Union and Nonunion in Cancer Patients," *Clin Orthop Rel Res*, Vol. 256, 1990, pp. 280–285.

[40] Ohgushi H., Goldberg V. M., and Caplan A. I., "Heterotopic Osteogenesis in Porous Ceramics Induced by Marrow Cells," *J Orthop Res*, Vol. 7, 1989, pp. 568–578.

[41] Grundel R. E., Chapman M. W., Yee T., and Moore D. C., "Autogenic Bone Marrow and Porous Biphasic Calcium Phosphate Ceramic for Segmental Defects in the Canine Ulna," *Clin Orthop Rel Res*, Vol. 26, 1991, pp. 244–258.

[42] Tiedeman J., Connolly J., Strates B., and Lippiello L., "Treatment of Nonunion by Percutaneous Injection of Bone Marrow and Demineralized Bone Matrix: An Experimental Study in Canines," *Clin Orthop Rel Res*, Vol. 268, 1991, pp. 294–302.

[43] Connolly J. F., Guse R., Tiedeman J., and Dehne R., "Autologous Marrow Injection as a Substitute for Operative Grafting of Tibial Nonunions," *Clin Orthop Rel Res*, Vol. 266, 1991, pp. 259–270.

[44] Goshima J., Goldberg V. M., and Caplan A. I., "The Origin of Bone Formed in Composite Grafts of Porous Calcium Phosphate Ceramic Loaded with Marrow Cells," *Clin Orthop Rel Res*, Vol. 269, 1991, pp. 274–283.

[45] Sharma S., Garg N., Veliath A., Subramanian S., and Srivastava K., "Percutaneous Bone Marrow Grafting of Osteotomies and Bony Defects in Rabbits," *Acta Orthop Scand*, Vol. 63, 1992, pp. 166–169.

[46] Garg N., Gaur S., and Sharma S., "Percutaneous Autogenous Bone Marrow Grafting in 20 Cases of Ununited Fracture," *Acta Orthop Scand*, Vol. 64, 1993, pp. 671–672.

[47] Wolff D., Goldberg V. M., and Stevenson S., "Histomorphometric Analysis of the Repair of a Segmental Diaphyseal Defect with Ceramic and Titanium Fibermetal Implants: Effects of Bone Marrow," *J Orthop Res*, Vol. 12, 1994, pp. 439–446.

[48] Connolly J. F., "Injectable Bone Marrow Preparations to Stimulate Osteogenic Repair," *Clin Orthop Rel Res*, Vol. 313, 1995, pp. 8–18.

[49] Garg N. K. and Gaur S., "Percutaneous Autogenous Bone-Marrow Grafting in Congenital Tibial Pseudoarthrosis," *J Bone Joint Surg Br*, Vol. 77, 1995, pp. 830–831.

[50] Werntz J. R., Lane J. M., Burstein A. H., Justin R., Klein R., and Tomin E., "Qualitative and Quantitative Analysis of Orthotopic Bone Regeneration by Marrow," *J Orthop Res*, Vol. 14, 1996, pp. 85–93.

[51] Bruder S. P., Kurth A. A., Shea M., Hayes W. C., Jaiswal N., and Kadiyala S., "Bone Regeneration by Implantation of Purified, Culture-Expanded Human Mesenchymal Stem Cells," *J Orthop Res*, Vol. 16, 1998, pp. 155–162.

[52] Richards M., Huibregste B. A., Caplan A. I., Goulet J. A., and Goldstein S. A., "Marrow-Derived Progenitor Cell Injections Enhance New Bone Formation During Distraction," *J Orthop Res*, Vol. 17, 1999, pp. 900–908.

[53]   Lee J. Y., Qu-Petersen Z., Cao B., Kimura S., Jankowski R., Cummins J., et al., "Clonal Isolation of Muscle-Derived Cells Capable of Enhancing Muscle Regeneration and Bone Healing," *J Cell Biol*, Vol. 150, 2000, pp. 1085–1100.

[54]   Bosch P., Musgrave D. S., Lee J. Y., Cummins J., Shuler F., Ghivizzani S. C., et al., "Osteoprogenitor Cells Within Skeletal Muscle," *J Orthop Res*, Vol. 18, 2000, pp. 933–944.

[55]   Zuk P. A., Zhu M., Mizuno H., Huang J., Futrell J. W., Katz A. J., Benhaim P., Lorenz H. P., and Hedrick M. H., "Multilineage Cells from Human Adipose Tissue: Implications for Cell-Based Therapies," *Tissue Engineering*, Vol. 7, 2001, pp. 211–228.

[56]   Lieberman J. R., Le L. Q., Wu L., Finerman G. A., Berk A., Witte O. N., and Stevenson S., "Regional Gene Therapy with a BMP-2-Producing Murine Stromal Cell Line Induces Heterotopic and Orthotopic Bone Formation in Rodents," *J Orthop Res*, Vol. 16, 1998, pp. 330–339.

[57]   Boden S. D., Titus L., Hair G., Liu Y., Viggeswarapu M., Nanes M. S., et al., "Lumbar Spine Fusion by Local Gene Therapy with a cDNA Encoding a Novel Osteoinductive Protein (LMP-1)," *Spine*, Vol. 23, 1998, pp. 2486–2492.

[58]   Lieberman J. R., Daluiski A., Stevenson S., Wu L., McAllister P., Lee Y. P., et al., "The Effect of Regional Gene Therapy with Bone Morphogenetic Protein-2-Producing Bone-Marrow Cells on the Repair of Segmental Femoral Defects in Rats," *J Bone Joint Surg Am,* Vol. 81, 1999, pp. 905–917.

[59]   Lou J., Xu F., Merkel K., and Manske P., "Gene Therapy: Adenovirus-Mediated Human Bone Morphogenetic Protein-2 Gene Transfer Induces Mesenchymal Progenitor Cell Proliferation and Differentiation In Vitro and Bone Formation In Vivo," *J Orthop Res*, Vol. 17, 1999, pp. 43–50.

[60]   Viggeswarapu M., Boden S. D., Liu Y., Hair G. A., Louis-Ugbo J., Murakami H., et al., "Adenoviral Delivery of LIM Mineralization Protein-1 Induces New-Bone Formation In Vitro and In Vivo," *J Bone Joint Surg Am*, Vol. 83, 2001, pp. 364–376.

[61]   Musgrave D. S., Bosch P., Lee J. Y., Pelinkovic D., Ghivizzani S. C., Whalen J., et al., "Ex Vivo Gene Therapy to Produce Bone Using Different Cell Types," *Clin Orthop Rel Res*, Vol. 378, 2000, pp. 290–305.

[62]   Lee J. Y., Musgrave D., Pelinkovic D., Fukushima K., Cummins J., Usas A., et al., "Effect of Bone Morphogenetic Protein-2-Expressing Muscle-Derived Cells on Healing of Critical-Sized Bone Defects in Mice," *J Bone Joint Surg Am*, Vol. 83, 2001, pp. 1032–1039.

[63]   Scaduto A. A. and Lieberman J. R., "Gene Therapy for Osteoinduction," *Orthop Clin North Am*, Vol. 30, 1999, pp. 625–633.

[64]   Oakes D. A. and Lieberman J. R., "Osteoinductive Applications of Regional Gene Therapy: Ex Vivo Gene Transfer," *Clin Orthop Rel Res*, Vol. 379S, 2000, pp. S101–S112.

[65]   Beresford J. N., "Osteogenic Stem Cells and the Stromal System of Bone and Marrow," *Clin Orthop Rel Res*, Vol. 240, 1989, pp. 270–280.

[66]   Muschler G. F., Nitto H., Boehm C. A., and Easley, K. A., "Age- and Gender-Related Changes in the Cellularity of Human Bone Marrow and the Prevalence of Osteoblastic Progenitors," *J Orthop Res*, Vol. 19, 2001, pp. 117–125.

[67]   Muschler G. F., Boehm C., and Easley, K. A., "Aspiration to Obtain Osteoblast Progenitor Cells from Human Bone Marrow: The Influence of Aspiration Volume," *J Bone Joint Surg Am*, Vol. 79, 1997, pp. 1699–1709.

[68]   Inoue K., Ohgushi H., Yoshikawa T., Okumura M., Sempuku T., Tamai S., et al., "The Effect of Aging on Bone Formation in Porous Hydroxyapatite: Biochemical and Histologic Analysis," *J Bone Mineral Res*, Vol. 12, 1997, pp. 989–994.

[69]   Kahn A., Gibbons R., Perkins S., and Gazit D., "Age-Related Bone Loss: A Hypothesis and Initial Assessment in Mice," *Clin Orthop Rel Res*, Vol. 313, 1995, pp. 69–75.

[70]   Tabuchi C., Simmon D. J., Fausto A., Russell J. E., Binderman I., and Avioli L. V., "Bone Deficit in Ovariectomized Rats: Functional Contribution of the Marrow Stromal Cell Population and the Effect if Oral Dihydrotachysterol Treatment," *J Clin Investigat*, Vol. 78, 1986, pp. 637–642.

[71]   Bruder S. P., Jaiswal N., and Haynesworth S. E., "Growth Kinetics, Self-Renewal and the Osteogenic Potential of Purified Human Mesenchymal Stem Cells During Extensive Subcultivation and Following Cryopreservation," *J Cell Biochem,* Vol. 64, 1997, pp. 278–294.

[72]   Haynesworth S. E., Baber M., and Caplan A. I., "Cell Surface Antigens on Human Marrow-Derived Mesenchymal Cells Are Detected by Monoclonal Antibodies," *Bone*, Vol. 13, 1992, pp. 69–80.

[73]   Maniatopoulos C., Sodek J., and Melcher A. H., "Bone Formation In Vitro by Stromal Cells Obtained from Marrow of Young Adult Rats," *Cell Tissue Res*, Vol. 254, 1988, pp. 317–330.

[74]   Yoshikawa T., Ohgushi H., and Tamai S., "Immediate Bone Forming Capability of Prefabricated Osteogenic Hydroxyapatite," *J Biomed Mater Res*, Vol. 32, 1996, pp. 481–492.

[75]   Breitbart A. S., Grande D. A., Kessler R., Ryaby J. T., Fitzsimmons R. J., and Grant R. T., "Tissue Engineered Bone Repair of Calvarial Defects Using Cultured Periosteal Cells," *Plastic Reconstruc Surg*, Vol. 101, 1998, pp. 567–574.

[76]   Okumura M., Ohgushi H., Dohi Y., Katuda T., Tamai S., Koerten H. K., and Tabata S., "Osteoblastic Phenotype Expression on the Surface of Hydroxyapatite Ceramics," *J Biomed Mater Res*, Vol. 37, 1997, pp. 122–129.

[77]   Katagiri T., Yamaguchi A., Komaki M., Abe E., Takahashi N., Ikeda T., et al., "Bone Morphogenetic Protein-2 Converts the Differentiation Pathway of C2C12 Myoblasts into the Osteoblast Lineage," *J Cell Biol*, Vol. 127, 1994, pp. 1755–1766.

[78]   Anderson W. F., "Human Gene Therapy," *Nature*, Vol. 392, 1998, pp. 25–30.

[79]   Baumgartner I., Pieczek A., Manor O., Blair R., Kearney M., Walsh K., et al. "Constitutive Expression of phVEGF165 After Intramuscular Gene Transfer Promotes Collateral Vessel Development in Patients with Critical Limb Ischemia," *Circulation*, Vol. 97, 1998, pp. 1114–1123.

[80]   Fang J., Zhu Y. Y., Smiley E., Bonadio J., Rouleau J. P., Goldstein S. A., et al., "Stimulation of New Bone Formation by Direct Transfer of Osteogenic Plasmid Genes," *Proc Nat Acad Sciences, USA,* Vol. 93, 1996, pp. 5753–5758.

[81]   Goldstein S. A. and Bonadio J., "Potential Role for Direct Gene Transfer in the Enhancement of Fracture Healing," *Clin Orthop Rel Res*, Vol. 355S, 1998, pp. S154–S162.

[82]   Felgner P. L., Gadek T. R., Holm M., Roman R., Chan H. W., Wenz M., et al., "Lipofection: A Highly Efficient, Lipid-Mediated DNA-Transfection Procedure, *Proc Nat Acad Sciences, USA,* Vol. 84, 1987, pp. 7413–7417.

[83]   Nakamura N., Shino K., Natsuume T., Horibe S., Matsumoto N., Kaneda Y., et al., "Early Biological Effect of In Vivo Gene Transfer of Platelet-Derived Growth Factor

(PDGF)-B into Healing Patellar Ligament," *Gene Therapy*, Vol. 5, 1998, pp. 1165–1170.

[84]   Cheng L., Ziegelhoffer P. R., and Yang N. S., "In Vivo Promoter Activity and Transgene Expression in Mammalian Somatic Tissues Evaluated by Using Particle Bombardment, *Proc Nat Acad Sciences, USA,* Vol. 90, 1993, pp. 4455–4459.

[85]   Benn S. I., Whitsitt J. S., Broadley K. N., Nanney L. B., Perkins D., He L., Patel M., Morgan J. R., Swain W.F., and Davidson J. M., "Particle-Mediated Gene Transfer with Transforming Growth Factor-Beta 1 cDNAs Enhances Wound Repair in Rats," *J Clin Investigat,* Vol. 98, 1996, pp. 2894–2902.

[86]   Wu G. Y. and Wu C. H., "Receptor-Mediated In Vitro Gene Transformation by a Soluble DNA Carrier System," *J Biolol Chem,* Vol. 262, 1987, pp. 4429–4432.

[87]   Perales J. C., Ferkol T., Beegen H., Ratnoff O. D., and Hanson R. W., "Gene Transfer In Vivo: Sustained Expression and Regulation of Genes Introduced into the Liver by Receptor-Targeted Uptake, *Proc Nat Acad Sciences, USA,* Vol. 91, 1994, pp. 4086–4090.

[88]   Engstrand T., Daluiski A., Bahamonde M. E., Melhus H., and Lyons K. M., "Transient Production of Bone Morphogenetic Protein 2 by Allogeneic Transplanted Transduced Cells Induces Bone Formation," *Human Gene Therapy*, Vol. 11, 2000, pp. 205–211.

[89]   Miller D. G., Adam M. A., and Miller A. D., "Gene Transfer by Retrovirus Vectors Occurs Only in Cells that are Actively Replicating at the Time of Infection," *Molec Cell Biol,* Vol. 10, 1990, pp. 4239–4242.

[90]   Donahue R. E., Kessler S. W., Bodine D., McDonagh K., Dunbar C., Goodman S., et al., "Helper Virus Induced T Cell Lymphoma in Nonhuman Primates After Retroviral Mediated Gene Tranfer," *J Experiment Med,* Vol. 176, 1992, pp. 1125–1135.

[91]   Mulligan R. C., "The Basic Science of Gene Therapy," *Science*, Vol. 260, 1993, pp. 926–932.

[92]   Rosenfeld M. A., Siegfried W., Yoshimura K., Yoneyama K., Fukayama M., Stier L.E., et al., "Adenovirus-Mediated Transfer of a Recombinant α1-Antitrypsin Gene to the Lung Epithelium In Vivo," *Science*, Vol. 252, 1991, pp. 431–434.

[93]   Kozarsky K. F., Jooss K., Donahee M., Strauss J. F. III, and Wilson J. M., "Effective Treatment of Familial Hypercholesterolemia in the Mouse Model Using Adenovirus-Mediated Transfer of the VLDL Receptor Gene," *Nature Genetics*, Vol. 13, 1996, pp. 54–62.

[94]   Rosenfeld M. A., Yoshimura K., Trapnell B. C., Yoneyama K., Rosenthal E. R., et al., "In Vivo Transfer of the Human Cystic Fibrosis Transmembrane Conductance Regulator Gene to the Airway Epithelium," *Cell*, Vol. 68, 1992, pp.143–155.

[95]   Wilson J. M., "Adenoviruses as Gene-Delivery Vehicles," *N Engl J Med*, Vol. 334, 1996, pp.1185–1187.

[96]   Mitani K., Graham F. L., and Caskey C. T., "Transduction of Human Bone Marrow by Adenoviral Vector," *Human Gene Therapy*, Vol. 5, 1994, pp. 941–948.

[97]   Yang Y., Nunes F. A., Berencsi K., Furth E. E., Gonczol E., and Wilson J. M., "Cellular Immunity to Viral Antigens Limits E1-Deleted Adenoviruses for Gene Therapy," *Proc Nat Acad Sci, USA*, Vol. 91, 1994, pp. 4407–4411.

[98]   Bett A. J., Haddara W., Prevac L., and Graham F. L., "An Efficient and Flexible System for Construction of Adenovirus Vectors With Insertions or Deletions in Early Regions 1 and 3," *Proc Nat Acad Sci, USA*, Vol. 91, 1994, pp. 8802–8806.

[99]   Morsy M. A., Gu M., Motzel S., Zhao J., Lin J., Su Q., et al., "An Adenoviral Vector Deleted for all Viral Coding Sequences Results in Enhanced Safety and Extended

Expression of a Leptin Transgene," *Proc of Nat Acad Sci, USA,* Vol. 95, 1998, pp. 7866–7871.

[100] Kotin R. M., "Prospects for the Use of Adeno-Associated Virus as a Vector for Human Gene Therapy," *Human Gene Therapy,* Vol. 5, 1994, pp. 793–801.

[101] Pan R. Y., Chen S. L., Xiao X., Peng H. J., and Tsao Y. P., "Therapy and Prevention of Arthritis by Recombinant Adeno-Associated Virus Vector with Delivery of Interleukin-1 Receptor Antagonist," *Arthrit Rheumat,* Vol. 43, 2000, pp. 289–297.

[102] Mosca J. D., Hendricks J. K., Buyaner D., Davis-Sproul J., Chuang L. C., Majumdar M. K., et al., "Mesenchymal Stem Cells as Vehicles for Gene Delivery," *Clin Orthop Rel Res,* Vol. 379S, 2000, pp. S71–S90.

[103] Lee K., Majumdar M. K., Buyaner D., Hendricks J. K., Pittenger M. F., and Mosca J. D., "Human Mesenchymal Stem Cells Maintain Transgene Expression During Expansion and Differentiation," *Molecular Therapy: J Am Soc Gene Therapy,* Vol. 3, 2001, pp. 857–866.

[104] Dragoo J. L., Choi J., Hedrick M., Lieberman J. R., and Benhaim P., "Bone Production by BMP-2 Transduced Stem Cells Derived from Human Fat," *Tissue Eng,* Vol. 7, 2001, p. 615.

[105] Praemer A., Furner S., and Rice D. P., "Costs of Musculoskeletal Conditions," *Musculoskeletal Conditions in the United States,* American Academy of Orthopedic Surgeons, Park Ridge, IL, 1992, pp. 145–170.

[106] Micheli L. J., Browne J. E., Erggelet C., Fu F., Mandelbaum B., Moseley J. B., and Zurakowski D., "Autologous Chondrocyte Implantation of the Knee: Multicenter Experience Minimum 3-Year Follow-Up," *Clin J Sports Med,* Vol. 11, 2001, pp. 223–228.

[107] Peterson L., Brittberg M., Kiviranta I., Akerlund E. L., and Lindahl A., "Autologous Chondrocyte Transplantation. Biomechanics and Long-Term Durability," *Am J Sports Med,* Vol. 30, 2002, pp. 2–12.

Preclinical, Clinical, and Regulatory Issues in Cell-Based Therapies

by T. Livingston Arinzeh, [1] *Ph.D.*

INTRODUCTION

CELL OR CELL-BASED TISSUE ENGINEERING therapy is a rapidly growing and evolving technology that can include a broad range of products, e.g., processed, selected, or expanded human or other mammalian cells, stem or progenitor cells, genetically engineered cell therapies, alone or in combination with a synthetic or biological biomaterial. The United States Food and Drug Administration (FDA) reviews and regulates these products to assure safety and effectiveness. Beginning in the 1990s, the FDA has set forth a considerable amount of resources to improve the review and regulation of these products to ensure the protection of the public health while permitting significant innovation and keeping regulatory burden to a minimum. Currently, the FDA has approved some cell-based tissue engineered products for use, whereas others are still in preclinical development or undergoing regulatory evaluation.

This chapter will discuss, in general, the procedures and guidelines created and/or proposed by the FDA for market approval and regulation of cell-based therapies. Before initiating clinical studies, sponsors/companies must have the appropriate preclinical data, and demonstrate that their nonclinical and clinical facilities follow good laboratory practices (GLP) and good manufacturing practices (GMP), respectively. The FDA is divided into centers that work in concert for premarket review and regulation of these products. These centers will be discussed with respect to their requirements for market approval. New proposals for regulation of human cellular and tissue-based products will also be discussed.

REQUIREMENTS FOR INITIATING A CLINICAL STUDY

Preclinical Studies

The FDA requires that preclinical studies be performed to assess the risks and potential benefits of a product prior to the evaluation in humans. Although developing in vitro models that mimic a tissue or system of interest is becoming increasingly popular in order to reduce the number of animals used in medical research, the FDA currently expects testing to ensure a product is safe and effective to be performed in animals. Testing should be performed in two or more species, one rodent and one non-rodent

---

[1] Department of Biomedical Engineering, New Jersey Institute of Technology, University Heights, Newark, NJ 07102.

species, since the product may affect one species differently than another. For cell-based therapies, animal testing can be used to measure toxicity, to determine dosage to achieve a positive outcome, to demonstrate effectiveness in an application, to determine feasibility of a cell-based approach, and to define a clinical model.

First and foremost, the Institutional Animal Care and Use Committee (IACUC) must approve all animal studies. This committee must be established at an institution performing animal research, as mandated by the United States Department of Agriculture (USDA) and the Public Health Service who publish rules, regulations, and policies on the care of use of laboratory animals, as detailed in Title 21 of the Code of Federal Regulations (CFR), section 58.90 (21 CFR 58.90) [1]. The purpose of this committee is to ensure humane and proper care of animals while ensuring that all procedures suggested (surgical or non-surgical) are optimal for the intended objective. The committee, consisting primarily of investigators, reviews animal use protocols, the entire animal care and use program, inspects laboratories where animals are used, and inspects the animal housing facilities.

A proposal involving animals must contain a rationale for involving animals, and for the appropriateness of the species and numbers of animals to be used. In order to determine the risk of an adverse systemic response to administered cells and the effectiveness of the therapy, in vivo studies are essential due to the complex interactions occurring in the body. Determining the appropriate animal species for a study should be based on routinely used or published animal models, anatomic and physiological features that have similarities to humans, and/or the inability to extrapolate the results of theoretical models/in vitro studies for direct use in humans.

The appropriate number of animals to be used in a study can be determined based on statistical tests. These tests should be chosen independently of the results of the experiment and should precede the experiment. In general, to obtain statistically significant results, animal numbers are determined by performing a pilot study, analyzing the variance of the data, and conducting a power analysis [2]. Power-based assessment of the adequacy of the sample size should be conducted before performing the experiment. Previously published or reported animal models of the same species and having similar outcome measures of interest can also be cited and used as support for determining numbers.

To establish safety of a cell therapy, toxicity studies in rodents (i.e., rats) are acceptable. These studies are similar to routinely performed drug and chemical toxicity tests [3]. Animals are administered cells, of varying concentrations, through a designated route of exposure, typically, intravenously. Animals may be exposed for acute (14 consecutive days) or chronic durations, depending on the indication/application, and then, sacrificed. Animals are weighed and observed daily for clinical signs of pain or distress, moribundity, and death. A complete necropsy is performed on all animals that either die or are sacrificed. A histopathologic evaluation on over 40 different tissues must be conducted. Other analyses, such as clinical testing of blood for hematology and clinical chemistry determinations, should also be performed.

For the approval to use cell-based therapies in human studies, preclinical data are gathered and submitted in the form of an Investigational New Drug Application (IND) to the FDA, which is explained in greater detail in sections to follow. The FDA recommends that in preparation for submitting an IND (i.e., Pre-IND), advice should be requested for issues related to therapy development plans; data needed to support the rationale for testing a therapy in humans; the design of nonclinical toxicology and activity studies; data requirements for an IND application; and regulatory requirements for demonstrating safety and efficacy. Potential cell-tissue engineering sponsors/developers should initiate contact with the FDA as early in the development process as possible, so that they will have the opportunity to consider recommendations in planning preclinical and clinical development programs.

Good Laboratory Practices

The FDA established Good Laboratory Practice (GLP) Regulations, 21 CFR Part 58, on December 22, 1978, to institute standards for the conduct and reporting of nonclinical laboratory studies and to assure the quality and integrity of safety data submitted to the FDA in support of research and/or marketing approval [4]. The FDA inspects and audits safety studies of sponsors who've submitted applications for research or marketing of their products. The FDA inspections include the assessment of the personnel involved in the studies, ensuring study protocols exist and are accurately followed, assessing data collection is documented, determining an independent Quality Control Unit (QCU) exists and monitors significant studies, evaluating the facilities and equipment are of adequate design and size, and ensuring adequate animal care and housing. In addition to the inspection, the FDA will also audit one complete study to verify that protocol requirements are met and that findings are accurately reported.

Good Manufacturing Practices

All products to be investigated in clinical trials must be of the identity, strength, quality, and purity that they claim, as detailed in 21 CFR 211.100 [5]. The sponsor must comply with Current Good Manufacturing Practices (CGMP), as described by the FDA. This entails written procedures for the production and process control of the product. These procedures provide documented evidence that assures that a specific process will consistently produce a product that meets its predetermined specifications and quality characteristics. These procedures are to be drafted, reviewed, and approved by the appropriate organizational units and reviewed and approved by the quality control unit. The protocols are to be followed during production and process control functions and documented at the time of performance. Personnel performing these tasks should have the appropriate education, training, and experience, or any combination thereof. Buildings and facilities should be of the appropriate design and construction features for manufacturing, processing, packing and holding products. The equipment should be of the appropriate design and size and sufficiently maintained.

Companies should have a structure and operational system in place that is in accordance with CGMP manufacturing, quality control and quality assurance prior to initiating clinical trials. Sponsors who are unfamiliar with CGMP procedures should seek advice from professional consultants, manufacturers, professional bodies such as the International Society of Professional Engineering (ISPE), and other regulatory bodies.

Investigational New Drug Application

As stated in the Federal Food, Drug, and Cosmetic (FD&C) Act, all new drugs and biological products must demonstrate safety, purity, and efficacy before beginning interstate commerce. Sponsors must submit an application to the FDA for approval to use new therapies in human studies. For cell-based therapies used in vivo, preclinical data are gathered and submitted in the form of an Investigational New Drug Application (IND) to the FDA. The FD&C considers both drugs and biologics to be drugs. For a device, the application is called Investigational Device Exemption (IDE). Guidelines concerning IDEs are described in 21 CFR 812 [6]. Excluding *ex vivo* organ assist devices utilizing cellular components, in vivo cell-based therapies to date have been primarily reviewed and regulated as a biologic drug. Hence, the IND application will be discussed in greater detail in this section. The FDA guidelines describing the Investigational New Drug Application are listed in 21 CFR 312.1 [7]. It describes "procedures and requirements governing the use of investigational new drugs, including procedures and requirements for the submission to, and review by, the Food and Drug Administration of investigational new drug applications (INDs)." An IND is a request for an exemption from the Federal statute that prohibits an unapproved drug from being shipped in interstate commerce. Current Federal law requires that a drug be the subject of an approved marketing application before it is transported or distributed across state lines.

The IND application consists of a investigation plan describing the rationale for the research study, the indication(s) to be studied, the general approach to be followed in evaluating the therapy, the kinds of clinical trials to be conducted in the first year following the submission, the estimated number and type of patients to be given the product in those studies, and any risks on the basis of the toxicological data in animals or prior studies in humans. Detailed protocols for each planned study are submitted. These protocols describe the indication to be treated, proposed patient population, patient inclusion or exclusion criteria, treatment regimen study end points, patient follow-up methods, and clinical trial stopping rules. Information concerning the composition of the product and the manufacturing processes and methods to ensure proper identification, quality, purity, and strength of the investigational therapy must also be provided to assure product safety. This information is assessed so as to ensure that the company submitting the IND application can adequately produce and supply consistent batches of the proposed therapy. Preclinical studies are submitted that demonstrate the product is reasonably safe to perform studies in humans (e.g., toxicology studies) and its effectiveness in a particular indication. The FDA requires that all clinical investigations have approval from the Institutional Review Board (IRB) before conducting the studies. The FDA will approve of the IND exemption and the start of clinical investigations when there is adequate information provided in the areas described above.

CLINICAL INVESTIGATION AND PREMARKET SUBMISSIONS

In general, the first investigation in humans is a safety/feasibility study, termed Phase I clinical trial. These studies are closely monitored and are performed in patients or sometimes in healthy volunteer subjects depending on the type of study. These studies are designed mainly to determine product safety, and if possible, to gain early evidence of effectiveness. This trial is typically conducted in a small number of subjects (generally in the range of 20–80 subjects). If these early studies indicate the product to be reasonably safe, Phase 2 studies can be developed to investigate proper and safe dosing and potential efficacy for a particular indication or indications in patients with the disease or condition. Phase 2 studies are typically well controlled, closely monitored, and conducted in a relatively large number of patients (when compared to Phase I), usually involving several hundred people. Phase 3/pivotal studies are expanded controlled and uncontrolled trials. They are performed after preliminary evidence suggesting effectiveness of the therapy has been obtained in Phase 2, and are intended to gather the additional information about effectiveness and safety that is needed to evaluate the overall benefit-risk relationship of the therapy (http://www.fda.gov/cder/handbook). Phase 3 studies usually include several hundred to several thousand people. After the completion of the Phase 3 trial, this typically leads to an application to the FDA for premarket approval of the product. The FDA inspects and audits the conduct and reporting of clinical trials to ensure that Good Clinical Practice (GCP) standards are followed.

Exceptions occur when human studies have been performed overseas or in a different patient population [8]. Under such circumstances, some or all of the clinical trials mentioned above may not be required before marketing approval. The FDA reviews the clinical data performed outside of the US in the IND process and/or in an application for marketing approval. Other exceptions occur when the product demonstrates significant benefit over existing therapy, or for serious or life-threatening illnesses for which no therapy exists, and it shows the potential to address unmet medical needs for such conditions. In this case, the product would undergo a fast-track development program (as published in November 18, 1998, Guidance for Industry: Fast Track Development Program, http://www.fda.gov/cber/gdlns/fsttrk.pdf), which allows for expedited approval based on surrogate end points, submission and review of portions of an application, and priority review. The FDA encourages that sponsors meet with the agency to discuss the clinical protocol, study results and statistical analyses prior to submitting a Premarket Approval (PMA), Biologics License Application (BLA), or New Drug Application (NDA).

The type of application that a sponsor must submit for premarket approval is dependent upon how the FDA designates the cell therapy, as a drug, biologic, medical device or combination product. This will be discussed further in the next section on regulation. If the cell-based therapy is regulated as a biologic, then this will require review and approval of a BLA that demonstrates safety and effectiveness of the product prior to marketing. If the therapy is regulated as a device, then it requires a PMA demonstrating safety and efficacy, or a premarket notification (510K) that must receive clearance [8]. In order to receive a 510K clearance, the product must demonstrate equivalence to a legally marketed predicate device. If the cell-based therapy will be regulated as a drug, then an NDA is required prior to market approval. The data gathered during the animal studies and human clinical trials of an IND become part of the NDA.

During the premarket approval process, the FDA can inspect the sponsor's manufacturing facilities and clinical trial sites to evaluate the manufacturer's compliance with Current Good Manufacturing Practices (CGMP) and manufacturing-related commitments made in the premarket application. Samples of the product may be collected for analysis by the FDA field and center laboratories. In general, pre-approval inspections are performed if the product is, or is composed of, a new chemical, has a narrow therapeutic range, represents the first approval for the applicant, or is sponsored by a company with a history of CGMP problems. The results of an inspection can affect the final approval decision if there are significant CGMP problems discovered that could affect the safety and efficacy of the product. The sponsor must address these issues prior to market approval.

The Regulatory Process

There are three main agencies within the FDA that regulate medical therapies for humans. The Center for Biologics Evaluation and Research (CBER) regulates biologics. The Center for Drug Evaluation and Research (CDER) regulates drugs. The Center for Devices and Radiological Health (CDRH) regulates medical devices and radiation-emitting electronic products. In general, one center will have the main responsibility and jurisdiction of reviewing a particular product based on its designated category. However, other agencies may contribute to the product's regulation.

A cell-based therapy is regulated based on its designation as a biologic, drug, medical device, or combination product. The term "biologic product" is defined as blood or blood components, virus, therapeutic serum, toxin, antitoxin, vaccine, allergenic product or analogous product, or arsphenamine or its derivatives (or any trivalent organic arsenic compound), applicable to the prevention, treatment, or cure of diseases or injuries in humans [42 U.S.C. 262(a)] [9]. A drug is an article intended for use in the diagnosis, cure, mitigation, treatment, or prevention of disease in humans or other animals, and an article (other than food) and other articles intended to affect the structure or any function of the body of human or other animals [21 U.S.C. 321(g)] [10]. A device is an instrument, apparatus, implement, machine, contrivance, implant, in vitro reagent, or other similar or related article, including any component, part or accessory, which is intended for use in the diagnosis of disease or other conditions, or in the cure, mitigation, treatment or prevention of disease, in human or other animals, or intended to affect the structure or any function of the body of humans or other animals, and which does not achieve any of its principal intended purposes through chemical action within or on the body of human or other animals, and which is not dependent on being metabolized for the achievement of any of its principal intended purposes [21 U.S.C. 201(h)] [11].

Currently, CBER reviews and regulates products that consist of manipulated, cultured, or expanded human cells, xenotransplants, encapsulated cells, and gene therapies. In the case where cells are combined with biomaterials, these products are designated as combination products and are reviewed and regulated by CBER and CDRH [8]. In this case, the FDA Office of Chief Mediator and Ombudsman (OCMO) will determine the product's primary mode of action and categorize it accordingly. The Tissue Reference Group (TRG), which is an intercenter committee composed of representatives from CBER, CDRH, and OCMO, established in 1997, also assists the OCMO in determining product designation. One center will be designated as the lead center and be responsible for product premarket review and determining which type of submission is appropriate, as described in Section 16 of the Safe Medical Devices Act (SMDA) of 1990 [21 U.S.C. 353(g)] [12]. Other centers will be asked to assist in the review in collaboration. The guidelines regarding the regulation of combination products are described in 21 CFR Part 3 and implements section 16 [13]. The sponsor should obtain an agency determination before submission of premarket applications and determine which agency will perform the premarket review and regulation of the product.

Additional intercenter working groups were established at the FDA to address scientific concerns and to provide input on regulatory issues for these cell-based tissue engineering products [8]. The Wound Healing Clinical Focus Group (WHCFG) was established for the development and assessment of products for wound healing. The group ensures consistency in review across centers and acts as a liason from the FDA to academic and industry organizations. Tissue Engineering Working Group (TEWG), consisting of members from five centers in the FDA, similarly addresses scientific and regulatory issues concerning tissue-engineering products. This center also communicates with other federal agencies, such as the National Institute of Health (NIH), National Science Foundation (NSF), and National Institute of Standards and Technology (NIST), and professional societies and academia regarding scientific and regulatory issues. The Intercenter FDA Transmissible Spongiform Encephalopathies (TSE) Working Group guides industry in the safe sourcing, processing, and end-product use of animal and human materials for the protection of animal and human health. This group evaluates the risks posed by animal and human TSE agents in regulated products.

Recent Regulatory Developments

Guidelines for regulating human cellular and tissue-based products were introduced on February 28, 1997 as described in 62 FR 9721 (http://www.fda.gov/cber/gdlns/celltissue.pdf) [14]. The regulation focuses on three areas: 1) preventing unwitting use of contaminated tissues with the potential of transmitting an infectious disease; 2) preventing improper handling or processing that might contaminate or damage tissues; 3) ensuring that clinical safety and efficacy are demonstrated for therapies that are highly processed, are used for other than normal function, are combined with non-tissue components, and are used for metabolic purposes.

Human cellular and tissue-based products are defined as products containing or consisting of human cell or tissues that are intended for implantation, transplantation, infusion, or transfer into a human recipient, e.g., musculoskeletal, ocular, skin tissue, hematopoietic stem cells, reproductive cells and tissues, human dura mater, human heart valve allografts, somatic cell therapy products, and combination products. The term does not include vascularized human organs for transplantation, whole blood, blood components or derivatives, secreted or excreted human products, minimally manipulated bone marrow, ancillary products used in the manufacture of cellular tissue-based products, cells, tissues and organs derived from animals other than humans, and in vitro diagnostic products.

The FDA defined the principal public health and regulatory concerns: prevention of the transmission of communicable disease; processing controls that prevented the contamination and preserved the integrity and function of the product; assurance of clinical safety and effectiveness; labeling and promotion of the product for proper use; monitoring and communicating with the cell and tissue industry. With these concerns, the FDA differentiated cells and tissues and their uses based on their risk relative to each concern. So, the degree of risk is dependent upon the source of cells, e.g., autologous or allogeneic, cell and tissue viability, homologous or nonhomologous function, degree of manipulation—minimal or nonminimal, systemic or local effect, storage—in a bank or not stored (unbanked) and combination of cells or tissue with a drug or device. The least amount of risk would be a product that has minimal manipulation, homologous function, not combined with a drug or device component, and having a local effect. This type of product could be regulated without an actual premarket submission to the FDA under the authority of the Public Health Service Act (PHS Act). The type of product that imposes a greater risk, such as more than minimal manipulation, promoted or labeled for a nonhomologous function, combined with a drug or device component, or having a systemic effect, would be regulated as a biological drug or device requiring a premarket submission to the FDA for evaluation of clinical safety and efficacy.

As part of the implementation of the proposed approach, the FDA has also issued additional rulings concerning human cellular and tissue-based products. In the Federal Register of May 14, 1998, sponsors are required to register with the agency, and list their products in an electronic database (63 FR 26744) [15]. Proposed on September 30, 1999, manufacturers are to screen and test the donors of cells and tissue used in those products for risk factors and for clinical evidence of relevant communicable disease agents and diseases (63 FR 52696) [16]. As of January 8, 2001, the FDA has proposed new regulations for manufacturers of human cellular and tissue-based products to follow current good tissue practices (CGTP), as detailed in 66 FR 1507 [17]. CGTP includes methods, facilities and controls used for the manufacture of human cellular and tissue-based products; record keeping; and the establishment of a quality program. It also includes labeling, reporting, inspections, and enforcement that will apply to manufacturers of those human cellular and tissue-based products that the agency has designated to be regulated solely under the authority of the PHS Act and not as biological drugs or as devices. Under Section 361 of the PHS Act (42 U.S.C. 264), it authorizes the agency to issue regulations to prevent the introduction, transmission, or spread of communicable diseases [18]. The agency's actions are intended to improve protection of the public health while permitting significant innovation and keeping regulatory burden to a minimum.

FUTURE DEVELOPMENTS IN THE REGULATION OF CELL-BASED THERAPIES

Developing standards for cell-based therapies is of critical importance to the FDA in order to achieve a more efficient and effective product approval process and to facilitate industry in its product development. The FDA is working with organizations such as the ASTM International to develop standards, such as test methods, specifications, practices, guides, classifications, or terminology that are scientifically sound. As more and more cell therapies are developed and are submitted for marketing approval, the FDA will continue to build on initiatives and perform the appropriate review and assessment of the therapies through further communications with other federal agencies, academia, industry, and other scientific organizations.

REFERENCES

[1]   Title 21 of the Code of Federal Regulations, Section 58.90 [21 CFR 58.90]: "Animal Care," Title 21: Food and Drugs, Chapter I: Food and Drug Administration, Department of Health and Human Services.

[2]   Mann M. D., Crouse D. A., and Prentice E. D., "Appropriate Animal Numbers in Biomedical Research in Light of Animal Welfare Considerations," *Lab Animal Soc*, Vol. 41, 1991, pp. 6–14.

[3]   National Toxicology Program Good Science for Good Decisions, URL: http://ntp-server.niehs.nih.gov/htdocs/Overviews/GenProtocolsPg.html, National Toxicology Program, Research Triangle, NC, 30 Nov 2001.

[4]   Title 21 of the Code of Federal Regulations, Section 58 [21 CFR 58], "Good Laboratory Practice for Nonclinical Laboratory Studies," Title 21: Food and Drugs, Chapter I: Food and Drug Administration, Department of Health and Human Services.

[5]   Title 21 of the Code of Federal Regulations, Section 211.100 [21 CFR 211.100]. "Current Good Manufacturing Practice for Finished Pharmaceuticals," Title 21: Food and Drugs, Chapter I: Food and Drug Administration, Department of Health and Human Services.

[6]   Title 21 of the Code of Federal Regulations, Section 812 [21 CFR 812]. "Investigational Device Exemptions," Title 21: Food and Drugs, Chapter I: Food and Drug Administration, Department of Health and Human Services.

[7]   Title 21 of the Code of Federal Regulations, Section 312 [21 CFR 312]. "Investigational New Drug Application," Title 21: Food and Drugs, Chapter I: Food and Drug Administration, Department of Health and Human Services.

[8]   Hellman K. B., Solomon R. R., Gaffey C., Durfor C. N., and Bishop J. G., "Regulatory Considerations," *Principles of Tissue Engineering*, 2nd ed., R. P. Lanza, R. Langer and J. P. Vacanti, Eds., Academic Press, San Diego, CA, 2000, pp. 915–928.

[9]   Title 42 of the United States Code, Section 262(a) [21 USC 262(a)]. "Regulation of Biological Products," Title 42: The Public Health and Welfare, Chapter 6A: Public Health Service.

[10] Title 21 of the United States Code, Section 321(g) [21 USC 321(g)]. "Definitions," Title 21: Food and Drugs, Chapter 9: Federal Food, Drug, and Cosmetic Act.

[11] Title 21 of the United States Code, Section 321(h) [21 USC 321(h)]. "Definitions," Title 21: Food and Drugs, Chapter 9: Federal Food, Drug, and Cosmetic Act.

[12] Title 21 of the United States Code, Section 353(g) [21 USC 353(g)]. "Exemptions and Consideration for Certain Drugs, Devices, and Biologic Products," Title 21: Food and Drugs, Chapter 9: Federal Food, Drug, and Cosmetic Act.

[13] Title 21 of the Code of Federal Regulations, Section 3 [21 CFR 3]. "Product Jurisdiction," Title 21: Food and Drugs, Chapter I: Food and Drug Administration, Department of Health and Human Services.

[14] Federal Register, Volume 62, Issue 9721 [62 FR 9721], "A Proposed Approach to the Regulation of Cellular and Tissue-Based Products."

[15] Federal Register, Volume 63, Issue 26744 [63 FR 26744], "Establishment Registration and Listing for Manufacturers of Human Cellular and Tissue-Based Products."

[16] Federal Register, Volume 63, Issue 52696 [63 FR 52696], "Suitability Determination of Donors for Human Cellular and Tissue-Based Products."

[17] Federal Register, Volume 66, Issue 1507 [66 FR 1507]. "Current Good Tissue Practice for Manufacturers of Human Cellular and Tissue-Based Products."

[18] Title 42 of the United States Code, Section 264 [21 USC 264]. "Regulations to Control Communicable Disease," Title 42: The Public Health and Welfare, Chapter 6A: Public Health Service.

Review of State of the Art: Growth Factor-Based Systems for Use as Bone Graft Substitutes

by Emilie V. Cheung, [1] M.D., Dhirendra S. Katti, [2] Ph.D.,
Randy N. Rosier, [3] M.D., Ph.D., and Cato T. Laurencin, [1,2] M.D., Ph.D.

INTRODUCTION

IN 1965 MARSHALL R. URIST [1] FIRST demonstrated that osteoinductive substances led to the formation of bone at extraskeletal sites, by observing that a new ossicle had formed after the implantation of demineralized bone matrix in a muscle pouch of a rat. Less than two decades later, Sampath and Reddi [2] in an in vivo bioassay separated insoluble demineralized bone matrix from the soluble morphogenetic protein responsible for this effect, which was named *bone morphogenetic protein*. Seven years later, Wozney et al. [3] identified the genetic sequence of bone morphogenetic protein, leading to the discovery of its different isoforms and later, in 1990 osteogenetic protein (OP-1) was cloned by Ozkaynak et al. [4].

Through extensive work on the molecular mechanisms of osteoinduction, we now know that the osteoinductive capacity of proteins such as bone morphogenetic protein may be enhanced by other cytokines and growth factors that influence cellular responses. These factors include those that enhance cellular proliferation, migration, attachment to extracellular matrix molecules, and differentiation.

The ability of growth factors to regulate cellular activity, has led to their being intensely investigated as substances that can augment fracture healing. Various bone growth factors, fabricated using gene therapy, show tremendous promise for use in therapeutic applications [5,6]. The current focus of growth factor application to skeletal injuries is to accelerate the healing process. With the advent of new technology, Reddi [7] has suggested that in the future, the possibility may exist of producing prefabricated biological spare parts of the human body, based on the correct combination of growth factors implanted on a template of computer-assisted designed matrix of biomimetic materials in the shape of the desired structure. This would be a true symbiosis of biotechnology, biomaterials, cell biology, and tissue engineering.

The four basic requirements for successful tissue engineering of bone are a suitable scaffold, an appropriate microenvironment, capable responding cells, and soluble osteoinductive signals [7–9]. A carrier matrix is required for local delivery of the growth

---

[1] Department of Orthopedic Surgery, School of Medicine, Drexel University, Philadelphia, PA 19104.
[2] Department of Orthopaedic Surgery, School of Medicine, University of Virginia, Charlottesville, VA 22908.
[3] Department of Orthopaedics, University of Rochester, Rochester, NY 14642.

factors, which are essentially soluble signaling molecules. The factors then act in a sequence of events that recapitulates those occurring during embryonic development [7].

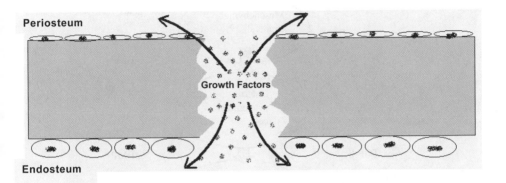

FIG. 1— During bone healing, growth factors are released from the fracture callus and local fracture site. Growth factors then stimulate osteoblast precursor cells on both the endosteal and periosteal surfaces to differentiate and proliferate, initiating a healing response. Among the important growth factors contained in bone matrix are TGF-βs, BMPs, IGFs, PDGFs, and FGFs.

Growth factors are proteins secreted by a cell that bind to specific receptors and affect cell function such as migration, proliferation, and differentiation during normal growth and development, as well as in injury, disease, and repair (Fig. 1). They have two types of effects, a *paracrine effect*, meaning that they stimulate neighboring cells to proliferate and increase matrix protein synthesis, as well as an *autocrine effect*, meaning that they can stimulate themselves for additional metabolic activity. The spectrum of growth factors, which affect proliferation, differentiation, and secretory function of bone cells is not completely known at this time. However with the advent of novel techniques in molecular biology, new factors are being identified and their relative importance will be able to be determined.

All musculoskeletal tissues produce and respond to growth factors, as they initiate the cascades of cellular events that lead up to fracture healing. Some of the most popular growth factors that have been associated with fracture healing include the transforming growth factor family (TGF-β), bone morphogenetic proteins (BMPs), insulin-like growth factors (IGFs), fibroblastic growth factors (FGFs), and platelet-derived growth factors (PDGFs).

Although osteoblasts-like cells produce many other growth factors, such as epidermal growth factors (EGFs), interleukins (IL-1, IL-3, IL-6) and colony stimulating factors (M-CSF, GM-CSF), in this review we will focus on the previously mentioned factors because

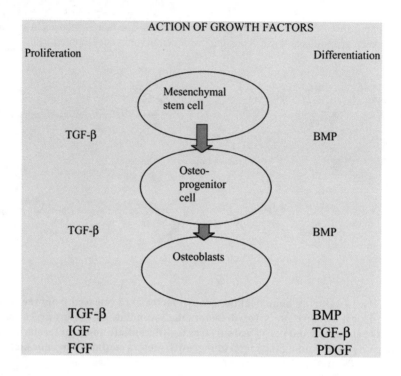

FIG. 2—**TGF-βs affect the proliferation of mesenchymal stem cells, osteoprogenitor cells, and osteoblasts, whereas BMPs primarily affect the differentiation of these cells into osteoblasts. After the stem cells are differentiated into osteoblasts, TGF-βs, IFGs, PDGFs, and FGFs have a role in their subsequent proliferation.**

they have clear functions in the regulation of bone formation and their actions on bone formation have been examined extensively in vivo (Fig. 2).

Transforming Growth Factor Beta (TGF-β)

TGF-β is present in many tissues, but is found in highest quantities in platelets, mesenchymal stem cells, osteoblasts, chondrocytes in callus formation following fracture, and in hypertrophic chondrocytes. TGF-β is also present in fracture hematoma within the first 24 hours after injury. The discovery of large amounts of TGF-β in bone matrix, its effect on protein synthesis by chondrocytes and osteoblasts in vitro, and its release into fracture hematoma by platelets, led to the belief that TGF-β is a major cytokine involved in regulating cartilage and bone formation following injury and during normal growth and remodeling [3,7].

Early attempts to purify bone-derived growth factors resulted in the purification of TGF-β1 and TGF-β2 [10]. The TGF-β isoforms (Types 1–5) are dimeric, disulfide-bonded molecules [10]. TGF-β is secreted in a latent form, which requires activation through enzymatic cleavage, acidic pH or heat [10].

TGF-βs comprise a superfamily of proteins that mediate many key elements in growth and development. This family has grown over the past few decades to include over 40 different proteins. There are four mammalian TGF-β isoforms as well as subfamilies, which include activins, Mullerian inhibitory substance, growth differentiation factors (GDFs), and the bone morphogenetic proteins (BMPs) [10].

It has been shown that TGF-β suppresses the formation of mineral in osteoid despite its stimulation of osteoid formation [11]. TGF-β inhibits markers of calcified bone matrix such as osteocalcin. In in vivo models, injections of TGF-β over murine calvaria, osteoid became mineralized only after the injections had ceased. Noda et al. [12] demonstrated that TGF-β1 and TGF-β2 inhibit osteocalcin gene expression, a marker of calcification, through transcriptional control. Although TGF-β initiates new bone formation, it must be removed before mineralization can occur [13].

Three TGF-β receptors have been identified: I, II, and III. Type III is a cell surface proteoglycan, and is not regarded as a true receptor because although it has high affinity binding, ligand binding is not associated with transduction of intracellular signaling. Types I and II receptors effect biologic signaling via heterodimeric serine/threonine kinases. TGF-β heterodimeric receptor complexes initiate intracellular signaling by dimerizing, with subsequent autophosphorylation of the receptor. Transcription factors called SMADS mediate downstream signaling. SMADS are phosphorylated upon activation, then form heterodimeric complexes that are translocated to the nucleus and regulate gene transcription. The downstream signaling pathways responsible for gene transcription have not been fully elucidated, but it is known that other molecules, such as steroid hormone receptors, may modulate SMAD activation of gene transcription through protein-protein interactions. The SMADS have selectivity for the TGF-β and BMP receptor signals, with SMADS 2 and 3 mediating TGF-β-stimulated gene transcription and SMADS 1, 5, and 8 mediating BMP-stimulated gene transcription. These SMADS all dimerize with a common partner, SMAD4, to form the active transcription factor that is translocated to the nucleus to regulate gene expression. In addition, SMADs 6 and 7 are inhibitory SMADS, which block signaling by the other SMADS (Fig. 3). A second level of complexity in TGF-β/BMP signaling control is mediated by two ubiquitin ligases, SMURF1 and SMURF2, which function to ubiquitinate SMADS 1, 2, 3, 5, and possibly 8, targeting these proteins for degradation by the proteasome within the cell. The SMURFS also can target the TGF-β receptors themselves for degradation.

The Type I receptor has higher affinity than Type II for the TGF-β isoforms. All three receptors have been identified on chondrocytes. A latent TGF-β binding protein exists, which prevents receptor activation by sequestering TGF-β and maintaining it in a latent form. Latent TGF-β can be activated by acid, heat, or specific proteolytic cleavage. The activation of TGF-β by acidic pH may have particular importance in bone remodeling, where the acidic microenvironment of osteoclasts may release and activate TGF-β, providing one of the mechanisms whereby bone resorption is coupled with subsequent bone formation.

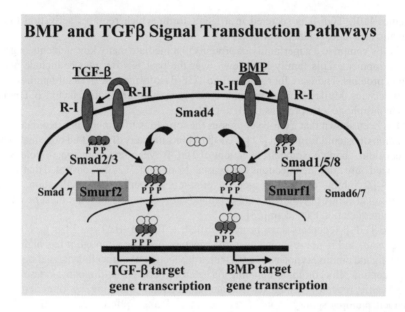

FIG. 3—The TGF-β and BMP family members use SMAD signaling pathways. The ligand binds to the Type I receptor. This results in the Type II receptor dimerizing and phosphorylating the Type I receptor. The SMADs are then activated and phosphorylated. Next, the SMADs associate with SMAD4, resulting in translocation to the nucleus, where gene transcription is regulated.

TGF-βs have different effects depending on tissue and receptor expression. For example, Opperman et al. [13] demonstrated in an in vitro rat calvaria model that the removal of TGF-β3 by neutralizing antibodies leads to obliteration of the cranial suture. However, with the removal of TGF-β2 by neutralizing antibodies, those sutures were rescued from osseous obliteration. In a more recent study Opperman et al. [14] added TGF-β3 to cultured calvaria cells, and the number of TGFβ-I receptor positive cells within the suture were measured. Addition of TGF-β3 to calvaria in culture decreased the number of TGFβ-I receptor expressing cells in both fusing and non-fusing sutures, with dramatic decreases in the numbers of osteoblasts expressing TGF-βI receptor. It was concluded that TGF-β3 binds to and down-regulates TGF-βI receptor expression by suture cells. This down-regulation thus limits the ability of cells to respond to all TGF-βs.

TGF-βs induce mesenchymal stem cells to produce cartilage-specific proteoglycans and Type II collagen. TGF-β also acts on osteoblasts to proliferate and produce collagen. However, the ability of TGF-β to stimulate or inhibit proliferation of osteoblasts in culture depends on the stage of differentiation of the osteoblast population and the growth conditions. The major effect of TGF-β on the osteoblast is to cause the cell to produce matrix and proliferate [15].

Agents that help regulate bone formation and maintenance of bone mass appear to increase the amount of TGF-β in bone. Bones from ovarectomized rats have less TGF-β than normal rats [16]. Vitamin D-deficient rats have less TGF-β than vitamin-repleted rats [17]. Parathyroid hormone studies showed that increased bone mass also coincided with increased TGF-β [18].

Isoforms

Dramatic differences in tissue distribution suggest that each isoform has a distinct function. Marra et al. [19] characterized the latent TGF-β complexes secreted by liver fat-storage cells (FSC) and kidney glomerular mesangial cells (GMC). Human liver FSC produce predominantly the TGF-β-1 isoform, whereas kidney GMC secrete predominantly the latent TGF-β1 and 2 isoforms. In bone, 80–90% of TGF-β exists as the TGF-β1 isoform. The prostate produces 30–70 times more TGF-β2 than TGF-β1 [20]. The TGF-β isoforms are also regulated differently. It has been shown that the promoter regions for TGF-β1, 2, and 3 show little similarity [21–23]. Furthermore, the various isoforms bind with different affinities to TGF-β receptors.

Recent Studies of TGF-β1 as an Osteoinductive Substance

TGF-β as a potentially osteoinductive substance has been studied in various animal models, using subperiosteal injections in the femur, calvaria, critical-sized defects, and bone-ingrowth into prosthetic devices. Joyce et al. [24] demonstrated that injections of TGF-β in the rat femur could stimulate periosteal cells to undergo endochondral ossification. Hock et al. [25] showed that when calvarial osteoblasts are incubated in vitro with TGF-β, there is an increase in bone matrix formation as well as the number of osteoblasts observed. In addition, TGF-β2 has been found to be autoregulatory, increasing the production of TGF-β1 in osteoblasts and chondrocytes [26]. These actions suggest potential therapeutic applications for osseous defects.

Lind et al. [27] delivered continuous infusion of TGF-β (with either 1 or 10 μg per day for six weeks) on rabbit tibial diaphyseal fractures fixed with a plate, and found that there was significant increase in callus formation, as well as a significant increase in bending strength, in comparison to non-treated control specimens. The group receiving 1 μg per day demonstrated superior mechanical strength in three-point bending as compared to both the untreated and the higher-dosed groups.

Nielsen et al. [28] also evaluated mechanical strength of a rat fracture model that received a local treatment of TGF-β (either 4 or 40 μg every other day for 40 days), and demonstrated that the fractures with TGF-β had superior amount of callus formation and strength. The group receiving the 40 μg dose demonstrated a significant increase in ultimate load to failure than the lower-dosed and untreated groups.

Critchlow et al. [29] investigated the effect of TGF-β2 injected around the developing callus of rabbit tibial fractures healing under stable (fixed with a dynamic compression plate), or unstable (without plate fixation) mechanical conditions 4 days after fracture. It was concluded that TGF-β2 cannot stimulate fracture healing under unstable mechanical conditions, but it can increase bony callus under stable mechanical conditions.

Although these studies [27–29] confirm that TGF-β enhances cellular proliferation, its potential as an osteoinductive substance may be limited [3]. Different isoforms and doses of TGF-β have been used in various studies by means of different animal models. The positive effects of TGF-β in the studies by Lind et al., Nielsen et al., and Critchlow et al. suggest that relatively large dosages are required to enhance bone repair [27–29]. Large dosages may not be possible in the clinical setting, as TGF-β enhances proliferation in a variety of cell types, which may cause undesired side effects. Based on studies thus far, it can be concluded that TGF-β has potential for being developed as an agent for clinical use, but further preclinical studies need to elucidate dosing parameters, safety, and appropriate methods of applications.

Bone Morphogenetic Protein (BMP)

BMP was discovered in demineralized bone material to have the unique ability to induce bone formation ectopically [1,2]. BMPs are localized to developing skeletal structures during development, as well as during the process of bone remodeling. The BMPs are a subfamily of the TGF-β superfamily, consisting of 15 known members. Purification of DBM by Sampath and Reddi [2] in 1981 has led to the isolation and identification of several members of the BMP family.

BMP-1 is a procollagen C-proteinase, which has the ability to cleave the carboxy terminals of procollagens I, II, and III [30]. BMP-2 and BMP-4 are osteoinductive factors that stimulate chondrogenic differentiation of mesenchymal stem cells, inducing enchondral bone formation. BMP-3 is a bone-inductive protein also known as osteogenin. Osteogenin has potent ability to induce the rapid differentiation of extraskeletal mesenchymal tissue into bone. BMPs 5, 6, and 7 are also effective osteoinductive agents. BMPs 6 and 7 are found in hypertrophic cartilage, and stimulate cartilage maturation. Other members of the BMP family include growth and differentiation factors (GDFs), also termed cartilage-derived morphogenetic proteins (CDMPs), which induce the formation of cartilage and tendon-like tissues. Myostatin (also known as GDF-8) plays a central role in muscle formation, but probably not in bone formation [31].

It has been shown that the presence of one BMP can enhance the expression of other BMPs. For example, combinations of BMP-2 with BMP-7 and BMP-2 with BMP-6 has been reported to be five to ten times more potent than BMP-2 alone in inducing cartilage and bone formation [32]. In addition, intracellular regulatory proteins such as Lim Mineralization Protein 1 (LMP1) may stimulate production of multiple BMP isoforms by bone and mesenchymal cells.

BMPs are dimeric disulfide-bonded hydrophobic glycoproteins, and are secreted in their active form, unlike the TGF-β isoforms, which are secreted in a latent form. Specific extracellular binding proteins, including chordin and noggin, control BMP activity by sequestering BMPs, thus preventing receptor interaction [4]. BMPs initiate their cellular action by binding transmembrane serine/threonine kinases, known as Type I and Type II receptors. Downstream activation and regulation of transcription is mediated by SMAD signaling proteins, similar to that of TGF-β (Fig. 3).

Boden et al. [33] found that physiologic levels of the glucocorticoid triamcinolone acetonide increased BMP-6 production by 5 to 8-fold, with subsequent osteoblast differentiation in fetal calvarial cells. In contrast, BMPs -2, -4, -5, -7, and TGF-β1 messenger RNA levels increased by less than two-fold. It was therefore postulated that the glucocorticoid may be the early signaling molecule during bone formation, and that it initiates a signal amplification cascade beginning with BMP-6. Thus, BMP-6 shows promise as an osteoinductive protein for investigation in clinical trials [26].

The use of BMP in humans is currently restricted to spinal arthrodesis trials and treatment of nonunions [34,35]. BMP-2 and BMP-7 (also known as osteogenic protein 1, OP-1) have been studied extensively for their ability to induce bone regeneration. The delivery method for these growth factors uses recombinant gene therapy to produce large quantities of the protein, and the protein is incorporation into a collagen sponge or collagen gel that acts as a reservoir for the growth factor. This is then implanted into the site of bone induction.

Sheehan et al. [36] demonstrated the effectiveness of Type I collagen gel combined with autogeneous iliac-crest bone and rhBMP-2, when compared to bone formation at the sites implanted without rhBMP-2. Furthermore, biomechanical testing of the harvested specimens showed superior strength of the rhBMP-2 treated sites in comparison to the untreated control group.

Fischgrund et al. [37] combined rhBMP-2 with autograft plus either a collagen "sandwich" made of collagen sheets, collagen "morsels" made of collagen sheets cut into small pieces, open-pore polylactic acid, or a polylactic acid-glycolic acid sponge sandwich, in a canine lumbar spine model. There was no significant difference between the carrier models, but the specimens treated with rhBMP-2 had greater bone mass volume and demonstrated greater bone maturity.

Recent studies of BMP-2 in spinal fusions have used genetically transformed marrow cells that are implanted directly to the desired site, where they continue to produce BMP-2. Boden et al. [38] used local delivery of bone marrow cells containing cDNA of an osteoinductive protein in posterior lumbar spine fusion of rats. They had a 100% fusion rate, compared with 0% for untreated controls. Adenoviral vector-transformed BMP-2-producing marrow cells have also shown similar results [39–42].

Recombinant DNA technology for the manufacturing of genetically engineered BMPs [2] has led to an abundant supply of recombinant human BMPs (rhBMPs), such as rhBMP-2, 4, and 6 (Genetic Institute, Cambridge, MA), and rhBMP-7 (OP-1) (Stryker Biotech, Natick, MA) for use in research and clinical trials [43]. Recombinant human BMP-2, when combined with a demineralized bone matrix carrier, and recombinant human BMP-7, when combined with a bovine collagen carrier, have been found to induce enchondral bone formation in segmental bone defects in a number of species.

Geesink et al. [44] were the first to report on rhBMP-7/OP-1 in humans. During high tibial osteotomy for degenerative joint disease of the knee, critical sized defects were created in the fibula. OP-1 was combined with a Type I collagen carrier, and placed into the defect. At six weeks, the OP-1 treated group showed radiographic evidence of bone formation, whereas the group receiving only collagen without OP-1 did not. This study validates the osteogenic activity of OP-1 in a critically sized human bony defect.

Friedlaender et al. [43] in a prospective, randomized, multicenter study of tibial nonunions treated with intramedullary nailing showed that OP-1 implanted with a Type I collagen carrier was comparable to autografts. Parameters measured were radiographic assessment, immunologic assessment, complications, and clinical assessment by patient and physician satisfaction. In 124 tibial nonunions at the 9-month follow-up time point, 75% of those in the OP-1 treated group and 84% of those in the autograft-treated group had radiographic union. By clinical criteria, 81% of the OP-1 treatment patients and 85% of the autograft treatment patients had achieved union. At the 2-year follow-up, these results continued at similar levels. OP-1 proved to be safe and effective for the treatment of tibial nonunions at 2 years following the operative procedure, with the benefit of lack of donor site morbidity (Fig. 4).

In a recent study by Salkeld et al. [45] using a canine ulna defect model, the OP-1 device was mixed with either freeze-dried allograft or autograft. Using radiographic, mechanical, and histologic criteria, the use of OP-1 alone, or any combination of autograft or allograft with OP-1, demonstrated improved healing compared with the used of autograft or allograft alone. They sought to determine the optimal volume ratio of the OP-1 device to allograft and autograft bone. It was noted that the highest radiographic and histological grades and greatest mechanical strength were achieved with the use of 33% allograft and 67% OP-1, although there were no significant differences among the groups containing OP-1.

The OP-1 device has little intrinsic biomechanical strength, but can be combined with various internal fixation devices. As with other bone graft materials, OP-1 requires a healthy host bed, which is capable of providing vascularity and cell populations necessary for cell regeneration and repair. The new bone induced by OP-1 continues to be remodeled in the same manner as that in the surrounding skeleton.

Gene therapy entails the transport of a gene into cells with its subsequent integration and transcription, leading to synthesis of the desired protein product of the gene. Because expression of BMPs are desirable for bone induction, gene therapy using BMPs has potentially valuable clinical applications. Gene therapy studies in animal models have shown direct introduction of a BMP gene (BMP-2, BMP-7, or BMP-9) carried by adenoviral vectors to enhance fracture healing and spinal arthrodesis [46–49]. In addition, bone marrow mesenchymal cells have been infected *ex vivo* using BMP-carrying adenoviral vectors. After reintroduction of the transfected cells into the animals, these cells were shown to aid in repair of bony and cartilaginous defects [50–52]. Adenoviral vectors induce an immune reaction, which ultimately limits the expression of the gene by transduced cells to a few weeks. Therefore, bone healing is in many ways an ideal potential application for this type of vector, since only transient expression of BMPs is needed to induce bone formation by host mesenchymal stem cell differentiation. A number of studies are currently underway to explore the potential of BMP gene therapies in bone healing.

These studies and others have demonstrated the beneficial effect of using recombinant human BMP-7 (rhBMP-7)/osteogenic protein (OP-1) for accelerated healing of bone defects. The clinical trial by Friedlander et al. [43] conducted under a Food and Drug Administration approved Investigational Device Exemption has established both the safety and efficacy of OP-1 for the treatment of tibial nonunions. Therefore, the United States Food and Drug Administration has recently approved the use of BMP-7/OP-1 in humans in tibial nonunions, and BMP2 in spinal arthrodesis under specific limited clinical circumstances.

One question concerning the use of recombinant BMPs in stimulating bone healing in animals or humans remains unanswered: why are huge doses required to have an osteoconducive efficacy? The effective doses are orders of magnitude greater than the endogenous amounts of BMPs during normal bone repair or in normal bone remodeling. Presumably the combined action of other factors may be required for maximal efficacy of BMP-mediated osteoinduction, including possibly other BMPs. The experimental complexity of combining multiple factors currently makes exploration of this hypothetical explanation difficult.

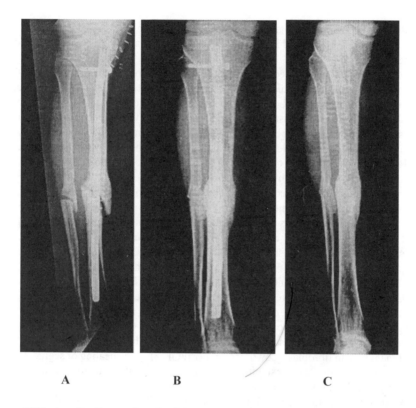

A   B   C

FIG. 4— Radiographs of a 34-year-old male patient treated with osteogenic protein-1 (OP-1) and 33 months following a closed, comminuted tibial fracture sustained in a motor vehicle accident. Prior treatment included intramedullary rod fixation, fresh bone autograft, a fibulectomy, and external electrical stimulation. The clinical and radiographic results were considered successful at both 9 and 24 months following treatment with an intramedullary rod and OP-1. A: Immediate postoperative radiograph. B: Radiograph 9 months following treatment with OP-1. C: Radiograph 24 months following treatment with OP-1. (Reproduced with permission from Friedlaender et al., *J Bone Joint Surg Am*, Vol. 83, pp. S1-151-158.)

Fibroblast Growth Factor (FGF)

FGFs are a family of growth factors, including 23 known members. FGF-1 (acidic) and FGF-2 (basic) are the most abundant of the FGF family. Both forms are present and active in cartilage matrix and bone, although FGF-2 is the more powerful of the two. They have been shown to be mitogenic under in vivo conditions for endothelial cells, fibroblasts, chondroblasts, and osteoblasts [5].

During the early stages of fracture-healing, including angiogenesis, chondrocyte, and chondroblast activation, both FGF-1 and FGF-2 have been identified to play a role. In vivo, administration of exogenous FGF-1 and FGF-2 increases bone formation. Their effects are mediated by TGF-β and prostaglandins, as the production of these factors are likewise regulated by FGFs. FGF-1 and FGF-2 under some circumstances are also able to stimulate bone resorption [53].

Four FGF receptors have been identified. They are membrane-spanning tyrosine-kinase receptors, activating intracellular signaling pathways. Mutations in these FGF receptors result in abnormalities in enchondral ossification and intramembranous ossification. For example, mutations in fibroblast growth factor receptor-2 (FGFR-2) have been identified in Apert syndrome, and also have been associated with the premature fusion of calvaria sutures resulting in skull abnormalities [45]. Mutations in fibroblast growth factor receptor-3 (FGFR-3) have been linked to achondroplasia, the most common form of dwarfism, thanatorphoric dysplasia, and hypochondroplasia [54].

In vivo studies show that exogenous FGF stimulates proliferation of osteoblastic cells. Local injection of FGF-1 promotes calvarial bone formation [55]. In rabbits, intraosseous application of FGF-2 increases bone formation and bone mineral density [56]. Exogenous FGF-1 and FGF-2 are thought to act by increasing the recruitment of osteoblast precursor cells, which differentiate into osteoblasts. TGF-β increases FGF-2 mRNA in cells, thus some of its cellular effects could be related to its regulation of other growth factors [57].

FGF also plays an important role during fracture repair. Scully et al. [58] demonstrated that FGF-1 and FGF-2 are expressed in the granulation tissue following fracture, suggesting that FGFs may stimulate cell migration and angiogenesis at the early stages of fracture healing. During callus formation, FGF-1 levels were found to increase [59].

Exogenous FGF-2 can also accelerate bone repair. The effect of local injection of recombinant human fibroblast growth factor-2 (rhFGF-2) on the healing of segmental 3 mm tibial defects in rabbits was investigated by Kato et al. [60]. After osteotomy and subsequent fixation by an external fixator, each animal in the treatment group received either 0, 50, 100, 200, or 400 µg at the fracture site. Injection of the growth factor increased the volume and mineral content of the regenerated bone at the defect in a dose-dependent manner. Significant effects were observed at concentrations of 100 µg or greater, as assessed by X-ray, dual energy X-ray absoptiometry (DEXA), and histological evaluation at five weeks. It was concluded that a single local injection of FGF-2 is capable of stimulating the healing of segmental defects.

Zellin et al. [61] found an increased number of osteocytes at newly formed bone sites in transosseous rat mandibular defects. Three different doses of rh FGF-2 (10 ng, 100 ng, and 1 µg) were delivered in an absorbable collagen sponge carrier. The higher 1 µg dose decreased bone formation, whereas the lower doses had a mild stimulatory effect on osteogenesis after 24 days.

In a nonhuman primate fracture model, Radomsky et al. [62] injected rhFGF-2 into 1 mm fibula osteotomy defects of baboons. The osteotomy sites treated with rhFGF-2 had larger callus, greater bone volume, and increased osteoblastic activity when compared to untreated controls. In addition, significant differences between energy to failure and load at failure between the treated and untreated groups was observed.

The results of these studies suggest that FGF-2 shows potential to be used in the future as an adjunct to bone healing. As with TGF-β, the effects of the FGFs on increasing bone formation or induction are modest compared with those of the BMPs.

Platelet-derived Growth Factor (PDGF)

PDGF is found in higher concentrations in platelets and vascular endothelial cells, although it is present in many different cell types. PDGF synthesis is often increased in response to external stimuli, such as low oxygen tension, thrombin, or stimulation by other growth factors.

The main functions of PDGF are chemotactic. It is released by platelets and monocytes in fracture callus and sites of injury, and induces mesenchymal stem cell proliferation, thus recruiting reparative cell populations [63]. PDGF is mitogenic for osteoblasts in vitro [64], as this is its primary effect on bone.

PDGF is a protein made of two polypeptide chains. The two subunits, PDGF-A and PDGF-B, can form either homodimers or heterodimers. Each chain is synthesized independently, and their synthesis is regulated by different pathways. For example, PDGF-A is overexpressed in certain Wilm's tumors [65]. PDGF-AA and PDGF-AB have similar effects on osteoblast cells. PDGF-BB is more potent than AA, and PDGF-AB has intermediate activity. The PDGF protein stimulates replication in bone cell cultures in vitro and increase Type I collagen synthesis.

Due to its mitogenic activity, it is unlikely that PDGF will be a suitable agent for the systemic therapy of skeletal disorders. Since PDGF increases the number of cells synthesizing collagen, PDGF administered systemically causes fibroblast replication and fibrosis at extraskeletal sites [55]. However, when normalized for cell number, PDGF does not increase collagen synthesis. Local application of PDGF has shown promise to promote bone formation via its mitogenic effect on osteoblasts in some animal models.

TABLE 1 — Effect of PDGF on skeletal cells.
Increases cell replication
Decreases collagen synthesis by the osteoblast
Decreases bone matrix apposition rates
Increases bone resorption
Increases collagen degradation and collagenase expression

Systemic administration of PDGF to estrogen-deficient rats was shown to prevent bone loss in the spine by Mitlak et al. [66]. These results concur with the mitogenic effects of PDGF in vitro. In addition, in the treated animals, there was fibrosis noted in extraskeletal tissues, demonstrating a potential problem with use of PDGF systemically in the clinical setting. Marden et al. [67] reported that topical administration of PDGF to rat craniotomy defects shows an increase in soft tissue repair. However, no increase in osteogenesis was observed, and these findings were attributed to nonspecific effects of PDGF.

In a study on the effect of PDGF on tibial osteotomies of rats, Nash et al. [68] found that PDGF-BB has a stimulatory effect on fracture healing. Radiographically, there was a clear increase in callus density and volume in the treated tibiae when compared to the untreated group. Histologically, the PDGF-treated tibiae displayed a more advanced stage of osteogenic differentiation. However, no significant increase in biomechanical strength was observed.

Although PDGF may have some potential usefulness in fracture healing, at the present time its role remains unclear.

Insulin-like Growth Factor (IGF)

Two IGFs have been identified: IGF-I and IGF-II. IGF-I is more potent than IGF-II, and has been localized to healing fracture sites, although IGF-II is more abundant [3,69,70]. IGF-I is a low molecular weight polypeptide, produced by the liver in response to growth hormone. IGF-I and IGF-II stimulate osteoblastic cell proliferation and Type I collagen expression, and interference with IGF function by use of antibodies to the ligands or receptors inhibits these effects [71].

IGFs are abundant in the bone microenvironemnt acting in both an autocrine and paracrine manner to regulate bone formation. Along with growth hormone, IGF is actively involved during fetal skeletal development, and plays a major role in the repair and remodeling of the adult skeleton. IGF expression is increased in cells of developing periosteum, growth plate, healing fracture callus tissue, and developing ectopic bone tissue.

The half-life of systemically administered IGFs are relatively short, due to their relatively small size. In vivo, IGFs are bound to larger protein complexes known as IGF binding proteins (IGFBPs). Six IGFBPs have been identified (Types 1-6); Types 2 through 6 are produced by osteoblasts. IGFBPs have been shown to modulate IGF activity. For example, IGFBP-3 and IGFBP-5 potentiate IGF stimulation of osteoblasts, whereas the other IGFBPs inhibit IGF activities. Bagi et al. [72] administered IGFBP-3 and IGF-I alone and in combination in ovarectomized, osteopenic rats. The two agents in combination were more effective than either agent alone for increasing bone formation in osteopenic bone. IGFBP-5 is unique in that IGFBP-5 alone or in combination with IGF-I or IGF-II can bind to hydroxyapetite [73]. Thus it serves to incorporate IGFs into mineralized bone matrix.

Animal studies show that IGF administered systemically can augment bone repair. Using a rat calvarial critical defect model, Thaller et al. [74] evaluated the role of IGF-I in stimulating intramembranous bone formation. Bone healing in the animals with continuous systemic administration of IGF-I via a subcutaneous pump was compared to saline-treated control. Within the experimental group, they observed repair commenced at approximately 1 week and the critical-size calvarial bone defects were completely obliterated by 6 weeks, whereas in the control group, the surgical defects remained at 8 weeks. These results suggest that IGF-I does enhance the healing of intramembranous bony defects.

In a more recent study, Thaller et al. [75] examined the effects of recombinant IGF-1 on standardized, critical-size calvarial defects in 25 adult, male streptozocin-induced diabetic rats. It appeared that IGF-1 exerted a potentiating effect on the repair of bony defects in diabetes-induced rats. Diabetic patients have an increased frequency of infection, delayed scar formation, and poor bony union. Thus, IGF-I may be useful in this population with clinically documented problems in bone healing.

In a rabbit tibial osteotomy model Carpenter et al. [76] found that intramuscular injections of human growth hormone increased serum IGF-I levels, but did not have a significant effect on bone healing. The fracture sites were stabilized with external fixation, and the animals received either recombinant human growth hormone (150 µg/kg) or saline (control group). Radiographic and biomechanical assessment was performed at four, six, and eight weeks. There was a correlation between higher serum levels of IGF-I and higher does of growth hormone, but this increase in IGF was not statistically significant. Moreover, with the higher serum levels of IGF, there was no improvement in radiographic evidence of healing, or increased strength using the four-point bending method in the treated animals.

Interestingly, IGF-I has been found within osteoclasts, and has been reported to increase osteoclast formation, thus having an autocrine effect during bone resorption [47]. IGF-I is thought to be released from bone during the resorption phase and function to increase osteoblast precursors [77]. During the remodeling cycle, resorption is balanced by an equal amount of bone formation. Therefore, bone formation and bone resorption are coupled, and IGFs play a role in the mediation of both these processes.

IGFs have an important role in bone remodeling, but the effects depend on interactions with IGFBPs. Therapeutic potential for bone healing exists for IGFs, but the role needs to be better defined by further study.

Summary

This is an exciting time in the development of growth factor-based therapies for the enhancement of bone healing because progress is being observed in the clinical arena. Areas of application for new technologies include: acceleration of fracture healing, treatment of nonunions, enhancement of spinal fusion, and treatment of significant bone loss. Comprehensive strategies for therapeutic applications will combine concepts of tissue-engineering for a suitable delivery mechanism and biologic scaffold, and gene therapy for transformation of cellular expression towards desirable bone healing effects.

BMP-7/OP-1 and BMP-2 are already being used therapeutically for augmentation of bone healing. Other BMPs are actively being investigated for similar purposes. TGF-βs have been shown in animal models to be effective in augmentation of bone healing, but dosing recommendations and safety assessments using large doses still need to be elucidated. IGFs, PDGFs and FGFs show potential as adjuncts to bony healing as shown in animal models, but their effects need to be further studied before conclusions can be made regarding their therapeutic role.

REFERENCES

[1] Urist M. R., "Bone: Formation by Autoinduction," *Science*, Vol. 150, 1965, pp. 893–899.

[2] Sampath T. K. and Reddi A. H., "Dissociative Extraction and Reconstitution of Bone Matrix Components Involved in Local Bone Differentiation," *Pro Natl Acad Sci USA*, Vol. 78, 1981, pp. 7599–7603.

[3] Wozney J. M., Rosen V., Celeste A. J., Mitsock L. M., Whitters M. J., Kriz R. W., et al., "Novel Regulators of Bone Formation: Molecular Clones and Activities," *Science*, Vol. 242, 1988, pp.1528–1534.

[4]   Ozkaynak E., Ruger D. C., Drier E. A., Corbett C., Ridge R. J., Sampath T. K., et al., "OP-1 cDNA Encodes an Osteogenic Protein in the TGFβ Family," *Eur Mol Biol Organ J*, Vol. 9, 1990, pp. 2085–2093.

[5]   Lieberman J. R., Daluiski A., and Einhorn T. A., "The Role of Growth Factors in the Repair of Bone," *J Bone Joint Surg Am*, Vol. 84, 2002, pp. 1033–1044.

[6]   Rosier R. N., Reynolds P. R., and O'Keefe R. J., "Molecular and Cell Biology in Orthopedics," *Orthopedic Basic Science*, 2nd ed., American Academy of Orthopedic Surgeons, Rosemont, IL, 2000, pp. 19–76.

[7]   Reddi A. H., "Morphogenesis and Tissue Engineering of Bone and Cartilage: Inductive Signals, Stem Cells, and Biomimetic Biomaterials," *Tissue Eng*, Vol. 6, 2000, pp. 351–359.

[8]   Ripamonti U., Ramoshebi L. N., Matsaba T., Tasker J., Crooks J., and Teare J., "Bone Induction by BMPs/OPs and Related Family Members in Primates," *J Bone Joint Surg*, Vol. 83, 2001, pp. S1-116-S1-126.

[9]   Reddi A. H., "Bone Morphogenetic Proteins and Biomaterials: Applications in Tissue Engineering of Bone and Cartilage," *J Cell Biochem*, Vol. 56, 1994, pp. 192–195.

[10]   Bonewald L. F., "Transforming Growth Factor-β," *Principles of Bone Biology*, 2nd ed., Academic Press, San Diego, CA, 2002, pp. 903–918.

[11]   Bonewald L. F. and Dallas S. L., "Role of Active and Latent Transforming Growth Factor Beta in Bone Formation," *J Cell Biochem*, Vol. 55, 1994, pp. 350–357.

[12]   Noda M. and Camilliere J. J., "In Vivo Stimulation of Bone Formation by Transforming Growth Factor-beta," *Endocrinology*, Vol. 124, 1989, pp. 2991–2994.

[13]   Opperman L. A., Chhabra A., Cho R. W., and Ogle R. C., "Cranial Suture Obliteration is Induced by Removal of Transforming Growth Factor (TGF)-beta 3 Activity and Prevented by Removal of TGF-beta 2 Activity from Fetal Rat Calvaria In Vitro," *J Craniofac Genet Dev Biol*, Vol. 19, 1999, pp. 164–173.

[14]   Opperman L. A., Galanis V., Williams A. R., and Adab K., "Transforming Growth Factor-beta3 (Tgf-beta3) Down-regulates Tgf-beta3 Receptor Type I (Tbetar-I) During Rescue of Cranial Sutures from Osseous Obliteration," *Orthod Craniofac Res*, Vol. 5, 2002, pp. 5–16.

[15]   Bonewald L. F. and Mundy G. R., "Role of Transforming Growth Factor-beta in Bone Remodeling," *Clin Orthop Rel Res*, Vol. 250, 1990, pp. 261–276.

[16]   Finkelman R. D., Bell N. H., Strong D. D., Demers L. M., and Baylink D. J., "Ovariectomy Selectively Reduces the Concentration of Transforming Growth Factor Beta in Rat Bone: Implications for Estrogen Deficiency-Associated Bone Loss," *Proc Natl Acad Sci USA*, Vol. 89, 1992, pp. 12190–12193.

[17]   Finkelman R. D., Linkhart T. A., Mohan S., Lau K. H., Baylink D. J., and Bell N. H., "Vitamin D Deficiency Causes a Selective Reduction in Deposition of Transforming Growth Factor Beta in Rat Bone: Possible Mechanism for Impaired Osteoinduction," *Proc Natl Acad Sci USA*, Vol. 88, 1991, pp. 3657–3660.

[18]   Pfeilschifter J., Wolf O., Nautmann A., Minnie H. W., Mundy G. R., and Ziegler R., "Chemotactic Response of Osteoblastlike Cells to TGFβ," *J Bone Miner Res*, Vol. 5, 1990, pp. 825–830.

[19] Marra F., Bonewald L. F., Park-Snyder S., Park I. S., Woodruff K. A., and Abboud H. E., "Characterization and Regulation of the Latent Transforming Growth Factor-beta Complex Secreted by Vascular Pericytes," *J Cell Physiol*, Vol. 166, 1996, pp. 537–546.

[20] Zhao S., Dallas S. L., Peehl D., Cramer S., and Bonewald L. F., "Prostate-specific Antigen is a Potent Activator of the 100kDa Latent TGVβ," *J Bone Miner Res*, Vol. 12, 1997, p. S397.

[21] Kim S. J., Glick A., Sporn M. B., and Roberts A. B., "Characterization of the Promoter Region of the Human Transforming Growth Factor-beta 1 Gene," *J Biol Chem*, Vol. 264, 1989, pp. 402–408.

[22] Malipiero U., Holler M., Werner U., and Fontana A., "Sequence Analysis of the Promoter Region of the Glioblastoma Derived T Cell Suppressor Factor/Transforming Growth Factor (TGF)-beta 2 Gene Reveals Striking Differences to the TGF-beta 1 and -beta 3 Genes," *Biochem Biophys Res Commun*, Vol. 171, 1990, pp. 1145–1151.

[23] Lafyatis R., Lechleider R., Kim S. J., Jakowlew S., Roberts A. B., and Sporn M. B., "Structural and Functional Characterization of the Transforming Growth Factor Beta 3 Promoter. A cAMP-responsive Element Regulates Basal and Induced Transcription," *J Biol Chem*, Vol. 265, 1990, pp. 19128–19136.

[24] Joyce M. E., Jingushi S., and Bolander M. E., "Transforming Growth Factor-beta in the Regulation of Fracture Repair," *Orthop Clin North Am*, Vol. 21, 1990, pp.199–209.

[25] Hock J. M., "Transforming Growth Factor-beta Stimulates Bone Matrix Apposition and Bone Cell Replication in Cultured Fetal Rat Calvariae," *Endocrinology*, Vol. 126, 1990, pp. 421–426.

[26] Joyce M. E., "Transforming Growth Factor-beta and the Initiation of Chondrogenesis and Osteogenesis in the Rat Femur," *J Cell Biol*, Vol. 110, 1990, pp. 2195–2207.

[27] Lind M., Schumacker B., Soballe K., Keller J., Melsen F., and Bunger C., "Transforming Growth Factor-beta Enhances Fracture Healing in Rabbit Tibiae," *Acta Orthop Scand*, Vol. 64, 1993, pp. 553–556.

[28] Nielsen H. M., Andreassen T. T., Ledet T., and Oxlund H., "Local Injection of TGF-beta Increases the Strength of Tibial Fracture Healing in Rabbit Tibiae," *Acta Orthop Scand*, Vol. 65, 1994, pp. 37–41.

[29] Critchlow M. A., Bland Y. S., and Ashhurst D. E., "The Effect of Exogenous Transforming Growth Factor-beta 2 on Healing Fractures in the Rabbit," *Bone*, Vol. 16, 1995, pp. 521–527.

[30] Rosen V. and Wozney J. M., "Bone Morphogenetic Proteins," *Principles of Bone Biology*, 2nd ed., Academic Press, San Diego, CA, 2002, pp. 919–928.

[31] Miyazono K., "Bone Morphogenetic Protein Receptors and Actions," *Principles of Bone Biology*, 2nd ed., Academic Press, San Diego, CA, 2002, pp. 929–942.

[32] Israel D. I., Nove J., Kerns K. M., et al., "Heterodimeric Bone Morphogenetic Protein-2 in Chinese Hamster Ovary Cells," *Growth Factors*, Vol. 7, 1992, pp. 139–150.

[33] Boden S. D., Hair G., Titus L., et al., "Glucocorticoid-induced Differentiation of Fetal Rat Calvarial Osteoblasts Is Mediated by Bone Morphogenetic Protein-6, *Endocrinology*, Vol. 137, 1996, pp. 3401–3407.

[34] Zlotolow D. A., Vaccaro A. R., Salamon M. L., and Albert T. J., "The Role of Human Bone Morphogenetic Proteins in Spinal Fusion," *J Am Acad Ortho Surg*, Vol. 8, 2000, pp. 3–9.

[35] Boden S. D., Zdeblick T. A., Sandhu H. S., and Heim S. E., "The Use of rhBMP-2 in Interbody Fusion Cages. Definitive Evidence of Osteoinduction in Humans: A Preliminary Report," *Spine*, Vol. 25, 2000, pp. 376–381.

[36] Sheehan J. P., Kallmes D. F., Sheehan J. M., et al., "Molecular Methods of Enhancing Lumbar Spine Fusion," *Neurosurgery*, Vol. 39, 1996, pp. 548–554.

[37] Fischgrund J. S., James S. B., Chabot M. C., et al., "Augmentation of Autograft Sing rhBMP-2 and Different Carrier Media in the Canine Spinal Fusion Model," *J Spinal Disord*, Vol. 10, 1997, pp. 467–472.

[38] Boden S. D., Titus L., Hair G., Lui Y., Viggeswarapu M., Nanes M. S., et al., "Lumbar Spine Fusion by Local Gene Therapy with a cDNA Encoding a Novel Osteoinductive Protein (LMP-1)," *Spine 1*, Vol. 23, 1998, pp. 2486–2492.

[39] Okubo Y., Bessho K., Fujimura K., Iizuka T., and Miyatake S. I., "In Vitro and In Vivo Studies of a Bone Morphogenetic Protein-2 Expressing Adenoviral Vector," *J Bone Joint Surg Am*, Vol. 83, Suppl 1 (Pt 2), 2001, pp. S99–S104.

[40] Partridge K., Yang X., Clarke N. M., Okubo Y., Bessho K., Sebald W., et al., "Adenoviral BMP-2 Gene Transfer in Mesenchymal Stem Cells: In Vitro and In Vivo Bone Formation on Biodegradable Polymer Scaffolds," *Biochem Biophys Res Commun*, Vol. 292, 2002, pp. 144–152.

[41] Okubo Y., Bessho K., Fujimura K., Kaihara S., Iizuka T., and Miyatake S., "The Time Course Study of Osteoinduction by Bone Morphogenetic Protein-2 via Adenoviral Vector," *Life Sci*, Vol. 70, 2001, pp. 325–336.

[42] Turgeman G., Pittman D. D., Muller R., Kurkalli B. G., Zhou S., Pelled G., et al., "Engineered Human Mesenchymal Stem Cells: A Novel Platform for Skeletal Cell Mediated Gene Therapy," *J Gene Med*, Vol. 3, 2001, pp. 240–251.

[43] Friedlaender G. E., "OP-1 Clinical Studies," *J Bone Joint Surg Am*, Vol. 83, Suppl 1(Pt 2), 2001, pp. S160–S161.

[44] Geesink R. G., Hoefnagels N. H., and Bulstra S. K., "Osteogenic Activity of OP-1 Bone Morphogenetic Protein (BMP-7) in a Human Fibular Defect," *J Bone Joint Surg Br*, Vol. 81, 1999, pp. 710–718.

[45] Salkeld S. L., Patron L. P., Barrack R. L., and Cook S. D., "The Effect of Osteogenic Protein –1 on the Healing of Segmental Bone Defects Treated with Autograft or Allograft Bone," *J Bone Joint Surg*, Vol. 83, 2001, pp. 803–816.

[46] Alden R. D., Pittman D. D., Beres E. J., Hankins G. R., Kallmes D. F., Wisotsky B. M., et al., "Percutaneous Spinal Fusion Using Bone Morphogenetic Protein-2 Gene Therapy," *J Neurosurg*, Vol. 90, 1999, pp. 109–114.

[47] Baltzer A. W., Lattermann C., Whalen J. D., Wooley P., Weiss K., Grimm M., et al., "Genetic Enhancement of Fracture Repair: Healing of an Experimental Segmental Defect by Adenoviral Transfer of the BMP-2 Gene," *Gene Therapy*, Vol. 7, 2000, pp. 734–739.

[48] Franceschi R. T., Wang D., Krebsbach P. H., and Rutherford R. D., "Gene Therapy for Bone Formation: In Vitro and In Vivo Osteogenic Activity of an Adenovirus Expressing BMP7," *J Cell Biochem*, Vol. 78, 2000, pp. 476–486.

[49] Helm G. A., Alden T. D., Beres E. J., Hudson S. B., Das S., Engh J. A., et al., "Use of Bone Morphogenetic Protein-9 Gene Therapy to Induce Spinal Arthrodesis in the Rodent," *J Neurosurg*, Vol. 92, 2000, pp. 191–196.

[50] Lieberman J. R., Daluiski A., Stevenson S., Wu L., McAllister P., Lee Y. P., et al., "The Effect of Regional Gene Therapy with Bone Morphogenetic Protein-2-producing Bone-marrow Cells on the Repair of Segmental Femoral Defects in Rats," *J Bone Joint Surg Am,* Vol. 81, 1999, pp. 905–971.

[51] Lieberman J. R., Le L. Q., Wu L., Finerman G. A., Berk A., Witte O. N., et al., "Regional Gene Therapy with a BMP-2-producing Murine Stromal Cell Line Induces Heterotopic and Orthotopic Bone Formation in Rodents," *J Orthop Res*, Vol. 16, 1998, pp. 330–339.

[52] Mason J. M., Breitbart A. S., Barcia M., Porti D., Pergolizzi R. G., et al., "Cartilage and Bone Regeneration Using Gene-enhanced Tissue Engineering," *Clin Orthop Rel Res*, Vol. 379, 2000, pp. S171–S178.

[53] Hurley M. M., Marie P. J., and Florkiewicz R. Z., "Fibroblast Growth Factor (FGF) and FGF Receptor Families in Bone," *Principles of Bone Biology*, Academic Press, San Diego, CA, 2002, pp. 825–851.

[54] Bellus G. A., Gaudenz K., Zackai E. H., Clarke L. A. A., Szabo J., Francomano C. A., et al., "Identical Mutations in Three Different Fibroblast Growth Factor Receptor Genes in Autosomal Dominant Craniosynostosis Syndromes," *Nature Genet*, Vol. 14, 1996, pp. 174–176.

[55] Mundy G. R., Garrett R., Harris S., Chan J., Chen D., et al., "Stimulation of Bone Formation In Vitro and in Rodents by Statins," *Science*, 1999, pp. 1946–1949.

[56] Nakamura K., Kurokawa T., Kato T., Ozakai H., Mamada K. K., et al., "Local Application of Basic Fibroblast Growth Factor into the Bone Increases Bone Mass at the Applied Site in Rabbits," *Arch Orthop Trauma Surg*, Vol. 115, 1996, pp. 344–346.

[57] Hurley M. M., Abreu C., Gronowicz G., Kawaguchi H., and Lorenzo L. J., "Expression and Regulation of Basic Fibroblast Growth Factor mRNA Levels in Mouse Osteoblastic MC3T3-E1 Cells," *J Biol Chem,* Vol. 269, 1994, pp. 9392–9396.

[58] Scully S. P., Joyce M. E., Abidi N., and Bolander M. E., "The Use of Polymerase Chain Reaction Generated Nucleotide Sequences as Probes for Hybridization," *Mol Cell Probes*, Vol. 4, 1990, pp. 485–495.

[59] Joyce M. E., Jingushi S., and Scully S. P., "Role of Growth Factors in Fracture Healing," *Clinical and Experimental Approaches to Dermal and Epidermal Repair*, Wiley-Liss, NY, 1991, pp. 391–416.

[60] Kato T., Kawaguchi H., Hanada K., Aoyama L., Hiyama Y., Nakamura T., et al., "Single Local Injection of Recombinant Fibroblast Growth Factor-2 in a Hyaluronan Gel Accelerates Fracture Healing of Segmental Bone Defects in Rabbits," *J Orthop Res*, Vol. 16, 1998, pp. 654–659.

[61] Zellin G. and Linda A., "Effects of Recombinant Human Fibroblast Growth Factor-2 on Ostegenic Cell Populations During Orthopedic Osteogenesis In Vivo," *Bone*, Vol. 26, 2000, pp. 161–168.

[62] Radomsky M. L., Thompson A. Y., Spiro R. C., and Poser J. W., "Potential Role of Fibroblast Growth Factor in Enhancement of Fracture Healing," *Clin Orthop Rel Res*, Suppl 355, 1998, pp. S283–S293.

[63] Canalis E. and Rydziel S., "Platelet-Derived Growth Factor and the Skeleton," *Principles of Bone Biology*, 2nd ed., Academic Press, San Diego, CA, 2002, pp. 817–824.

[64] Canalis E., McCarthy T. L., and Centrella M., "Effects of Platelet-derived Growth Factor on Bone Formation In Vitro," *J Cell Physiol*, Vol. 140, 1989, pp 530–537.

[65] Heldin C. and Westermark B., "Mechanism of Action and In Vivo Role of Platelet-Derived Growth Factor," *Physiol Rev*, Vol. 79, 1999, pp.1283–1316.

[66] Mitlak B. H., Finkelman R. D., Hill E. L., Li J., Martin B., Smith T. D., et al., "The Effect of Systemically Administered PDGF-BB on the Rodent Skeleton," *J Bone Miner Res*, Vol. 11, 1996, pp. 238–247.

[67] Marden L. J., Fan R. S. P., Pierce G. F., Reddi A. H., and Hollinger J. O., "Platelet-Derived Growth Factor Inhibits Bone Regeneration Induced by Osteogenin, a Bone Morphogenetic Protein in Rat Craniotomy Defects," *J Clin Invest*, Vol. 92, 1993, pp. 2897–2905.

[68] Nash T. J., Howlett C. R., Martin C., Steele J., Johnson K. A., and Hicklin D. J., "Effect of Platelet-derived Growth Factor on Tibial Osteotomies in Rabbits," *Bone*, Vol. 15, 1994, pp. 203–208.

[69] Andrew J. G., Hoyland J., Freemont A. J., and Marsh D., "Insulin-like Growth Fracture Gene Expression in Human Fracture Callus," *Calcif Tissue Int*, Vol. 62, 1993, pp. 97–102.

[70] Bak B., Jorgensen P. H., and Andreassen T. T., "Dose Response of Growth Hormone on Fracture Healing in the Rat," *Acta Orthop Scand*, Vol. 61, 1990, pp. 54–57.

[71] Linkhart T. A., Mohan S., and Baylink D. J., "Growth Factors for Bone Growth and Repair: IGF, TGFβ and BMP," *Bone*, Vol. 19, Suppl, 1996, pp. 1S-11S.

[72] Bagi C. M., Brommage R., Deleon L., Adams S., Rosen D., and Sommer A., "Benefit of Systemically Administered rhIGF-I and rhIGF-I/IGFBP-3 on Cancellous Bone in Ovarectomized Rats," *J Bone Min Res*, Vol. 9, 1994, pp. 1301–1312.

[73] Mohan S. and Baylink D. J., "Bone Growth Factors," *Clin Orthop Rel Res*, Vol. 263, 1991, pp. 30–48.

[74] Thaller S. R., Dart A., and Tesluk H., "The Effects of Insulin-like Growth Factor-1 on Critical Size Calvarial Defects in Sprague-Dawley Rats," *Ann Plast Surg*, Vol. 31, 1993, pp. 429–433.

[75] Thaller S. R., Lee T. J., Armstrong M., Tesluk H., and Stern J. S., "Effect of Insulin-like Growth Factor Type 1 on Critical-size Defects in Diabetic Rats," *J Craniofac Surg*, Vol. 6, 1995, pp. 218–223.

[76] Carpenter J. E., Hipp J. A., Gerhart T. N., Rudman C. G., Hayes W. C., and Trippel S. B., "Failure of Growth Hormone to Alter the Biomechanics of Fracture-Healing in a Rabbit Model," *J Bone Joint Surg*, Vol. 74, 1992, pp. 359–367.

[77]   Mohan S., "IGF Binding Proteins in Bone Cell Regulation," *Growth Regul*, Vol. 3, 1993, pp. 67–70.

Bone Morphogenetic Protein (BMP) Implants as Bone Graft Substitutes—Promises and Challenges

by T. Kuber Sampath, [1] Ph.D. and A. Hari Reddi,[2] Ph.D.

INTRODUCTION

BONE MORPHOGENETIC PROTEINS (BMPS) ARE GROWTH and differentiation factors originally isolated from bone matrix based on their ability to induce new bone formation in vivo, and form a large family of proteins structurally related to TGF-βs and activins. Recombinant human BMP, when implanted with an appropriate carrier matrix at defect sites, is capable of inducing new bone formation and restoring the lost bone by initiating a cellular process that mirrors embryonic bone formation. BMP containing osteogenic devices have been shown to be efficacious for the treatment of delayed and non-union fractures of long bone and anterior inter-body fusions of the spine and have been found to be equivalent to that of autograft in prospective, randomized, controlled and multi-centered clinical trials. Recently, regulatory agencies in USA, Europe, Canada, and Australia have approved BMP-7 (OP-1™) and BMP-2 (InFuse™) containing osteogenic devices as bone graft substites for the treatment of long bone fractures and inter-body fusions in the spine. BMP is the first recombinant protein approved for orthopedic use and thus offers significant promise in the field of regenerative medicine.

HISTORICAL PERSPECTIVE

Bone has an inherent capacity to regenerate itself by repeating a cellular process that mirrors embryonic bone development (Fig. 1). It has long been known that demineralized bone matrix, when implanted in subcutaneous or intramuscular sites, initiates a cascade of cellular and molecular events, which results in the formation of new bone containing functional bone marrow elements both spatially and temporally [1,2]. Urist postulated that bone matrix contains "bone morphogenetic proteins" (BMPs), which are responsible for normal bone growth and natural bone healing [3]. The progress in identifying a BMP was initially slow due to difficulty in isolating these proteins from insoluble bone matrix and ill-defined bioassays to quantify bone-inducing activity.

[1]Orthopaedic Research Laboratory, Cell and Protein Therapeutic Division, Genzyme Corporation, Framingham, MA 01701.
[2]Center for Tissue Regeneration and Repair, Department of Orthopaedic Surgery, School of Medicine, University of California at Davis, Sacramento, CA 95817.

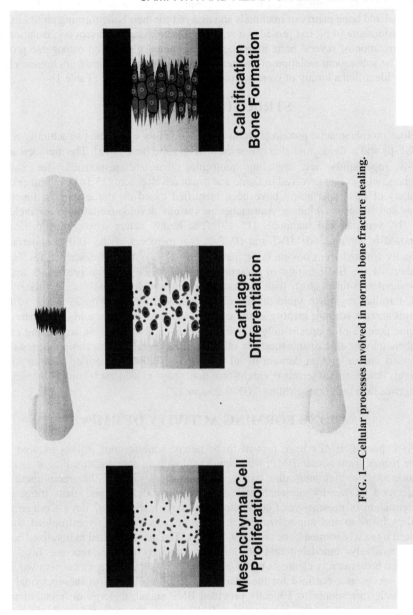

FIG. 1—Cellular processes involved in normal bone fracture healing.

Mesenchymal Cell
Proliferation

Cartilage
Differentiation

Calcification
Bone Formation

However, the demonstration that osteogenic proteins could be extracted from the demineralized bone matrix of mammals and assayed for their bone forming ability in a rat subcutaneous site [4,5], has provided a reproducible bioassay for discovery, isolation and characterization of several bone morphogenetic proteins, also called osteogenic proteins [6–8]. The subsequent isolation of the genes encoding these proteins from human cDNA libraries identified a family of bone morphogenetic proteins [9–11] (Table 1).

STRUCTURE OF A BMP

Bone morphogenetic proteins belong to a large family of proteins structurally related to TGF-βs and activins, and also called the TGF-β superfamily [12]. The members of the TGF-β superfamily are signaling molecules that are responsible for specific morphogenetic events involved in tissue and organ development [13,14]. A number of the members of this superfamily have been identified based on tissue-specific functional assays and molecular cloning approaches in various developmental systems including fruit fly, xenopus and mammals [15–19]. The highly active osteogenic proteins are composed of dimers of BMP-7 and BMP-2, two members of the TGF-β superfamily, originally isolated from bovine bone matrix (Fig. 2) [8]. As first described for TGF-β, members of the BMP family of proteins are synthesized as large precursors that are approximately 3 times larger than the mature protein and are proteolytically processed at the C-terminal region to yield mature disulfide-linked dimers (Fig. 3). Some of these proteins share a striking identity in the carboxy-terminal, which is a highly conserved 7 cysteine domain of approximately 100 amino acids (TGF-β domain), suggesting certain members may be able to substitute for others in their specific tissue morphogenesis. The processed mature protein domain of all the family members identified to date contain relatively short amino-terminal extensions that show considerably more evolutionary divergence than the corresponding TGF-β domain [20].

BONE FORMING ACTIVITY OF BMPs

As expected, BMPs have proven to be potent bone-forming agents in vivo [21]. Single recombinant human BMP, when implanted with an appropriate collagen carrier at subcutaneous or intramuscular sites in mammals, initiates the recruitment and proliferation of nearby mesenchymal stem cells by 3 days and then triggers the differentiation of mesenchymal cells into chondrocytes within 5–7 days. Concurrent to capillary invasion and mineralization, the chondrocytes become hypertrophied and are replaced by newly formed bone within 9–11 days. The newly formed mineralized bone is then extensively remodeled and becomes occupied by ossicles that are filled with functional bone marrow elements by 14–28 days (Fig. 4). The collagen carrier used in the implant serves as a scaffold for the attachment and proliferation of mesenchymal stem cells which, in response to a locally provided BMP signal, undergo differentiation into endochondral bone. In the absence of a BMP signal, the collagen implants become surrounded by fibrous tissue and are slowly resorbed. Further studies have shown that recombinant BMP alone can induce new bone formation provided responding cells and a proper microenvironment are made available; the collagen carrier that is required for optimal bone formation can be substituted with bioresorbable synthetic biopolymers and/

TABLE 1— BMP family of proteins.

BMPs	Other names	Bone Forming Potential*
BMP-1	Procollagen C proteinase (not a BMP - mistakenly named)	
BMP-2	BMP-2a	+ + + +
BMP-3	Osteogenin	
BMP-3b	GDF-10	
BMP-4	BMP-2b	+ + + + +
BMP-5		+ + +
BMP-6	Vgr-1	+ + + + +
BMP-7	OP-1	+ + + +
BMP-8	OP-2	+ +
BMP-8b	OP-3	
BMP-9	GDF-2	
BMP-10	...	
BMP-11	GDF-11	
BMP-12	GDF-7/CDMP-3	
BMP-13	GDF-6/CDMP-2	+ +
BMP-14	GDF-5/CDMP-1/MP-52	+ +
BMP-15	GDF-9b	

*Bone forming potential of specific BMP was assayed in the rat subcutaneous implant model (4).

or inert ceramic particles [22–25].

The bone morphogenetic potential of BMPs has been further confirmed by their ability to restore large segmental defects by forming normal weight-bearing bone containing functional bone marrow elements in small and larger animal models [26–31]. In these studies, a recombinant human BMP-7/OP-1 containing collagen matrix preparation (OP-1^{TM} Implant) was placed into surgically created, large diaphyseal segmental defects and the device was contained by wrapping muscle flaps over the implant material. The sites were stabilized mechanically either by intact radius in an ulna defect model or by an intramedullary rod in a mid shaft-tibial defect model (Fig. 5). The union of segmental gaps by the OP-1^{TM} Implant was monitored biweekly by radiographs and evaluated by histology and biomechanical testing after sacrifice. The results demonstrate that the quantity and the rate of bone formation depended on the concentration of BMP-7/OP-1 in the implant. Similar results have also been demonstrated using recombinant BMP-2 containing devices in various animal models [32–35]. The first recombinant BMP-7 containing osteogenic device (OP-1^{TM}) was implanted in a 23-year-old male who had an open comminuted Type II fracture of the left tibia. The patient had previously underwent treatment with autograft, intramedullary rod fixation, skin flap placement and multiple irrigation and debridements to treat an infection of his leg and was scheduled for an amputation as all treatments had failed. The OP-1 device (3.5 mg of

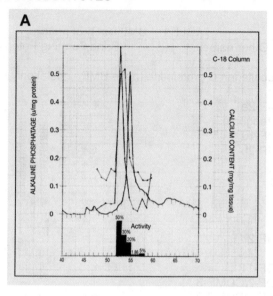

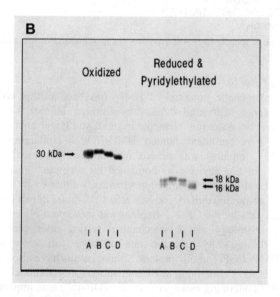

FIG. 2—The purification of native bone morphogenetic protein (BMP) from bovine bone matrix. (A) Final step in the purification of BMP involves a C_{18}-HPLC (high pressure liquid chromatography) column. Each fraction eluted was assayed for bone forming activity in the rat subcutaneous implantation model. (B) SDS gels showing the mobility of purified BMP fraction is ~ 30 kDa and is composed of an 18 kDa protein subunit (BMP-7 (OP-1)) and a 16 kDa protein subunit (BMP-2) [8].

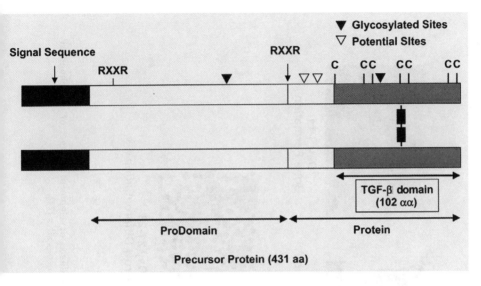

FIG. 3—Structure of a BMP (BMP-7) [21].

protein in 1 gram of Type I collagen) was implanted at his tibial non-union site and intramedullary nail fixation was performed for mechanical stability. He became pain free upon 9 months following OP-1 device implantation [36,37]. Figure 6 shows the radiographic analyses of the repair site at 6 months, 5 and 10 years following OP-1 implantation. BMP containing osteogenic devices are currently being tested in human clinical studies for acute and delayed fracture healing, periodontal repair, spinal fusion and cranio-facial augmentation and repair.

DELIVERY BIOMATERIALS FOR BMPs

The carrier plays an important biological role as a component of the BMP device in effecting new bone formation. The carriers used in the device should have certain biological properties: (1) they must be biocompatible and biodegradable, and absorbed naturally with minimal immunological and inflammatory response in vivo; (2) they must act as a delivery vehicle for the in vivo sustained release of BMP at the appropriate time and in the proper dose; (3) they must present a substratum/scaffold for migration, proliferation, and differentiation of anchorage-dependent osteoprogenitor cells (mesenchymal stem cells); and (4) should have a geometrical structure with void space sufficient to allow cellular ingrowth and scaffold resorption appropriate for its function.

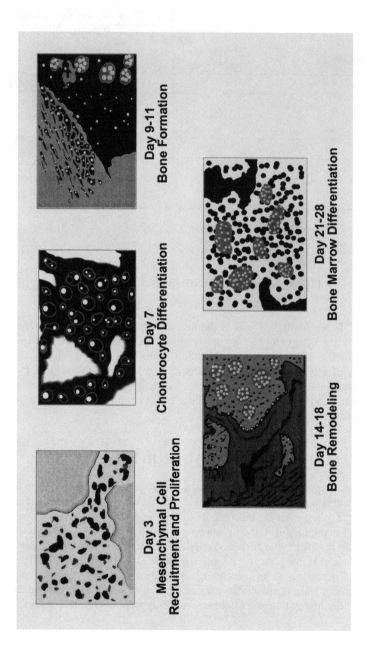

FIG. 4—Schematic representation of the recombinant BMP induced developmental stages of endochondral bone differentiation on days 3, 7, 9-11, 14-18 and 21-28 in the rat subcutaneous sites [21].

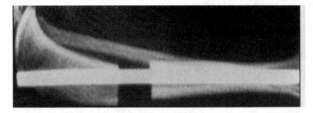

2 cm Defect in Tibia (Post-Op)

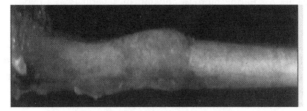

OP-1 Device (16 weeks)

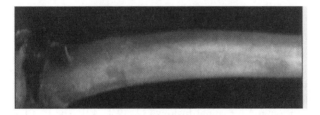

Untreated Control

FIG. 5—Bone regeneration in segmental defect by BMP-7/collagen device (OP-1) in nonhuman primates [28].

Several carriers and delivery systems have been used to deliver BMP in preclinical and clinical studies to effect osteogenesis. They include, Type I collagen (prepared from bovine bone, tendon and skin), mineral (hydroxyapatite, tricalcium phosphate, coral and cements), synthetic polymers (polylactide and polyglycolide, hydrogels), extracellular matrix components (hyaluronic acid, glycosaminoglycans, fibrin), and bone graft materials (autograft and allograft). Type I collagen is currently a preferred carrier for BMP as it is a natural component of bone and undergoes resorption comparable to that of extracellular matrix components and is considered a "gold standard" for comparison [21].

The BMP devices used in clinical trials have all employed Type I collagen [38,39]. A fibril acid soluble Type I collagen prepared from bovine Achilles tendon has been used to deliver BMP-2 (also called InFuse[TM]). Bovine diaphyseal bone derived particulate Type I collagen has been used to deliver BMP-7 (also called OP-1[TM]) [21,37]. The next preferred carrier for BMP is mineral, which is the major component of bone. Studies using hydroxyapatite and BMP-2 or BMP-7/OP-1 are being evaluated currently in preclinical and clinical studies. The use of some synthetic polymers as carriers to deliver BMP and affect osteogenesis has been demonstrated in experimental animal models.

Although Type I collagen has been used successfully as a carrier for BMPs to effect osteogenesis, the amount of protein used in the device is a lot more than the amount of BMPs available naturally at the fracture site. Since bone formation is a biological cascade of mesenchymal cell recruitment, proliferation and differentiation, it is likely that BMP in combination with specific peptide growth factors may be more effective in inducing optimal bone formation. Furthermore, a cocktail of several BMPs may likely be more efficacious than a single BMP as it has been shown that more than one BMP is expressed at the fracture site at various times and at different levels.

Recent studies have used formulations that suspend recombinant BMPs without solid-phase matrices. In experimental animal models they are administered locally at the fracture site to speed up the natural repair process. Upon fracture, the newly formed callus could be used as a scaffold and BMP could be injected into the callus in suspension at a lower temperature and precipitated under physiological temperature. A wide variety of biomaterials to facilitate this type of delivery must be developed in the future.

BMP CLINICAL STUDIES

Preclinical testing has demonstrated that BMPs are potent bone forming agents and can restore lost bone in a variety of orthopedic defects. The native BMP preparations prepared from adult donor bone have been used to restore large bone defects in humans [40]. Several clinical trials have been conducted to assess the efficacy of recombinant BMP containing devices in the treatment of diaphyseal segmental bone defects, tibial nonunions, delayed union and for spinal fusions [37–39,41,42]. The first human clinical study was performed to assess the efficacy of recombinant human BMP-7 (OP-1) for the treatment of tibial nonunions in a prospective, randomized and controlled clinical trail involving 122 patients with 124 tibial nonunions in 17 centers within United States [37]. The OP-1 device composed of approximately 3.5 mg of recombinant BMP-7 was dispersed with one gram of bone Type I collagen and lyophilized in a vial. The device was sterilized through radiation using 2.5 MRAD. The treatment consisted of intramedullary nail fixation for mechanical stability and implantation of either the OP-1 device (61 patients) or autologous iliac bone graft (61 patients). The conclusion of this clinical study demonstrated that OP-1 implant was a safe and effective treatment modality for tibial nonunion, and the outcome was comparable to the use of bone autograft. Furthermore, the OP-1 device demonstrated advantages over autograft bone, including a reduction in the amount of operative blood loss, decreased incidence of osteomyelitis at the surgical site, elimination of donor site complications and pain as well as a decrease in the use of post-operative pain medication.

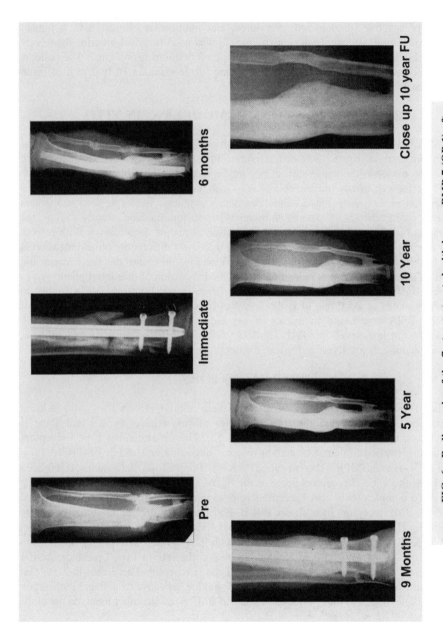

FIG. 6—Radiographs of the first man treated with human BMP 7 (OP-1) after having sustained a closed comminuted tibial fracture in a motor-vehicle accident. Prior to this he had 2 autograft failures and 1 plate failure [36,37].

In a prospective, randomized, controlled, and multicenter clinical trial, a human BMP-2 containing osteogenic device (InFuse™) was used to affect anterior inter-body fusion of lumbar vertebrae with the use of a tapered titanium fusion cage. The patients were treated with a cage filled with either 10 mg of recombinant BMP-2 in a collagen carrier or with autologous bone graft [38,39].

Bmps AFFECTS BONE REMODELING IN VIVO

BMPs have been shown to stimulate the migration and proliferation of osteoblast progenitors, and to trigger their differentiation into the osteoblast lineage [21,43–45]. BMPs also maintain the expression of phenotype of mature osteoblasts in cultures [21, 45]. The effects of BMP-7 on osteoblasts vary with their stage of differentiation (induces proliferation in early osteoblasts, stimulates matrix synthesis and expression of markers that are characteristic of osteoblast phenotype at intermediate stages during the maturation process, and increases nodule formation in mature osteoblasts). With respect to bone resorption, BMP-7 appears to modulate osteoclast differentiation and maturation [46]. Given that BMP-7 induces new bone formation, promotes the recruitment and growth of osteoblast progenitors, and maintains the expression of osteoblast phenotype in cultures, BMP-7 may be centrally involved in overall bone homeostasis. In studies to identify the sites of synthesis of BMP-7 in post-fetal life analysis, the highest level of BMP-7 mRNA was found in tissues of the kidneys and urogenital system [47,48]. Detectable, but low, levels of BMP-7 mRNA were also seen in the brain and calvaria, whereas the lung, heart, liver, and spleen did not present detectable levels.

BMP RECEPTORS

Like TGF-β, all members of BMP elicit their cellular effects by ligand induced association of specific heterodimeric complexes of two related Type I and Type II serine/threonine kinase receptors (Table 2) [49–52]. Three mammalian Type I receptors have been identified to date, i.e., activin receptor-like kinase (ALK)-2, BMPR-1A (also called ALK-3) and BMPR-1B (also called ALK-6). For TGF-βs and activins, it has been shown that the Type II receptors serve as the ligand recognition and binding site, which then form a complex with Type I receptors prior to initiating signal transduction. Original studies on BMP receptors have shown that BMP-7 and BMP-4 can bind directly to Type I receptors, BMPR-1A (ALK-3), and BMPR-1B (ALK-6) in the presence of DAF-4, a BMP Type II receptor from *C.elegans*. Although TGF-βs and activins do not bind to BMPRs and DAF-4, BMP-7 is also shown to bind to the activin Type I receptor, ActR-I in the presence of DAF-4 or ActR-II, activin Type II receptor. These data indicate that BMP-7 and activin have overlapping receptor-binding specificity and exhibit certain common biological activities [49,50]. BMP-2 and BMP-4, on the other hand, do not bind

TABLE 2— Cell Surface Receptor for BMP family proteins.

Ligand	Type I Receptor	Type II Receptor
BMP-2 and BMP-4	BMPR-IA /ALK-3, BMPR-IB /ALK-6 BMPR-IA /ALK-3	BMPR-II
BMP-6 and BMP-7/ OP-1	ActR-I /ALK-2 BMPR-IA/ALK-3, BMPR-IB/ALK-6	BMPR-II, ActR-II, ActR-IIB

to activin receptors. Three different Type II receptors have been implicated in BMP signaling: BMPR-II, and the activin Type II receptors, ActR-II and ActR-IIB. The binding affinities of ActR-II/IIB are lower than those for activin. These findings imply that proteins in the TGF-β superfamily may have broader biological function than previously contemplated [51,52].

Both Type I and Type II receptors are required for BMP signaling (Fig. 7). BMPs bind with weak affinity to either a Type I or Type II receptor alone and with high affinity to heterodimeric complexes of the two receptors types. Upon BMP-induced heterodimeric complex formation, the constitutively active Type II receptor kinase phosphorylates a Type I receptor and subsequently activates intracellular signaling by phosphorylating down stream components, including nuclear effector proteins known as Smads [53,54]. Smads can be divided into three distinct subclasses: signal transducing receptor regulated Smads (R-Smads, i.e., Smad1, Smad5 and Smad8) and common mediator Smads (C-Smads, i.e., Smad4) and inhibitory Smads (I-Smads, i.e., Smad6 and Smad7) [55].

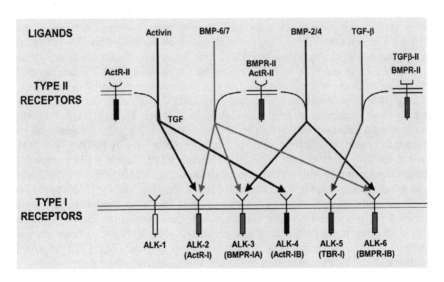

FIG. 7—Schematic illustration of binding of BMPs, TGF-β and activin to Type I and Type II receptors [52].

Upon BMP receptor activation, BMPR-Smad1/5/8 forms heterodimeric complexes with C-Smad4 and then translocates to the nucleus. Within the nucleus, R-Smad/C-Smad complexes act directly and/or in cooperation with other transcription factors, to regulate transcription of target genes. Inhibitory Smad6/7 specifically inhibits BMP and TGF-β signaling thus a negative regulation is controlled to keep the activation in balance.

Bmps BEYOND BONE

Tissue morphogenesis in the developing embryo occurs as a result of a reciprocal interaction between a thin layer of epithelium and a condensed mass of mesenchyme [13, 56,57]. Such an inductive event gradually culminates in the migration, proliferation, differentiation and apoptosis of responding cells at various developmental stages leading to a process of budding morphogenesis as observed in limbs, branchial arches, genitalia and feathers or branching morphogenesis as observed in mammary and salivary glands, lungs and kidney. There is a growing body of evidence to suggest that the cellular processes involved in tissue morphogenesis are induced by secreted proteins of conserved multigene families in particular *fgfs, bmps, hedgehogs, wnts,* and *egfs.*

Although BMPs are expressed at the earliest stages of skeletal development and are required for formation of specific skeletal structure, high levels of mRNA transcripts for BMPs are observed in several extra skeletal organs during embryogenesis, suggesting BMPs may play a morphogenic role in tissues beyond bone. These organs include the myogenic layer of the atrioventricular cushions of the developing heart, developing hair and whisker follicles, tooth buds, developing central nervous system, branching organs including mammary and salivary glands, lung and kidney, craniofacial tissue and reproductive organs, ovary, and testis. Loss of function studies have shown that while there is an apparent redundancy among BMPs with respect to bone formation, specific BMPs are required for a specific organ development during embryonic growth and tissue morphogenesis. For example, loss of BMP-2 function in mice displays a defective cardiac morphogenesis and amniotic fold closure [58] and in contrast BMP-7 mutant mice die at birth due to defective kidney and eye [59–61]. Targeted mutation of the murine genes encoding BMP-4 (a closely related member of BMP-2) results in defects in mesoderm formation and patterning during gastrulation [62]. Mice lacking BMP-5 or BMP-6 (closely related members of BMP-7) on the other hand, are viable and fertile and show perturbance in certain selective skeletal structure, short ears in BMP-5 (-/-) [63] and sternal defects in BMP-6 (-/-) mice [64]. Double BMP mutant studies among some members demonstrate additional uncovered defects (e.g., BMP-5/GDF-6; BMP-5/BMP-7) and in other cases display exacerbation of the defect (e.g., BMP-5/BMP-6) [65,66]. In accordance with these findings, BMPs have been shown to induce cardiac myocyte differentiation [67] inhibit vascular smooth muscle proliferation in vitro [68], and reduce intima thickening in rat baloon angioplastic models [69]. BMPs have been observed in ovaries as a putative leutinizing factor for the action of FSH [70]. Biochemical, histochemical and functional studies indicate that in addition to their morphogenic role in the musculoskeletel system, BMPs serve as mediators of overall tissue development during embryogenesis, suggesting BMPs may have therapeutic utility beyond bone in post-natal life.

PROMISES AND CHALLENGES

Demineralized bone matrix (DBM) has been widely used as a bone graft substitute to induce new bone formation during reconstructive surgery as it supports both osteoinduction and osteooconduction properties. Demineralized bone matrix is composed of predominantly Type I collagen (95%). The remaining non-collagenous proteins include small amounts of growth factors and naturally occurring bone morphogenetic proteins. The osteoinductive property of DBM has been attributed to BMPs that are present within the matrix. BMPs are an evolutionarily conserved family of proteins from *Drosophila* to Man. The human equivalent of BMP-2, *DPP* and BMP-7, *60A* proteins have been shown to induce bone in mammals when implanted with an appropriate carrier, indicating the biological activity of BMPs is dictated by the microenvironment and the responding cells [71].

Local bone formation induced by the demineralized matrix of bone serves as a prototype for tissue engineering, in that the collagenous matrix acts as a substratum for migration and proliferation of mesenchymal cells and morphogenetic proteins resided within the bone matrix to signal the differentiation of mesenchymal cells into endochondral bone (Fig. 8). Thus, this biological principle of bone formation enable us to identify a family of BMPs, which then led to the development of therapeutic osteogenic devices for use in the repair and regeneration of bone. The availability of human BMP in an unlimited quantity through recombinant technology has now made it possible to evaluate its clinical utility for bone repair in various indications, including normal, delayed and non-union fractures. No doubt, our future generation will have the benefit of using off-the shelf recombinant BMP devices instead of harvesting iliac crest bone and thus avoiding associated donor site morbidity.

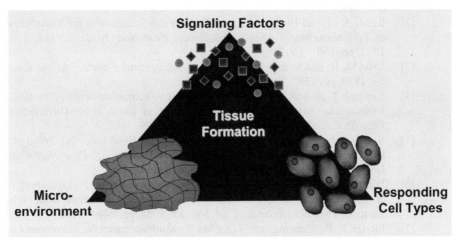

FIG. 8—Biology of tissue engineering.

Although BMP devices offer tremendous promises as bone graft substitutes, there are still numerous challenges we are faced with. The current BMP devices—though they can induce bone readily—do not impart mechanical stability of the graft during the procedure. There is a need for optimal delivery systems for BMPs with varying geometry and resorptive times depending on location and mechanical loading of the defects. The handling properties of the device are also important as is the surgical approximation and retention of the BMP device at the site of repair. Because the availability of vascular components and responding cells along with the mechanical stability at the repair site determine the efficacy of BMP-induced bone formation, efforts should be taken to provide appropriate microenvironments during the procedure. Furthermore, internal and/or external fixation has to be modernized according to the rate of osteogenesis induced by BMP devices.

Recombinant BMP containing osteogenic devices are currently very expensive and faced with reimbursement issues for their wider usage. In the future, autologous bone marrow derived mesenchymal cells could be engineered in the surgical suite to deliver the BMP via ex vivo gene therapy with an appropriate carrier matrix to induce new bone formation [72]. Such a therapy would be very cost effective as compared to the use of recombinant protein. The "cell-gene-matrix" device exploits the donor site to make the protein for a period of time sufficient enough to induce the differentiation of adjacent mesenchymal stem cells from bone marrow, periosteum and muscle into bone and restore function.

Acknowledgments

We thank our colleagues from all over the world with whom we have had an opportunity to collaborate on BMPs.

REFERENCES

[1]   Urist M. R., "Bone Formation by Autoinduction," *Science,* Vol. 150, 1965, pp. 893–899.

[2]   Reddi A. H. and Huggins C. B., "Biochemical Sequence in the Transformation of Fibroblasts into Cartilage and Bone," *Proc Natl Acad Sci USA,* Vol. 69, 1972, pp. 1601–1605.

[3]   Urist M. R. and Strates B. S., "Bone Morphogenetic Protein," *J Dent Res,* Vol. 50, 1970, pp. 1392–1406.

[4]   Sampath T. K. and Reddi A. H., "Dissociative Extraction and Reconstitution of Extracellular Matrix Components Involved in Local Bone Differentiation," *Proc Natl Acad Sci USA,* Vol. 78, 1981, pp. 7599–7602.

[5]   Sampath T. K. and Reddi A. H., "Homology of Bone Inductive Proteins from Human, Monkey, Bovine and Rat Extracellular Matrix," *Proc Natl Acad Sci USA,* Vol. 80, 1983, pp. 6591–6595.

[6]   Wang E. A., Rosen V., Cordes P., Hewich R. M., Kriz, M. F., Luxenberg D. P., et al., "Purification and Characterization of Other Distinct Bone-inducing Factors," *Proc Natl Acad Sci USA,* Vol. 85, 1988, pp. 9484–9488.

[7]   Luyten F. P., Cunningham N. S., Ma S., Muthukumaran N., Hammonds R. G., Nevins W. B., et al., "Purification and Partial Amino Acid Sequence of Osteogenin, a Protein Initiating Bone Differentiation," *J Biol Chem,* Vol. 264, 1989, pp. 13377–13380.

[8]   Sampath T. K., Coughlin J. E., Whetstone R. M., Banach D., Corbett C., Ridge R. J., et al., "Bovine Osteogenic Protein is Composed of Dimers of OP-1 and BMP-2A, Two Members of the Transforming Growth Factor-β Superfamily," *J Biol Chem,* Vol. 265, 1990, pp. 13198–13205.

[9]   Wozney J. M., Rosen V., Celeste A. J., Mitsock L. M., Kriz R. W., Hewick R. M., et al., "Novel Regulators of Bone Formation: Molecular clones and activities," *Science,* Vol. 242, 1988, pp. 1528–1534.

[10]   Ozkaynak E., Rueger D. C., Drier E. A., Corbett C., Ridge, R. J., Sampath T. K., et al., "OP-1 cDNA Clones, an Osteogenic Protein in the TGF-β Family," *Eur Mol Biol Organ J,* Vol. 9, 1990, pp. 2085–2093.

[11]   Celeste A. J., Lannazzi J. A., Taylor R. C., Hewick R. M., Rosen V., Wang, E. A., et al., "Identification of Transforming Growth Factor-β Superfamily Presents in Bone Inductive Protein Purified from Bovine Bone," *Proc Natl Acad Sci USA,* Vol. 87, 1990, pp. 9843–9847.

[12]   Massague J., "The Transforming Growth Factor-β Family," *Ann Rev Cell Biol,* Vol. 6, 1990, pp. 597–641.

[13]   Hogan B. L., "Bone Morphogenetic Proteins in Development," *Curr Opin Genet Dev,* Vol. 6, 1996, pp. 432–438.

[14]   Reddi A. H., "Role of Morphogenetic Proteins in Skeletal Tissue Engineering and Regeneration," *Nat Biotechnol,* Vol. 16, 1998, pp. 247–252.

[15]   Padget R. W., St Johnson R. D., and Gelbart W. M., "A Transcript from a Drosophila Pattern Gene Predicts a Protein Homologous to the Transforming Factor-β Family," *Nature,* Vol. 325, 1987, pp. 81–84.

[16]   Wharton K. A., Thomsen G. H., and Gelbart W. M., "Drosophila 60A Gene, Another Transforming Growth Factor β Family Member, is Closely Related to Human Bone Morphogenetic Proteins," *Proc Natl Acad Sci USA,* Vol. 88, 1991, pp. 9214–9218.

[17]   Weeks D. L. and Melton, D. A., "A Maternal mRNA Localized to the Vegetal Hemisphere in Xenopus Eggs Codes for a Growth Factor Related to TGF-β," *Cell,* Vol. 51, 1987, pp. 861–867.

[18]   Jones C. M., Lyons K. M., Lapan P. M., Wright C. V. E., and Hogan B. L. M., "DVR-4 (bone morphogenetic protein-4) as a Posterior-ventralizing Factor in Xenopus Mesoderm Induction," *Development,* Vol. 115, 1992, pp. 639–647.

[19]   Martinovic S., Borovecki F., Sampath T. K., and Vukicevic S. "Biology of Bone Morphogenetic Proteins," *Bone Morphogenetic Proteins: From Laboratory to Clinical Practice* S. Vukicevic and T. Kuber Sampath, Eds., Birkhauser Verlag Basel/Switzerland, 2002.

[20]   Sampath T. K. and Rueger D. C., "Structure, Function and Orthopedic Application of Osteogenic Protein-1 (OP-1)," *Complications in Orthopedics,* Vol. 9, 1994, pp. 101–107.

[21]   Sampath T. K., Maliakal J. C., Hauschka P. V., Jones W. K., Sasak H., Tucker R. F., et al., "Recombinant Human Osteogenic Protein-1 (hOP-1) Induces New Bone Formation In Vivo with a Specific Activity Comparable with Natural Bovine Osteogenic Protein and Stimulates Osteoblast Proliferation and Differentiation In Vitro," *J Biol Chem,* Vol. 267, 1992, pp. 20352–20362.

[22] Behravesh E., Yasko A. W., Engel P. S., and Mikos A. G., "Synthetic Biodegradable Polymers for Orthopedic Applications," *Clin Orthop Rel Res,* Vol. 367, 1999, pp. S118–129.

[23] Salkeld S., Cook S. D., and Rueger D. C., "Synthetic Polymers as Carriers for Osteogenic Proteins," Abstract, *Transactions of the 21st Annual Meeting of the Society for Biomaterials and 27th International Biomaterials Symposium,* San Francisco, CA, 1995.

[24] Ripamonti U., Ma S., and Reddi A. H., "The Critical Role of Geometry of Porous Hydroxyapatite Delivery System in Induction of Bone by Osteogenin, a Bone Morphogenetic Protein," *Matrix,* Vol. 12, 1992, pp. 202–212.

[25] Hollinger J. O. and Leong K., "Poly(alpha-hydroxy acids): Carriers for bone morphogenetic proteins," *Biomaterials,* Vol. 17, 1996, pp. 187–194.

[26] Cook S. D., Baffes G., Wolfe M., Sampath T. K., Rueger D. C., and Whitecloud T., "The Effect of Recombinant Osteogenic Protein-1 on Healing of Large Segmental Bone Defects," *J Bone Joint Surg Am,* Vol. 76, 1994, pp. 27–28.

[27] Cook S. D., Baffes G., Wolfe M., Sampath T. K., and Rueger D. C., "Recombinant Human Bone Morphogenetic Protein-7 Induces Healing in a Canine Long Bone Segmental Defect Model," *Clin Orthop Rel Res,* Vol. 301, 1994, pp. 302–312.

[28] Cook S. D., Wolfe M., Salkeld S., and Rueger D., "Recombinant Human Osteogenic Protein-1 (rhOP-1) Heals Segmental Defects in Nonhuman Primates," *J Bone Joint Surg Am,* Vol. 77, 1995, pp. 734–750.

[29] Grauer J., Patel T., Erulkar J., Troiano N., Panjabi M., and Friedlander G., "Evaluation of OP-1 as a Bone Graft Substitute for Inter-transverse Process Lumbar Fusion," *Spine,* Vol. 26, 2001, pp. 127–133.

[30] Cook S. D. and Rueger D. C., "Preclinical Models of Recombinant BMP Induced Healing of Orthopedic Defects," *Bone Morphogenetic Proteins: From Laboratory to Clinical Practice,* S. Vukicevic and T. Kuber Sampath, Eds., Birkhauser Verlag Basel/Switzerland, 2002.

[31] Salkeld S., Patron L., Barrack R., and Cook S. D., "The Effect of Osteogenic Protein-1(OP-1:BMP-7) on the Healing of Segmental Defects Treated with Autograft or Allograft Bone," *J Bone Joint Surg Am,* Vol. 83, 2001, pp. 803–816.

[32] Yasko A., Lane J., Fellinger E., Rosen V., Wozney J., and Wang E., "The Healing of Segmental Defects Induced by Recombinant Human Morphogenetic Protein (rhBMP-2)," *J Bone Joint Surg Am,* Vol. 74, 1992, pp. 59–671.

[33] Gerhart T., Kirker-Head C., and Kriz M., "Healing Segmental Defects in Sheep Using Recombinant Human Bone Morphogenetic Protein," *Clin Orthop Rel Res,* Vol. 293, 1993, pp. 317–326

[34] Boden S., Moskovitz P., Morone M., and Toribitake Y., "Video-assisted Lateral Inter-trasverse Process Arthrodesis: Validation of a new minimally invasive lumbar spinal fusion technique in the rabbit and nonhuman primate (rhesus) models," *Spine,* Vol. 21, 1996, pp. 2689–2697.

[35] Santhu H., Kanim L., Kabo M., Toth J., Zeegen E., Liu D., et al., "Effective Doses of Recombinant Human Bone Morphogenetic Protein-2 in Experimental Spinal Fusion," *Spine*, Vol. 21, 1996, pp. 2115–2122.

[36] Cook S. D., "Preclinical and Clinical Evaluation of Osteogenic Protein-1 (BMP-7) in Bony Sites," *Orthopedics*, Vol. 22, 1999, pp. 669–671.

[37] Friedlaender G. E., Perry C. R., Cole J. D., Cook S. D., Clerny G., Muschler G. F., et al., "Osteogenic Protein-1 (bone morphogenetic protein-7) in the Treatment of Tibial Nonunions: A prospective randomized clinical trial comparing rhOP-1 with fresh bone autograft," *J Bone Joint Surg Am*, Vol. 83, Suppl 1, 2001, pp. S151–158.

[38] Wozney J. M., "Overview of Bone Morphogenetic Proteins," *Spine*, Vol. 73, 2002, pp. 1020–1209.

[39] Uludag U. M., Gao T., Porter T. J., Friess W., and Wozney J. M., "Delivery Systems for BMPs: Factors contributing to protein retention at an application site," *J Bone Joint Surg Am*, Vol. 83, 2001, pp. S128–135.

[40] Gao T., Lindholm T. S., Martinnen A., and Urist M. R. "Composites of Bone Morphogenetic Protein (BMP) and Type IV Collagen, Coral-derived Hydroxyapatite and Tricalcium Phosphate Ceramics," *Int Orthop*, Vol. 20, 1996, pp. 321–325.

[41] Johnson E. E., Urist M. R., and Finerman G. A., "Repairs of Segmental Defects of the Tibia with Cancellous Bone Grafts Augmented with Human Bone Morphogenetic Protein. A Preliminary Report," *Clin Orthop Rel Res*, Vol. 236, 1988, pp. 257–265.

[42] Geesink R. G., Hoefnagels N. H., and Bulstra S. K., "Osteogenic Activity of OP-1 Bone Morphogenetic Protein (BMP-7) in a Human Fibular Defect," *J Bone Joint Surg Br*, Vol. 81, 1999, pp. 710–718.

[43] Vukicevic S., Luyten F. P., and Reddi A. H., "Stimulation of the Expression of Osteogenic and Chondrogenic Phenotypes in Vitro by Osteogenin," *Proc Natl Acad Sci*, Vol. 86, 1989, pp. 8793–8797.

[44] Knutsen R., Wergedal J. E., Sampath T. K., Baylink D. J., and Mohan S., "Osteogenic Protein-1 Stimulates Proliferation and Differentiation of Human Bone Cells in Vitro," *Biochem Biophys Res Commun*, Vol. 194, 1993, pp. 1352–1358.

[45] Maliakal J. C., Asahina I., Hauscha P. V., and Sampath T. K., "Osteogenic Protein-1 (BMP-7) Inhibits Cell Proliferation and Stimulates the Expression of Markers Characteristic of Osteoblast PhenoType In Rat Osteosarcoma (17/2.8) Cells," *Growth Factors*, Vol. 11, 1994, pp. 227–234.

[46] Hentunen T. A., Lakkakorpi P. T., Tuukkanen J., Lehenkari P. P., Sampath T. K., and Väänänen H. K., "Effects of Recombinant Human Osteogenic Protein-1 on the Differentiation of Osteoclast-like Cells and Bone Resorption," *Biochem Biophys Res Commun*, Vol. 209, 1995, pp. 433–443.

[47] Ozkaynak E., Schnegelsberg P. N. J., and Oppermann H., "Murine Osteogenic Protein (OP-1): High levels of mRNA in kidney," *Biochem Biophys Res Commun*, Vol. 179, 1991, pp. 116–123.

[48] Ozkaynak E., Schnegelsberg P. N. J., Jin D. F., Clifford G. M., Warren F. D., Drier E. A., and Oppermann H., "Osteogenic Protein-2: A new member of the

transforming growth factor-β superfamily expressed early in embryogenesis," *J Biol Chem,* Vol. 267, 1992, pp. 25220–25227.

[49]　Ten Dijke P., Yamashita H., Sampath T. K., Reddi A. H., Estevez M., Riddle D. L., et al., "Identification of Type I Receptors for Osteogenic Protein-1 and Bone Morphogenetic Protein-4," *J Biol Chem,* Vol. 269, 1994, pp. 16985–16988.

[50]　Yamashita H., Ten Dijke P., Huylebroeck D., Sampath T. K, Andries M., Smith J. C., et al., "Osteogenic Protein-1 Binds to Activin Type II Receptors and Induces Certain Activin-like Effects," *J Cell Biol,* Vol. 130, 1995, pp. 217–226.

[51]　Massagué J., "TGF-β Signal Transduction," *Ann Rev Biochem,* Vol. 67, 1998, pp. 753–791.

[52]　Heldin C-H., Miyazono K., and Ten Dijke P., "TGF-β Signaling from Cell Membrane to Nucleus Via Smad Proteins," *Nature,* Vol. 390, 1997, pp. 465–471.

[53]　Macías-Silva M., Hoodless P. A., Tang S. J., Buchwald M., and Wrana J. L., "Specific Activation of Smad1 Signaling Pathways by the BMP7 Type I Receptor, ALK2," *J Biol Chem,* Vol. 273, 1998, pp. 25628–25636.

[54]　Derynck R., Zhang Y., and Feng X. H., "Smads: transcriptional activators of TGF-β responses," *Cell,* Vol. 95, 1998, pp. 737–740.

[55]　Imamura T., Takase M., Nishihara A., Oeda E., Hanai J., Kawabata M., et al., "Smad6 Inhibits Signaling by the TGF-β Superfamily," *Nature,* Vol. 389, 1997, pp. 622–626.

[56]　Vukicevic S., Latin V., Chen P., Batorsky R., Reddi A. H., and Sampath T. K., "Localization of Osteogenic Protein-1 (bone morphogenetic protein-7) During Guman Embryonic Development: high affinity to basement membrane," *Biochem Biophys Res Commun,* Vol. 198, 1994, pp. 693–700.

[57]　Helder M. N., Ozkaynak E., Sampath T. K., Luyten F. P., Latin V., and Oppermann H., et al., "Expression Pattern of Osteogenic Protein-1 (bone morphogenetic protein-7) in Human and Mouse Development, " *J Histochem Cytochem,* Vol. 43, 1995, pp. 1035–1044.

[58]　Zhang H. and Bradley A., Mice Deficient for BMP2 are Nonviable and Have Defects in Amnion/chorion and Cardiac Development," *Development,* Vol. 122, 1996, pp. 2977–2986.

[59]　Dudley A. T., Lyons K., and Robertson E. J., "A Requirement for Bone Morphogenetic Protein-7 During Development of the Mammalian Kidney and Eye, *Genes Dev,* Vol. 9, 1995, pp. 2795–807.

[60]　Luo G., Hofmann C., Bronckers A. L. J. J., Sohocki M., Bradley A., and Karsenty G., "BMP-7 is an Inducer of Nephrogenesis and is Also Required for Eye Development and Skeletal Patterning, *Genes Dev,* Vol. 9, 1995, pp. 2808–2820.

[61]　Vukicevic S., Kopp J. B., Luyten F. P., and Sampath T. K., "Induction of Nephrogenic Mesenchyme by Osteogenic Protein 1 (bone morphogenetic protein 7), *Proc Natl Acad Sci,* Vol. 93, 1996, pp. 9021–9026.

[62]　Winnier G., Blessing M., Labosky P. A., and Hogan B. L. M., "Bone Morphogenetic Protein-4 is Required for Mesoderm Formation and Patterning in the Mouse," *Gen Dev,* Vol. 9, 1995, pp. 2105–2116.

[63] Kingsley D. M., Bland A. E., Grubber J. M., Marker P. C., Russell L. B., Copeland N. G., and Jenkins N. A., "The Mouse *Short Ear* Skeletal Morphogenesis Locus is Associated with Defects in a Bone Morphogenetic Member of the TGFβ Superfamily," *Cell*, Vol. 71, 1992, pp. 399–410.

[64] Solloway M. J., Dudley A. T., Bikoff E. K., Lyons K. M., Hogan B. L., and Robertson E. J., "Mice Lacking BMPs Function," *Dev Genet*, Vol. 22, 1998, pp. 321–339.

[65] Solloway M. J. and Robertson E. J., "Early Embryonic Lethality in BMP5; BMP7 Double Mutant Mice Suggests Functional Redundancy Within the 60A Subgroup," *Development*, Vol. 126, 1999, pp. 1753–1768.

[66] Storm E. E. and Kingsley D. M., "Joint Patterning Defects Caused by Single and Double Mutations in Branchypodism Mice Due to Mutations in a New Member of the TGF-β Superfamily," *Development*, Vol. 122, 1996, pp. 3969–3979.

[67] Monzen K., Hiroi Y., Kudoh S., Akazawa H., Oka T., Takimoto E., et al., Smads, TAK1, and Their Common Target ATF-2 Play a Critical Role in Cardiomyocyte Differentiation," *J Cell Biol*, Vol. 153, 2001, pp. 687–698.

[68] Dorai H., Vukicevic S., and Sampath T. K., "Bone Morphogenetic Protein-7 (osteogenic protein-1) Inhibits Smooth Muscle Cell Proliferation and Stimulates the Expression of Markers that are Characteristic of SMC PhenoType *In vitro*," *J Cell Phys*, Vol. 184, 2000, pp. 37–45.

[69] Nakaoka T., Gonda K., Ogita T., Otawara-Hamamoto Y., Okabe F., Kira Y., et al., "Inhibition of Rat Vascular Smooth Muscle Proliferation In Vitro and In Vivo by Bone Morphogenetic Protein-2," *J Clin Invest*, Vol. 100, 1997, pp. 2824–2832.

[70] Shimasaki S., Zahow R. J., Li D., Kim H., Iemura S. I., Ueno N., et al., "A Functional Bone Morphogenetic System in Ovary," *Proc Natl Acad Sci USA*, Vol. 96, 1999, pp. 7282–7287.

[71] Sampath T. K., Rashka K. E., Doctor J. S., Tucker R. F., and Hoffmann F. M., "Drosophila Transforming Growth Factor β Superfamily Proteins Induce Endochondral Bone Formation in Mammals," *Proc Natl Acad Sci USA*, Vol. 90, 1993, pp. 6004–6008.

[72] Scaduto A. A. and Lieberman J. R., "Gene Therapy for Osteoinduction," *Orthop Clin North Am*, Vol. 30, 1999, pp. 625–633.

Bone Graft Substitutes: A Regulatory Perspective

12

by Sergio J. Gadaleta, [1] *Ph.D.*

INTRODUCTION

FOR MORE THAN 30 YEARS, the orthopedic community, including academic, industrial, and government sectors, has been investigating the use of synthetic-, growth factor-, and cell-based therapies as bone graft substitutes; the ultimate goal of which is to reduce or eliminate the use of autograft in healing bony defects. Synthetic bone graft substitutes, demineralized bone matrix, and bone morphogenetic proteins are legally marketed bone graft substitutes; however, each of these products has a distinct regulatory classification and, as such, requires a different regulatory path for approval prior to marketing.

The regulatory environment surrounding bone graft substitutes is complex and requires knowledge of device, biologic, and tissue regulations, as these products are regulated by different centers under different regulations within the Food and Drug Administration (FDA). Synthetic bone graft substitutes, when indicated for filling bony voids or gaps that are not intrinsic to the stability of the bony structure, require pre-market notification (also known as a 510k) before marketing. Bone graft substitutes incorporating morphogenetic proteins require pre-market approval (also known as a PMA), and thus clinical studies to show safety and effectiveness prior to marketing. Demineralized bone matrix, when provided without additives, is regulated as tissue for transplant and therefore does not require pre-market notification or approval prior to marketing. The degree of regulatory control imposed by the FDA is different for each of the aforementioned products according to the product's classification and regulatory status.

The goal of this manuscript is to provide the reader with a rudimentary review of the classification of medical devices, the mechanisms by which a manufacturer may commercialize a medical device, and the current regulatory status of various bone graft substitutes. Much of the text describing the FDA's programs such as pre-market notification (510k), pre-market approval (PMA), humanitarian device exemption, and product development protocols is taken directly from various publications available on the FDA's website and has been referenced as such. The reader is encouraged to review these documents in detail, as they provide more comprehensive information regarding these topics.

---

[1] MITEK Worldwide, a Division of Ethicon Inc., a Johnson & Johnson Company, Norwood, MA 02062.

CLASSIFICATION OF MEDICAL DEVICES

The Food, Drug, and Cosmetic Act defines a medical device as "an instrument, apparatus, implement, machine, contrivance, implant, in vitro reagent, or other similar or related article, including a component, part, or accessory, which is:

- Recognized in the official National Formulary, or the United States Pharmacopoeia, or any supplement to them,
- Intended for use in the diagnosis of disease or other conditions, or in the cure, mitigation, treatment, or prevention of disease, in man or other animals, or
- Intended to affect the structure or any function of the body of man or other animals, and which does not achieve any of its primary intended purposes through chemical action within or on the body of man or other animals and which is not dependent upon being metabolized for the achievement of any of its primary intended purposes..."

Medical devices may be classified into 3 general categories: Class I, Class II, and Class III. The classification of a device determines the type of application that must be submitted to the FDA before the product may be legally commercialized. Class I and II devices typically require pre-market notification to the FDA, unless they have been exempt from this requirement by regulation. A list of devices exempt from the pre-market notification requirement may be found in the Code of Federal Regulations. Medical devices categorized as Class III require the submission of a pre-market approval application.

Medical devices categorized as Class I are devices for which general controls are sufficient to provide reasonable assurance of safety and effectiveness. General controls consist of mandatory procedures to ensure proper registration, device listing, design and manufacture, labeling, and notification to the FDA before marketing the device. For certain Class I devices, however, general controls may not be sufficient to provide reasonable assurance of safety and effectiveness. These medical devices may remain Class I so long as they are not life-supporting, life-sustaining, and not for a use of substantial importance in preventing impairment of human health and which do not present a potential unreasonable risk of illness or injury to the patient. General controls apply to all devices, regardless of class, unless specifically exempted by regulation. General controls contain requirements for device manufacturers or other designated persons to: register their establishment with the FDA; list their devices with the FDA; comply with labeling regulation in 21 CFR Part 801, 809 or 812; submit a pre-market notification to the FDA; and design and produce devices under good manufacturing practices (GMP). Table 1 provides a description of general controls.

TABLE 1— General controls.

	General Controls
Registration and Listing	Section 510 of the FD&C Act requires that United States (U.S.) device manufacturers and distributors register their establishments with the FDA on form FDA-2891. All manufacturers are required to list the generic type of devices they have in U.S. commerce with the FDA on form FDA-2892. Establishment registration and medical device listing should be submitted prior to commercial distribution. Requirements for establishment registration and medical device listing can be found in 21 CFR Part 807.20.
Labeling	All medical devices in U.S. commerce must be properly labeled. Device labeling requirements of the FD&C Act are found in the following parts of Title 21: Part 801 General Device Labeling; Part 809, In Vitro Diagnostic Products; Part 812, Investigational Device Exemptions; Part 820, Good Manufacturing Practices; Part 1010, General Electronic Products. The FD&C Act, section 201 defines the terms "label" and "labeling" as they apply to medical devices as follows: Section 201(k) defines "label" as a "display of written, printed, or graphic matter upon the immediate container of any article..." The term "immediate container" does not include package liners. Any word, statement, or other information appearing on the immediate container must also appear "on the outside container or wrapper, if any there be, of the retail package of such article, or is easily legible through the outside container or wrapper." Section 201(m) defines "labeling" as: "all labels and other written, printed, or graphic matter (1) upon any article or any of its containers or wrappers, or (2) accompanying such article." The definitions of label and labeling apply to devices held for delivery for shipment or for sale after shipment in interstate commerce. The term "accompanying" is interpreted liberally to mean more than physical association with the product. It extends to posters, tags, pamphlets, circulars, booklets, brochures, instruction books, direction sheets, fillers, etc. "Accompanying" includes labeling that is brought together with the device held for delivery for shipment or after shipment in interstate commerce.
Pre-Market Notification	Most devices are cleared for commercial distribution in the U.S. by the premarket notification [510(k)] process. Most class I devices are exempt from the 510(k) requirement by regulation. However, they are not exempt from other general controls, such as establishment registration and device listing. Before marketing a medical device, which is not exempt from the marketing clearance process, the manufacturer must submit a premarket notification [510(k)] or a premarket approval (PMA) application to THE FDA. The manufacturer cannot market the device unless the firm receives a marketing clearance letter from THE FDA as stated in section 513(I)(1)(A) or section 515(d)(1)(A)(I) of the FD&C Act.
Good Manufacturing Practices	As required by section 520(f) of the Act, the Good Manufacturing Practices (GMP) regulation covers the methods used in, and the facilities and controls used for the design, manufacture, packaging, storage, and installation of devices. The GMP regulation is codified in 21 CFR Part 820. Some Class I devices, such as a manual surgical instruments for general use, 21 CFR section 878.4800, are exempt by regulation from most of the GMP requirements. The GMP regulation contains general quality assurance (QA) or quality system requirements in areas of concern to all manufacturers of finished devices. Among other requirements, it covers the following general areas: organization and personnel; design practices and procedures (proposed); buildings and environmental control; design of labeling and packaging; controls for components, processes, packaging and labeling; device holding, distribution and installation; device evaluation; device and manufacturing records; complaint processing; and QA system audits.

Medical devices categorized as Class II are devices for which general controls are *insufficient* to provide reasonable assurance of safety and effectiveness; however, special controls are sufficient to provide reasonable assurance of safety and effectiveness. Special controls may include labeling requirements, mandatory performance standards, post-market surveillance, patient registries, and/or guidance documents.

Medical devices categorized as Class III are devices for which insufficient information exists to assure safety and effectiveness of the device solely through general or special controls. Moreover, these devices generally support or sustain human life, are of substantial importance in preventing impairment of human health, and/or present a potential unreasonable risk of illness or injury to the patient.

ROUTES TO MARKET

Manufacturers of medical devices are required to go through one of two evaluation processes before marketing a medical device: pre-market notification or pre-market approval. In certain instances, devices legally on the market prior to May 28, 1976 may not require either a 510(k) or PMA submission. These products, known as pre-amendments products have unique regulatory status. Information regarding pre-amendments devices may be found in the Code of Federal Regulations. Additionally, most Class I and many Class II devices are exempt from the pre-market notification requirement and, as such, may be commercialized without notification to the FDA.

Pre-Market Notification [1]

Most medical devices are cleared for commercial distribution by the pre-market notification process. A pre-market notification is a marketing application demonstrating that the medical device is as safe and effective or substantially equivalent to a legally marketed device (i.e., predicate device) that was or is currently on the U. S. market and that does not require pre-market approval.

If the indication for use statement of a new device is shared with another legally marketed device (i.e., a predicate device) that was or is currently on the U. S. market and that does not require pre-market approval, the new device will require a pre-market notification submission, prior to marketing, unless exempt from this requirement by regulation. It is, however, important to fully understand the definition of a predicate device:

A predicate device is:

- A medical device that was legally marketed in the United States prior to May 28, 1976;

      OR

- A medical device that has been reclassified from Class II to Class I or II; OR
- A medical device found substantially equivalent through the pre-market notification process. The term predicate device only applies to devices undergoing review via pre-market notification and not to devices requiring pre-market approval (i.e., Class III). A medical device is substantially equivalent if, in comparison to a legally marketed

predicate device, has the same intended use and has the same technological characteristics of the predicate device OR has the same intended use and has the same technological characteristics of the predicate device AND does not raise new questions of safety and effectiveness AND demonstrates that the device is as safe and effective as the predicate.

If, however, the proposed Indication for Use statement of the new device is NOT shared with another legally marketed device (i.e., predicate device) that was or is currently on the U.S. market OR shares an Indication for Use statement with a product approved via a PMA, the new device will require a PMA submission, prior to marketing.

A medical device is substantially equivalent if, in comparison to a legally marketed predicate device:

- Has the same intended use; and
- Has the same technological characteristics of the predicate device

OR

- Has the same intended use as the predicate; and
- Has different technological characteristics of the predicate device; AND
- Does not raise new questions of safety and effectiveness AND demonstrates that the device is as safe and effective as the predicate.

Substantial equivalence is established with respect to: intended use, design, energy used or delivered, materials, performance, safety, effectiveness, labeling, biocompatibility, standards, and other applicable characteristics. A claim of substantial equivalence does not mean the devices must be identical. Figure 1 presents a decision tree used to determine substantial equivalence.

If the FDA finds the device to be substantially equivalent (SE), the FDA will send the manufacturer a marketing clearance letter, referred to as an "SE letter," and the device may be marketed as described in the 510(k). If the FDA finds the device not to be substantially equivalent (NSE), the FDA will send a not-substantially equivalent letter. In the latter instance, the firm may choose to resubmit another 510(k) with new information, may petition the FDA requesting the device be reclassified into Class I or II, as described in Section 513(f) of the Act, or may submit a PMA.

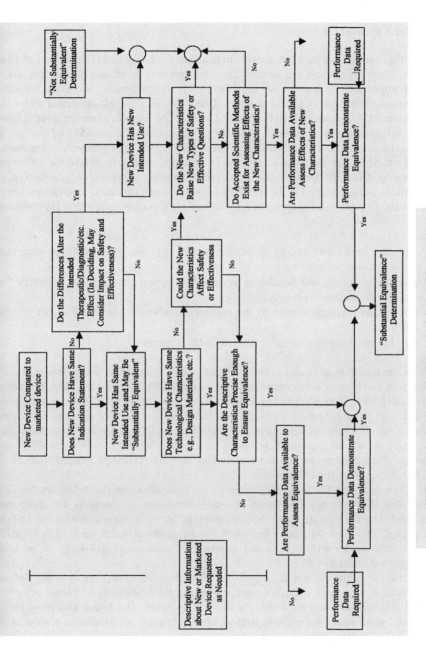

FIG. 1—Substantial equivalence decision-making process.

Pre-Market Approval [2]

Pre-market approval is the FDA process to evaluate the safety and effectiveness of Cla III devices. Class III devices are usually those that support or sustain human life, are substantial importance in preventing impairment of human health, or which present potential, unreasonable risk of illness or injury. Due to the level of risk associated with Cla III devices, the FDA has determined that general and special controls alone are insufficient assure the safety and effectiveness of Class III devices. Under Section 515 of the act, a devices placed into Class III are subject to pre-market approval requirements. Pre-mark approval by the FDA is the required process of scientific review to ensure the safety an effectiveness of Class III devices. An approved Pre-market Approval Application is, effect, a private license granted to the applicant for marketing a particular medical device.

The review of a pre-market approval application is a four-step review process consistir of:

- Administrative and limited scientific review by the FDA staff to determin completeness (filing review);
- In-depth scientific and regulatory review by appropriate the FDA scientific ar compliance personnel (in-depth review);
- Review and recommendation by the appropriate advisory committee (panel review and
- An FDA good manufacturing practices (GMP) inspection.

During the administrative and limited scientific review, the FDA determines whether PMA includes the type of information required by the FD&C Act and the PMA procedur regulations (21 CFR, Part 814) and is suitable for filing. The filing of a PMA applicatic means that the FDA has made a threshold determination that the application is sufficient complete to permit a substantive review. If the information or data are not presented clear or completely or are not capable of withstanding rigorous scientific review, the FDA ma consider the PMA incomplete and not file it. The 180-day review period provided by t FD&C Act begins when the PMA is filed.

Any PMA accepted for filing may undergo an in-depth scientific review by the FD personnel and may be presented to an advisory committee representing the appropria medical field. The FDA notifies the PMA applicant of any deficiencies. Within the 180-da review period, the FDA will send the applicant an approval order under 814.44(d), approvable letter under 814.44(e), a not approvable letter under 814.44(f), or an ord denying approval under 814.45.

The FDA will notify the applicant by letter of its decision to approve or deny, and in Federal Register notice will announce the decision and the availability of a summary of t safety and effectiveness data on which the decision is based. The notice also provides t applicant and other interested persons with an opportunity for administrative review of t FDA approval or denial action.

Product Development Protocol [3]

The 1976 Medical Device Amendments created a mechanism for the regulation of Cla III medical devices that would allow a sponsor to come to early agreement with the FDA to what would be done to demonstrate the safety and effectiveness of a new device. It was recognized that early interaction in the development cycle of a device could allow a sponsor to address the concerns of the FDA before expensive and time-consuming resources were expended. Many manufacturers already employ the concept of concurrent engineering, that is, they involve manufacturing and service personnel early in the design process to identify and address potential concerns. The Product Development Protocol (PDP) extends this concept to regulatory requirements. It is an attempt at "front loading" the approval process by considering all regulatory areas as well as product design and testing in the early concept and planning stages, since this will most efficiently solve most problems. Thereby, the regulatory oversight during product development is limited to administrative and conformance assessment.

The PDP describes the agreed upon details of design and development activities, the outputs of these activities, and acceptance criteria for these outputs. It establishes reporting milestones that convey important information to the FDA as it is generated, where they can be reviewed and responded to in a timely manner. The sponsor would be able to execute their Protocol at their own pace, keeping the FDA informed of their progress with these milestone reports.

As each device is unique, negotiations should be conducted to reach agreement as to what activities will be performed during the course of product development. This guidance document is designed to identify all potential areas for discussion of what the outputs of these activities will be and the acceptance criteria that can be used to assess these outputs. This "contract" establishes a predictable path to market with a potentially shorter review time frame when the device is ready for market. This document is intended to provide guidance throughout the life cycle of the device ("cradle-to-grave") on the engineering, pre-clinical, clinical, manufacturing and post-market content of the PDP contract.

The PDP process is initiated with an optional consultation with the FDA to determine if the device is appropriate for review as a PDP, PMA, or other regulatory pathway. This phase is referred to as the Proposal. Its purpose is to establish that both the FDA and the sponsor are willing to commit to activities, outputs, and acceptance criteria, which would support regulatory approval of the described device. The sponsor would prepare a submission based on the guidance promulgated by the FDA. The FDA has 30 days to review this information.

After it has been determined that the appropriate regulatory mechanism for approval is the Product Development Protocol, the sponsor may submit the Detailed Contents of the Protocol.

The Protocol generally consists of a table of contents, device requirements and description, details of proposed verification and validation activities, clinical trial data, quality systems and post-market information. It may have details and timing of milestones and reporting requirements, notices, and special requirements for Notice of Initiation of Clinical Trials and the last progress report before the Notice of Completion. The FDA has 120 days to review the Detailed Contents during which time it can request additional information. Following this review, the FDA can either accept the PDP or deny for lack of content.

Humanitarian Device Exemption [4]

On June 26, 1996, the FDA issued a final rule to perform provisions of the Safe Medical Devices Act of 1990 regarding humanitarian use devices (HUDs). This regulation became effective on October 24, 1996. An HUD is a device that is intended to benefit patients by treating or diagnosing a disease or condition that affects fewer than 4,000 individuals in the United States per year. A device manufacturer's research and development costs could exceed its market returns for diseases or conditions affecting small patient populations. The FDA, therefore, developed and published this regulation to provide an incentive for the development of devices for use in the treatment or diagnosis of diseases affecting these populations.

The regulation provides for the submission of a humanitarian device exemption (HDE) application, which is similar in both form and content to a pre-market approval (PMA) application, but is exempt from the effectiveness requirements of a PMA. An HDE application is not required to contain the results of scientifically valid clinical investigations demonstrating that the device is effective for its intended purpose. The application, however, must contain sufficient information for the FDA to determine that the device does not pose an unreasonable or significant risk of illness or injury, and that the probable benefit to health outweighs the risk of injury or illness from its use, taking into account the probable risks and benefits of currently available devices or alternative forms of treatment. Additionally, the applicant must show that no comparable devices are available to treat or diagnose the disease or condition and that they could not otherwise bring the device to market.

An approved HDE authorizes marketing of the Humanitarian Use Device and is tantamount to a PMA approval. However, a Humanitarian Use Device may only be used after IRB approval has been obtained for the use of the device for the FDA approved indication. The labeling for a Humanitarian Use Device must state that the device is a humanitarian use device and that, although the device is authorized by Federal Law, the effectiveness of the device for the specific indication has not been shown.

REGULATORY STATUS BONE GRAFT SUBSTITUTES

Synthetic Bone Graft Substitutes

At the time of the Medical Device Amendments of 1976, an FDA advisory panel was charged with the responsibility of recommending device classifications (Class I, Class II, or Class III) to the FDA for all devices known to have been sold in interstate commerce. Bone graft substitutes were not classified because, at that time, interstate commercialization of such devices was not known. Hence, new devices intended to be used as bone graft substitutes required pre-market approval before marketing the product. Consequently, the first bone graft substitute devices submitted to the FDA were Class III devices requiring Pre-market Approval Application (PMA). Two products were subsequently approved via PMA: ProOsteon™ 500 Porous Hydroxyapatite Bone Graft Substitute Blocks & Granules (Interpore Cross, Irvine, CA) and Collagraft™ (Collagen Corporation, Palo Alto, CA).

More recently, the existence of pre-amendments bone void filler for orthopedic use – U.S. Gypsum's calcium sulfate dihydrate bone void filler — was established. According to section 510(k) of the Food, Drug, and Cosmetic Act, post-amendments devices may be found substantially equivalent to pre-amendments devices if both devices have the same intended use and the same technological characteristics. The establishment of a pre-amendment device provided a new regulatory path, that is, pre-market notification, for products having the same intended use and technological characteristics as U.S. Gypsum's product. Wright

Medical Technology was the first company to obtain 510(k) clearance for a bone graft substitute for orthopedic use, namely, Plaster of Paris Pellets. The indication statement for the product reads:

> Wright Plaster of Paris Pellets are intended to be gently packed into non-load-bearing long bone voids. These bone voids may be surgically created osseous defects or osseous defects created from traumatic injury to the bone. The Wright Plaster of Paris Pellets provide a bone filler that resorbs and is replaced with bone during the healing process.

Since Wright Medical Technology's 510(k) clearance, numerous companies have used this approach to market synthetic bone graft substitutes having similar indications for use and technological characteristics. Products cleared for this indication include DePuy's α-BSM Bone Substitute Material, Synthes' Norian SRS Bone Void Filler, EBI's Osteostim Granules, and DePuy Acromed's Conduit TCP Granules.

Demineralized Bone Matrix

Demineralized bone matrix (DBM) has an interesting regulatory history and dynamic regulatory status. DBM is prepared by removing the mineral from human bone specimens by chelating the calcium phosphate mineral component of bone. The process of demineralization removes mineral and cellular components while preserving and exposing the endogenous proteins and growth factors of the bone specimen. The product can be formulated as a dry powder or with other additives to provide different physical and chemical characteristics.

DBM was regulated, originally, as a human tissue intended for transplant as defined by 21 CFR Part 1270:

"any tissue derived from a human body, which:

(1) Is intended for transplantation to another human for the diagnosis, cure, mitigation, treatment, or prevention of any condition or disease;

(2) Is recovered, processed, stored, or distributed by methods that do not change tissue function or characteristics;

(3) Is not currently regulated as a human drug, biological product, or medical device;

(4) Excludes kidney, liver, heart, lung, pancreas, or any other vascularized human organ; and

(5) Excludes semen or other reproductive tissue, human milk, and bone marrow."

In 1997, the Center for Biologics Evaluation and Research issued a document entitled: "Proposed Approach to the Regulation of Cellular- and Tissue-based Products." The purpose of the document was to provide a unified approach to the regulation of traditional and new products, to specify criteria for regulation, and to provide harmonized review of applications within different centers of the agency.

The proposal provided guidance in its regulatory approach regarding demineralized bone matrix:

"The FDA would consider demineralized bone (decalcified freeze dried bone allograft) to be an unclassified pre-Amendments device rather than a tissue under section 361 because the bone is more than minimally manipulated. The FDA would seek a classification recommendation from the Orthopedic/Dental Advisory Panels. The device to be classified would be defined as including allograft bone that is processed ONLY to demineralize and preserve the bone, and ONLY intended to be used as a bone filler in orthopedic and/or dental procedures.

Based on current information, the FDA expects to propose that demineralized allograft bone be regulated as a Class I medical device exempted from pre-market notification. In addition, the FDA expects that it would also propose to exempt demineralized allograft bone from the GMP requirements except for certain requirements consistent with those proposed for human tissues regulated under section 361."

Since 1997, no action was taken to formally classify DBM products; the FDA used enforcement discretion in its regulation of DBM. That is, the FDA has allowed DBM manufacturers to continue marketing DBM products without pre-market notification or pre-market approval. However, in March, 2002, the FDA's Office of Compliance issued a letter to DBM manufacturers announcing the requirement of pre-market notification for DBM products. In filing 510(k)s, the Center for Devices and Radiological Health has instructed sponsors to use resorbable calcium salt bone void filler devices as predicates for demonstrating substantial equivalence. Examples of DBM products include Osteotech's (Eatontown, NJ) Grafton® DBM and Gen-Sci's (Irvine, CA) DynaGraft® DBM.

Bone Morphogenetic Proteins

Bone morphogenetic proteins (BMPs), when provided with an osteoconductive scaffold, are a combination of a biologic and a device, respectively, and as such are regulated as combination products. Under section 503(g) of the Food, Drug, and Cosmetics Act, the FDA must designate a Center within the FDA to have primary jurisdiction over the pre-market review based on the primary mode of action of the combination product. Currently, pre-market review of combination products composed of bone morphogenetic proteins and osteoconductive scaffolds is performed by the Center for Devices and Radiological Health. These products are Class III and require pre-market approval.

Stryker Biotech was the first manufacturer to receive approval to market a bone morphogenetic protein bone graft material, namely, OP-1 Implant. OP-1 Implant is an osteoinductive and osteoconductive bone graft material containing recombinant human Osteogenic Protein 1 (also known as BMP-7) and bovine derived collagen (3.5mg OP-1:1gm collagen). This combination product device was approved as a Humanitarian Device for use as an alternative to autograft in recalcitrant long bone non-unions where use of autograft is unfeasible and alternative treatments have failed. OP-1 did not provide the agency with effectiveness data, as this device was approved under the HDE regulation.

More recently, Medtronic Sofamor Danek received a recommendation for marketing approval, with conditions, by the Orthopedic and Rehabilitation Devices Panel of the United States Food and Drug Administration (the FDA). The product, InFUSE Bone Graft, when used with the LT-CAGE Lumbar Tapered Fusion Device, is indicated to treat spinal degenerative disc disease, a common cause of low back pain. The FDA panel conditions for approval included three additional post-approval studies in the areas of antibody response during pregnancy, dosing and tumorogenicity. In addition, the panel recommended the product only be used with tapered cages.

CONCLUSION

Bone graft substitutes encompass a variety of formulations from synthetic calcium salts to demineralized human bone tissue to recombinant growth factor technology. These products differ in their technological characteristics and also in their indications for use. Generally, synthetic bone graft substitutes are indicated for filling bony voids or gaps that are not intrinsic to the stability of the bony structure require pre-market notification prior to commercialization of the product. That is, synthetic bone graft substitutes serve as osteoconductive matrices, allowing bone to grow on or within the products. Demineralized bone matrix and rhBMP are indicated as bone graft replacements as they provide osteoconductive and osteoinductive factors. This combination provides both a signal to the cells to generate new bone and offers a scaffold on which these cells may deposit the newly formed bone. As the regulatory status of the medical devices depends on the technological characteristics and indications for use, it follows that these products have different regulatory classifications and hence different levels of regulatory control.

REFERENCES

[1] HHS Publication FDA 95-4158; Pre-Market Notification 510(k): Regulatory Requirements for Medical Devices, 1995.

[2] HHS Publication FDA 97-4214; Pre-market Approval Manual, 1998.

[3] FDA Draft Guidance for Industry: Contents of a Product Development Protocol. Available at: http://www.the FDA.gov/cdrh/pdp/420.html, 1997.

[4] Humanitarian Use Device. Available at: http://www.the FDA.gov/cdrh/ode/hdeinfo.html, 2002.

Section III: Polymers, Ceramics, and Other Synthetic Materials for Bone Graft Substitutes

OVERVIEW

Every year several hundred thousand bone graft procedures are performed in the United States alone. Autograft remains the gold standard and hence is the most widely used. It is osteogenic and the risk of infection is minimal. However, there is significant patient morbidity associated with it, which can be a deterrent to its use especially in the case of the elderly.

Allograft is an often-used alternative to autograft. It too is osteogenic to a degree, but it carries an increased risk of infection. The rise in HIV and hepatitis infected cases in recent years has made this issue even more critical. Stringent sterilization techniques using radiation may decrease the infection risk but have detrimental effects on the structural properties (e.g., toughness or energy required for fracture) of bone. It has also been shown that the collagen component of bone is adversely affected due to these sterilization techniques.

Given these limitations, there has been a search for decades to find a suitable synthetic bone graft material. It would be ideal for a surgeon to pull off the shelf a packet of bone graft material that serves the function of an autograft material, has a low infection rate and whose supply is virtually unlimited. This section of the book sheds some light on the state of science related to polymeric and ceramic synthetic bone graft substitutes.

An overall summary of the different bone graft materials currently available has been provided by Boyan et al. The authors state that, "the ideal bone graft substitute material would be osteoinductive, osteoconductive, resorbable in a predictable manner, biologically acceptable and with a proven safety profile with no adverse local or systemic effects." They discuss the bone healing and the biologies of wound healing and bone grafting. This is followed by a comprehensive coverage of the different materials used for bone graft substitutes such as hydroxyapatite, coral-based materials, calcium sulfates, and polymers. This chapter provides an excellent overview from a biology and biomaterials point of view.

More specific information on calcium sulfate-based materials is provided in the chapter by Haggard et al. They provide a very logical and easy to comprehend progression of details in their chapter. First the chemistry and basics of the material are discussed, followed by a description of the preclinical and clinical performance of these materials. In the same vein, coralline porous ceramics are discussed by Shors. A brief history of the coralline process is provided followed by discussions of the manufacturing processes, the physical and chemical properties, animal studies (including different models for trauma and spinal fusion), and clinical results.

Dr. Bucholz, an orthopedic surgeon, discusses the clinical issues associated with bone graft substitutes. This includes the goals of clinical trials and the criteria used for judging the efficacy of different materials. And finally a section is devoted to the factors influencing the choice of clinical trials.

Lastly, Yaszemski et al. address the need for standards in the realm of bone graft substitutes. They discuss the existing standards, those under development, and the gaps that remain to be filled.

Overall, this section of the book provides a very comprehensive overview of the state of the art for the different synthetic materials considered for bone graft substitutes. We believe that it provides an excellent starting point for anyone new to the field and will serve as a valuable reference for those with more experience.

C. Mauli Agrawal, Ph.D.   *Dhirendra S. Katti, Ph.D.*

Section Leader   *Section Leader*

Bone Graft Substitutes: Basic Information for Successful Clinical Use with Special Focus on Synthetic Graft Substitutes

by Barbara D. Boyan, [1,2] *Ph.D., Jacquelyn McMillan,* [1] *M.B.Ch.B., F.R.C.S.Ed., F.R.C.S. (Tr & Orth), Christoph H. Lohmann* [2,3] *M.D., Don M. Ranly,* [1] *D.D.S., Ph.D., and Zvi Schwartz,* [1,2,4] *D.M.D., Ph.D.*

INTRODUCTION

BONE GRAFTING TECHNIQUES ARE USED in many fields of surgery including orthopedic and trauma surgery, periodontal surgery, and maxillofacial surgery. The need to replace bone lost in chronic disease, infection or trauma is clear, and the field has expanded considerably since substitutes were first used to supplement or replace autologous or allogeneic bone grafting. As a result, the number of choices continues to increase as new materials are developed. However, the rationale for selection of one material over another is not yet clear in many clinical situations. This is in part due to the lack of information on basic bone biology as it applies to implant materials in general, and to a particular clinical application. The purpose of this review is to introduce the variety of bone graft materials currently available, discuss some of the new materials under development, and provide a biological rationale for the outcome when these materials are used clinically in orthopedics.

The current accepted gold standard in bone grafting is autograft, which allows replacement with host bone. Although transmission of infection is minimal, autograft brings its own problems of donor site morbidity and limitation of supply [1]. The most common bone graft substitute in clinical use is allograft, including frozen, freeze-dried and demineralized. Cadaveric allograft bone has the advantage of being osteogenic, albeit to a lesser degree than autograft, and there is no donor site morbidity, but it is not in limitless supply, and the tissue processing it must undergo in order to reduce the risks of transmission of infection can cause changes in its structural integrity and its biological activity. Tissue banks distribute allografts, and there is lack of uniformity in the products of individual banks [2]. Thus there has been only little standardization of material when

[1] Wallace H. Coulter Department of Biomed Engineering at Georgia Tech and Emory University, 315 Ferst Drive NW, Atlanta, GA 30332.
[2] University of Texas Health Science Center at San Antonio, San Antonio, TX.
[3] University of Hamburg Eppendorf, Hamburg, Germany.
[4] Hebrew University Hadassah, Jerusalem, Israel.

performing experimental or clinical work using human material. This, coupled with the limits to supply of bone grafts, has stimulated the development of bone graft substitutes.

The ideal bone graft substitute material would be osteoinductive, osteoconductive, resorbable in a predictable manner, biologically acceptable and with a proven safety profile with no adverse local or systemic effects. As yet, the perfect material does not exist, although many materials address one or more of these features (Table 1). These descriptive terms have evolved as our understanding of bone biology has developed. They are now used in very specific ways in the current literature.

TABLE 1— Osteoinductive, osteoconductive, and osteogenic materials used as bone graft substitutes. In clinical practice, two or more of these materials may be used in combination. Generally, all of these materials are used with any available autologous bone and in some cases, with autologous bone marrow. Osteoinductive materials cause bone to form in tissues that would otherwise not support bone formation; osteoconductive materials provide a substrate that supports the migration of osteoprogenitor cells, their proliferation and differentiation into osteoblastic cells, and extracellular matrix synthesis and physiological calcification by these cells. Osteogenic materials permit bone formation to occur in an orthotopic site to a greater extent than would be expected in the presence of an osteoconductive substrate.

Osteoinductive	Osteoconductive	Osteogenic
DBM[1]	Ceramics	Autografts
BMPs[2]	Hydroxyapatite	Allografts
	Deproteinized bone	Xenografts
	Coral-derived products	MSCs[3]
	Calcium phosphates	Growth Factors
	Calcium Sulfates	Cytokines
	Polymer scaffolds	Enamel Matrix Proteins
	Bioglass	Attachment peptides[4]

[1]Demineralized bone matrix, demineralized freeze-dried bone allograft (DFDBA).
[2]Bone morphogenetic proteins including BMP-2, BMP-4 and BMP-7 (osteogenic protein-1, OP-1).
[3]Mesenchymal stem cells, marrow stromal cells, and osteoprogenitor cells.
[4]Peptides such as the arg-gly-asp (RGD) sequence in fibronectin; the attachment proteins themselves.

Osteoinduction is a specific term describing the ability of a material to cause bone to form in a tissue that would otherwise not form bone. This can only be shown in a heterotopic site, since it is not possible to distinguish osteoinduction from osteogenesis in an orthotopic site. However, materials that are osteoinductive tend to enhance or promote osteogenesis in bone defects over the bone formation that would occur in the absence of the material. Bone morphogenetic proteins (BMPs) are classic examples of osteoinductive agents; implantation of BMPs in muscle tissue results in formation of a complete ossicle consisting of cortical and trabecular bone and bone marrow. When BMPs are implanted in an orthotopic site, bone formation occurs more effectively. Demineralized bone matrix (DBM) also has osteoinductive characteristics, which are hypothesized to be due to the presence of BMPs.

Clearly, if BMPs are present in DBM, they are also present in autograft and allograft. However, unless autograft and allograft are demineralized, they are not osteoinductive by the definition above; rather they are osteoconductive. Osteoconduction is the ability to support new bone formation via the ingrowth of new host bone into/onto a scaffolding material. This may be a naturally occurring scaffold such as an organized haematoma or autograft, or a biomaterial such as synthetic polymeric foam. Agents that enhance osteogenesis but are not themselves osteoinductive can be thought of as osteogenic. These agents have the ability to enhance heterotopic bone formation by an osteoinductive agent or to enhance osteoconduction in an osseous site.

Different properties are required of bone graft materials in different clinical situations. Bone graft substitutes for use in long bone diaphyses may need to be weight bearing; mandibular grafts may not. Contained metaphyseal grafts may require different properties than grafts that bridge cortical defects. Some grafts will be placed with supportive internal or external fixation, while others will be placed in a defect with no additional structural support. The site of graft placement will determine the functional properties expected of the graft material. Although the clinical use may differ, however, all bone grafts are expected to perform one function in all sites—that of re-creating a bone-like material in an area of bone that has been damaged by either trauma or chronic disease.

BIOLOGY OF WOUND HEALING

All bone grafts are placed in a wound, and it is appropriate here to review briefly the events occurring in a fresh soft tissue wound. In most tissues, wound healing is a reparative process rather than a regenerative one, and results in a scar composed of fibrous tissue. The phases of wound healing provide an environment in which fibrous protein synthesis is facilitated. The first phase of healing includes haemorrhage, ultimately producing haematoma. As the fibrin polymerises, the edges of the wound become more closely approximated. Vasoconstriction also occurs. Platelets adhere to exposed endothelium and to the haematoma. Substances released from both the damaged tissue and from the platelets themselves mediate platelet aggregation. The coagulation and complement cascades are initiated, and platelets release mitogens for endothelial cells and fibroblasts, such as transforming growth factor beta (TGF-β), platelet derived growth factor (PDGF), and vascular endothelial factor (VEGF), as well as other cytokines, chemokines, and regulatory agents.

In the second phase, vasodilatation occurs with a consequent increase in local blood flow. Chemotactic agents attract polymorphonuclear leucocytes (PMNs) and endothelial permeability increases. The PMNs release proteolytic enzymes, which assist in remodeling of the haematoma. They also release chemokines and cytokines that modulate responses of the cells migrating to the haematoma. Circulating monocytes are attracted and are activated, becoming macrophages, which phagocytose the necrotic cell debris and produce factors to stimulate fibroblast proliferation and angiogenesis.

During the third phase of healing, the fibroblasts produce proteoglycans and structural proteins including collagen. Angiogenesis proceeds by capillary budding, and the wound edges contract. The wound is filled with vascular granulation tissue, in which fibroblasts proliferate and protein synthesis continues. Wound strength increases with the increase in collagen, and the fourth phase, that of scar formation, is entered.

In a wound in which healing conditions are compromised by low oxygen tension due to poor blood supply, by chronic pre-existing disease or drug effects, the healing process is slowed and the risk of infection increases. In wounds with infection or the presence of a continuing tissue irritant, chronic inflammation may supervene, and the process of inflammation will continue alongside the healing response.

BONE HEALING

Healing in a primary bone wound involves similar stages to healing in other wounds, with the initial formation of haematoma, followed by an inflammatory reaction and PMN infiltration. The clot is invaded by macrophages and chemotactic agents attract marrow stromal cells and stimulate angiogenesis. Marrow stromal cells contain a small number of mesenchymal stem cells (MSCs), which have the ability to differentiate into a variety of cell types depending on the local environment and regulatory factors. In addition, some of the marrow stromal cells are already in the osteochondral lineage, and in a bone environment they have the potential to differentiate into chondrocytes or osteoblasts, depending in part on the relative stability of the bone and oxygen tension. In sites that are stable and well vascularized, most of the cells will become osteoblasts, whereas in sites that are mechanically unstable and less well vascularized, the cells tend to become chondrocytes. Some of the marrow stromal cells may also differentiate into adipocytes, which is why regions of fat are frequently found in histological sections of healing bone.

MSCs are fibroblastic in appearance, as are many of the uncommitted or partially committed populations of marrow stromal cells. It is these cells that actually migrate to the wound site. If conditions are not optimal for bone or cartilage formation, the cells may differentiate along a default pathway and become fibroblasts. When this occurs, nonunion results. Fibrogenesis also is seen next to implant materials that are not osteogenic or osteoconductive, when there is an excessive immune response, and when infection is present.

As indicated above, when the ends of the bone are in close approximation and the bone is mechanically stable, osteochondroprogenitor cells are able to migrate across the haematoma and form bone directly. Following proliferation, these cells differentiate into osteoblasts, which synthesize and then calcify osteoid via a mechanism that involves matrix vesicles. Those osteoblasts that are surrounded by calcified osteoid become osteocytes. This rapidly forming bone is termed woven bone because it lacks structural organization. After it undergoes remodeling, it is replaced by lamellar bone, including Haversian canals. This process takes varying lengths of time depending on the site and whether the bone is in mechanical function. Generally, bone healing and remodeling require at least six months and this may be longer in complicated or large wounds.

If the wound site is mechanically unstable, callus formation occurs. In this situation, osteochondroprogenitor cells that have migrated to the wound site proliferate and differentiate into chondroblasts, which then synthesize cartilage matrix. This cartilage is similar to the cartilage found during embryonic bone formation, and in the growth plate. It undergoes endochondral differentiation, resulting in calcified cartilage. Once the cartilage matrix is calcified, it is remodeled by chondroclasts (osteoclasts that resorb calcified cartilage), leaving the newly formed underlying bone. The calcified cartilage serves as a scaffold for new bone formation and it acts as an internal fixation device. As a result, wounds and defects that heal by callus formation are mechanically stiffer during healing than those that heal by primary bone formation. Recent work has shown the role of growth factors in fracture healing. These factors are released by platelets aggregating at the wound site and by the injured bone itself, and include TGF-β, PDGF, insulin like growth factors (IGF-I and IGF-II), and acidic and basic fibroblast growth factors (FGF-1 and FGF-2) [3]. FGFs play a particular role in angiogenesis and act as mitogens for osteoblast precursors.

Design of graft substitutes must take into account the fact that, whatever material is used, it will be placed in a wound, often a wound in compromised tissue or where there has been a long-standing disease process. There will inevitably be interaction between the graft material and the local host tissue, which may affect the ability of the tissue to form living bone on the graft and to incorporate the graft. Therefore, experimental studies should take into account the differing environments in which the substitute compounds will be placed. The effect of age on the host bone and its ability to form new bone due to poorer vascularity or lower numbers of marrow stem cells and MSCs [4,5] must be considered, as should the effect of pharmacological agents such as steroids, anti-inflammatory drugs and chemotherapeutic agents. The presence of significant host disease such as diabetes, neoplastic conditions, infection, and vascular disease may all have a detrimental effect on bone formation [6], and models or clinical studies must be designed to address the specific questions posed by each of these circumstances.

BIOLOGY OF BONE GRAFTING

The gold standard in bone grafting is autograft. One of the reasons for this is the fact that autograft is osteogenic in addition to being osteoconductive. However, it can also be stated that no bone graft substitution procedure can be undertaken without some degree of local host bone debridement and preparation, so that there is always some autograft present at the graft site, even when substitutes are being used.

The synthetic bone graft substitutes include ceramics, polymers and substances such as calcium sulfate and de-organified coral or bovine bone. These materials are osteoconductive rather than osteoinductive. Methods already exist to alter the properties of these materials in order to enhance their osteoconductivity and these will be outlined. These substances can also be used with various growth factors to enhance the biologic activity of the local host tissues, resulting in increased bone formation. Moreover, addition of specific growth factors like the BMPs can cause the materials to become osteoinductive. These materials are increasingly being used in combination with each other, with or without the addition of osteogenic factors, either from the host tissues or manufactured by recombinant techniques. Bone marrow cells may be added to these graft materials, as will be described below.

In order for new bone to form at the site of bone grafting, whether autologous or allogeneic bone grafts or bone graft substitutes are used, cells must be present that have potential to become bone cells. These cells must be able to follow the osteoblastic lineage cascade, synthesizing and calcifying osteoid, and going on to become bone lining cells or osteocytes within newly-formed calcified matrix. These multipotent cells are present in adult human bone marrow [7,8]. Early experiments with rat bone marrow cells used with ceramic scaffolds show that they are capable of osteogenesis [9], even after culture expansion [10], and of healing bone defects [11]. This ability depends on local factors, including the presence of growth factors and other peptides [12,13], and on the oxygen tension of the local environment [14]. Other factors affecting their osteogenic potential include age and gender of the animal. The number of osteogenic cells is decreased in older rabbits and in humans, particularly in females [4,5].

Surface characteristics of any bone graft substitute material influence the adherence and differentiation of marrow stromal cells [15,16]. It is possible to alter these surfaces by the addition of various proteins such as fibronectin or laminin [17], or of peptides or growth factors [18], in order to promote cell attachment, proliferation, and osteoblastic differentiation.

SYNTHETIC BONE GRAFT SUBSTITUTES

Ceramics

Ceramics are highly crystalline structures formed by heating non-metallic mineral salts to high temperatures in a process known as sintering. Many ceramics are known to be biocompatible and are used in orthopedics in various applications. These include the resorbable ceramics such as tricalcium phosphate; ceramics with highly reactive surfaces such as bioactive glasses; and ceramics with surface chemistries that do not react with biological fluids to an appreciable extent [19]. The least reactive ceramics, for example alumina and yttrium-stabilized zirconia, are in use in arthroplasty components, while the more reactive ceramics have been used as bone graft substitutes in the form of granules, porous blocks and cements.

Bone growth behavior varies on different bioceramic materials. This is due in part to the morphological characteristics of the bone graft substitute. Granule size can alter the particle packing characteristics, and affect bone ingrowth through the resulting interstices [20]. The temperature at which porous ceramics are sintered can affect biological response by altering the chemical and topographical features of the material surface [21]. Crystallinity (crystal size and perfection) also influences cell and tissue response by affecting the adsorption of serum components to the surface, and ultimately the ability of osteogenic cells to attach, proliferate, and differentiate [22].

Ceramics can be modified to improve the tissue response. Porous ceramics have been shown to provide an osteogenic platform for bone marrow stromal cells [10,11], and the attachment of these cells is enhanced by fibronectin and laminin treatment of the ceramic surfaces [17]. Surface chemical modifications also influence cell reactions to ceramics [23].

Hydroxyapatite

Hydroxyapatite is one of the families of calcium orthophosphate molecules, and is one of the most biologically compatible substances used as a bone graft substitute material. Although synthetic hydroxyapatite materials share similarities with the mineral phase of bone, they are very different. Bone mineral is highly carbonated and exists as very small plate-like crystals in a three-dimensional matrix in dynamic arrangement with proteins and other extracellular matrix constituents. Moreover, it contains numerous ion substitutions that alter the chemical and physical characteristics of the crystals, how they interact with the organic phase of the extracellular matrix, and ultimately, the material properties of the bone. In contrast, synthetic apatites tend to be homogeneous in composition, with larger and more perfect crystals. Although organic constituents adsorb on the surface, they are generally not structural components of the biomaterial and do not modify the physical properties of the bone graft substitute.

Hydroxyapatites have been used in particulate form for over half a century [24]. Porous blocks prepared by sintering [25], enabled clinicians to use these materials to restore physical structure. Although this was an important advance, these materials tend to be highly crystalline and are resorbed very slowly—over decades rather than years. Other calcium phosphates are designed to be more soluble, such as tricalcium phosphate, but as a group, resorption is still relatively slow, certainly longer than the time needed to synthesize and remodel bone.

Ideally, a bone graft substitute should resorb as new bone is synthesized and remodeled (Fig. 1). If a ceramic implant remains after bone healing is complete, it has the potential to alter the material properties of the bone, and its mechanical resistance to stress. Most hydroxyapatite implant materials are osteoconductive, but when large blocks are used, even if they are highly porous, the ability of osteoprogenitor cells to migrate throughout the implant may be compromised, and fibrous connective tissue may result. To overcome these problems, hydroxyapatite and other calcium phosphates may be used as composites with a more resorbable material, such as collagen or a synthetic biodegradable polymer [26–29].

Pore size and porosity are also important characteristics of hydroxyapatite bone graft substitutes. Pore size was initially thought to be the most important factor [30]. No ingrowth occurred with small pore sizes and fibrous tissue formed with pore sizes from 15–40 microns, whereas osteoid formed with pores of around 100 microns. Pore sizes of 300–500 microns were thought to be ideal since vascular ingrowth could occur. Pore size may be less critical than the presence of interconnecting pores [31]. Interconnecting pores prevent the formation of "blind alleys" at the bottom of which is found low oxygen tension, which prevents osteoprogenitor cells from following the osteoblast lineage cascade, differentiating instead into cartilage, fibrous tissue or fat [32].

Porous hydroxyapatite ceramics have been used in treatment of bone defects following curettage of benign bone tumors [33], in part because they are osteoconductive, but also because they provide space-filling structural support. There is recent evidence from animal studies that hydroxyapatite may also be osteoinductive [34,35]. It is clear, however, that these are highly effective materials in many ways [36–38].

Coral-derived Products

Coralline bone graft substitutes are derived from marine corals. Natural corals have a highly porous exoskeleton, which is similar in structure to cancellous bone. Coral has been used in its natural mineral form of calcium carbonate [39]. More commonly, the replamineform process is used to convert calcium carbonate to calcium hydroxyapatite [40].

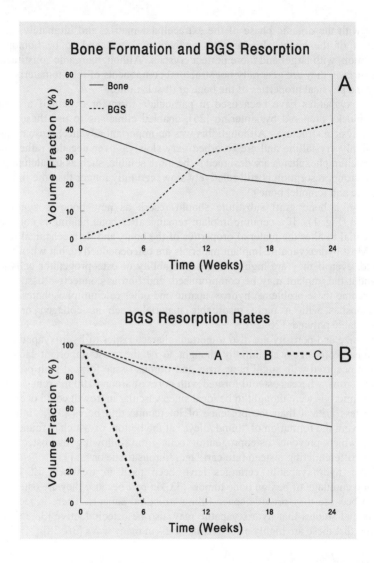

FIG. 1—Relationship between bone graft substitute (BGS) resorption and new bone formation. Ideally, bone graft substitutes are replaced by new bone (A). To accomplish this goal, the BGS formulations vary in their rate of resorption (B). Even when designed to resorb over the average healing period for most bone defects, many BGS materials do not meet this goal, and may remain in the tissue for relatively long periods of time, in some instances for the lifetime of the patient. In such instances, it is important to show that the retained material does not negatively impact the mechanical properties of the bone. It should be noted that even autograft and allograft might remain within newly formed bone for relatively long periods of time.

Hydroxyapatite is less resorbable than calcium carbonate, and hybrid forms of these compounds have been developed which have a core of calcium carbonate and a variable surface layer of calcium hydroxyapatite [41]. This allows manufacture of a product with variable and, more importantly, predictable, resorption rates, as the hydroxyapatite layer resorbs slowly with bone formation, but the carbonate core, once exposed, resorbs rapidly, again allowing bone substitution.

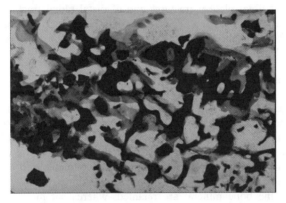

A

B

FIG. 2—**Bone formation within the pores of coral-derived bone graft substitutes.** (A) Low power micrograph of a human biopsy showing the ability of bone to grow throughout the interconnecting pores of an implant used as a bone graft substitute. Lack of blind alleys limits the formation of cartilage and adipose tissue. (B) Back scatter electron micrograph showing the close inter-relationship of the newly formed bone (dark gray) and the bone graft substitute (pale gray) and soft tissue including marrow and blood vessels (black).

Coral derived bone graft substitutes are available in granular and block form. Depending on the type of material, the pore sizes may vary. Two average pore sizes have emerged as the most common, 200 and 500 microns, and studies have shown that the rate of vascular ingrowth is comparable in both. One advantage of the coral-derived materials is that the pores are interconnected so that bone can grow throughout the interstices of the implants (Figs. 2a and b). Coralline implants have been used in lumbar spinal fusion, orbital reconstruction, and bone defect reconstruction in orthopedic oncology, in addition to the treatment of tibial plateau fractures and of distal radial fractures in conjunction with internal fixation [36,42–45]. These materials have been combined with growth factors and BMPs to enhance osteogenesis. When used without osteogenic factors, the coral derived products are osteoconductive only.

Deproteinized Bone

Similar to the concept underlying the use of coral-derived materials as bone graft substitutes, bovine bone can be processed to remove the organic component, leaving the structural properties of the mineral intact. This is an attractive concept because the pore size and porosity of the resulting material is biologically compatible with normal bone. Deproteinized bone has been developed as an alternative to autograft or allograft using a variety of processing methods. At lower temperatures, many of the physical characteristics of the bone mineral are retained, whereas at higher temperatures, the mineral becomes sintered hydroxyapatite. Recent studies have shown that bone processed at lower temperatures retains some organic material trapped within the mineral phase, including minute levels of biologically active osteogenic factors [46], which may contribute to the apparent clinical success of these bone graft substitutes. However, as with deproteinized bone processed at high temperatures, the attractive feature is the osteoconductive three-dimensional bone-like morphology.

Tricalcium Phosphates (TCP)

Tricalcium phosphate was first used as a bone graft substitute in 1920 [47]. Whereas hydroxyapatite has a Ca:P molar ratio of 1.67, TCP has a Ca:P molar ratio of 1.5. TCP is less crystalline than hydroxyapatite, and therefore, more soluble. Implants that contain TCP are both biocompatible and osteoconductive, but because of its relative solubility it is used in situations where structural support is less important. TCP has been used in the treatment of large cancellous defects in pigs and in humans [48,49], and has been used in spinal fusion mixed with allograft bone with results comparable to allograft alone [50].

Alpha and beta tricalcium phosphates are high-temperature tricalcium phosphates with a similar chemical composition to amorphous calcium phosphate but with increased crystallinity [51]. Alpha-TCP is more soluble than beta-TCP and is a major component in apatite cements. In addition to being more soluble than beta-TCP, alpha-TCP has been reported to be more easily degraded in vivo. However, recent reports examining resorption in mini-pigs, suggests that both forms of TCP degrade at comparable rates [52]. Alpha-TCP bone graft substitutes can be obtained in block, granular or powder form. Beta-TCP also has been used as a bone graft substitute as blocks or granules and is degradable by osteoclast activity [31].

Biphasic Calcium Phosphate

Biphasic calcium phosphate is a composite of hydroxyapatite and beta-TCP. It is more rapidly degradable than hydroxyapatite alone. Biphasic calcium phosphate is commercially available and has been used as a bone graft substitute in posterior lumbar fusion mixed with autograft [53]. Clinical results were good in 31 of 32 patients, and in three patients, solid fusion was noted at second surgery for hardware removal.

Calcium Phosphate Cements

Calcium phosphate cements form on mixing one of a range of calcium phosphates with an aqueous solution, resulting in dissolution of the calcium followed by a precipitation reaction in which the calcium phosphate crystals grow and the cement becomes rigid. Brown and Chow invented the first calcium phosphate cement that could be constituted at room temperature from calcium phosphate powder and water in 1985 [54]. Modern formulations enable surgeons to inject the cement directly into the defect because the set-up involves an endothermic rather than an exothermic reaction [55–57], limiting the potential for local tissue damage.

Calcium phosphate cements fall into one of two categories: apatite and brushite. Apatite cements form hydroxyapatite as an end product, although some have carbonates present and form carbono-apatites. They are more degradable than hydroxyapatite but still degrade slowly. Mechanical properties vary between the cements, and depend to some degree on the composition. Porosity is similarly variable, and has an inverse relationship with tensile strength. Mechanical strength increases over time in vivo. Apatite cements are biocompatible and few inflammatory reactions have been reported. Brushite cements degrade to form dicalcium phosphate dihydrate (DCPD), and are more degradable than apatite cements. They resorb more quickly in vivo, by dissolution as well as by osteoclast resorption. The mechanical properties of brushite cement decrease rapidly in vivo. However, as bone ingrowth occurs, the mechanical properties of the healing bone increase. Brushite cements are biocompatible, although inflammatory reactions have also been reported [58].

Calcium phosphate cements have been used as carriers for growth factors, antibiotics, and BMP. As a group, the calcium phosphate cements are strong in compression but have low tensile strength, making them most suitable for treatment of fractures and defects that are not weight bearing. Their use is reported in the treatment of fractures of the distal radius, the calcaneus, and the tibial plateau, with or without fixation [59–61]. These materials are generally unsuitable for diaphyseal fractures.

Bioactive Glasses

Bioactive glasses are surface-reactive ceramics formed by melt or sol-gel techniques and are available in sintered porous bulk or particulate form. The surface of a bioactive glass takes part in a reaction with host tissue on implantation, involving dissolution of the surface of the glass and release of mineral ions. In vitro studies have shown that initial reaction of some bioactive glasses cause a local increase in pH [62]. Other studies have confirmed this and proposed that this alkalinization is beneficial to cell activity and hydroxyapatite production [63]. A calcium phosphate layer forms [64], and this layer is thought to enhance protein adsorption to the surface of the implant [62] and to be involved in the surface reaction with host bone. Surface-treated bioglass has been shown to adsorb fibronectin more selectively than do hydroxyapatite ceramics [65]. Fibronectin is closely involved in the osteogenic function of bioglass ceramics [66]; this protein has been shown to increase cell attachment on bioactive glasses that have been pre-treated with calcium phosphate or hydroxyapatite surface layers [67]. The presence of both the calcium phosphate layer and serum proteins has been shown to influence the behavior of osteoblasts on the surface of the material [62].

Osteoblast responses to bioactive glasses are variable. In vitro studies show that the ionic products of glass dissolution increase osteoblast proliferation and up regulate many genes concerned with cell attachment, proliferation, and protein production in human osteoblasts [68–71], and confirm that osteoblastic differentiation occurs in the presence of bioactive glasses [72]. Moreover, bioactive glass ceramics are osteogenic even in osteopenic bone [73], suggesting that they not only support osteoblast differentiation, but enhance it as well. Recent reports suggest that bioglasses may have some osteoinductive properties [74].

Porous melt-derived glasses resorb very slowly in vitro, but the recent sol-gel glasses, which have higher specific surface area, are much more resorbable while having similar osteoconductive effects and no loss of structural characteristics [75,76]. This allows replacement of the resorbed implant by new bone, thereby eliminating the concern that their retention in bone may compromise the mechanical properties of the tissue. Sol-gel derived bioactive glasses have a number of properties that make them attractive materials as bone graft substitutes. They may be used as carriers for proteins such as BMP-2 and TGF-β in the bone graft setting, and they appear to act synergistically with the growth factors [77–79]. One compound of this family has been shown to have bacteriostatic properties as well [80].

Bioactive glasses have been studied for use in bone defects with good results in animal studies [81–83] and have been used clinically, particularly in restorative dentistry with varying results, [84–86] and in craniofacial surgery [87]. These materials are biocompatible, and in many clinical situations are as effective as hydroxyapatite or autologous bone graft, but some bioglass formulations are brittle and may form particular debris, contributing to the release of inflammatory cytokines [88].

Calcium Sulfate

Calcium sulfate is familiar to orthopedic surgeons as plaster of Paris, but its use as a bone graft material was first described in the late 19th century and over the ensuing years there have been reports of its use for this purpose [89]. Peltier described his experiences with this material in 1959 [90] and in 1978, he described the long-term follow-up of 26 patients with unicameral bone cysts, of whom 24 healed without complication [91]. Coetzee reported in 1980 on 100 patients in whom he had used calcium sulfate to treat cranial bone defects, and concluded that it was a safe and effective substitute for autologous bone graft, allowing deposition of cancellous host bone while the graft substance resorbed [92].

Calcium sulfate is a crystalline substance, which is osteoconductive. The variable crystallinity of the early plaster of Paris has been addressed in the manufacture of surgical-grade calcium sulfate, which has predictable structure and properties. This has been used in the form of pellets to treat bone defects with successful results. Kelly et al. [93] reported the use of calcium sulfate pellets alone or in combination with other substances in the treatment of 109 patients with contained bone lesions with radiographic and clinical follow-up showing that 88% of defects filled with trabecular bone. Turner et al. [94] described a study of canine humeral models in which calcium sulfate tablets were implanted into large medullary defects and compared with autograft and no graft. The calcium sulfate-grafted defects compared well with the autografted defects, and histological examination confirmed the resorption of the calcium sulfate as the defects healed with new bone. In a sheep vertebral fusion model, in which calcium sulfate was compared with autologous bone graft, frozen allograft, coral derived hydroxyapatite implants, and demineralized bone, there were no differences in the amount of new bone formed between the groups, and strength testing of the constructs was similar in autograft and calcium sulfate grafts [95,96].

Calcium sulfate has also been used as a bone graft expander with excellent results both experimentally in a canine spinal fusion model [97] and a canine femoral defect model [98], and clinically in the treatment of benign bone lesions [99] and human spinal fusion [100]. It has been used together with demineralized bone and with hydroxyapatite and bovine osteogenic protein-1 (BMP-7) [101,102]. In these studies, it was shown to be biocompatible and caused little inflammatory reaction, although this has been described [103]. However, its relatively rapid resorption means that it is not suitable for clinical applications where structural support is required of the graft material. Therefore, it can be used alone only in contained non-structural defects or combined with fixation and other materials to enhance bone formation. It may well prove to be a good carrier for growth factors and bone morphogenic proteins in appropriate clinical settings.

Demineralized Bone Graft

Bone graft that has been demineralized is osteoinductive, based on the definition that it can cause bone to form in tissues that would otherwise not form bone (Fig. 3). Dentists and oral and maxillofacial surgeons call this "demineralized freeze-dried bone allograft" (DFDBA), whereas orthopedic surgeons and neurosurgeons call it "demineralized bone matrix" (DBM). As a material, human DBM consists of cell remnants, extracellular matrix, and a small amount of residual mineral. Historical recognition of the value of DBM as a bone graft substitute dates from the time of Aristotle. More recently, Nicholas Senn reported on the use of cadaver bone that was "sterilized" using muriatic acid as a treatment for osteomyelitis in patients who needed bone graft during the United States' Civil War in the 1860s. Based on the studies of Marshall Urist, Hari Reddi, and Julie Glowacki [104–108], the use of DBM clinically is now well accepted, particularly in situations where the benefits of osteoinduction are desired but the mechanical stability of the bone graft substitute alone is not required.

Exactly why DBM is osteoinductive is not well understood. This property is ascribed to the presence of active BMPs and their release from the mineralized matrix of bone during the demineralization step, but other factors may play a role as well. When DBM is implanted in heterotopic sites, it attracts mesenchymal cells to the implant surface. There is some question as to whether the surface of the DBM is remineralized as an initial step, since tissues that are implanted with DBM exhibit radio-opaque masses on X-ray but histology may fail to show the presence of new bone [109]. If the DBM has retained its osteoinductive ability and a suitable responding cell population is present, the mesenchymal cells will proliferate and differentiate into chondroblasts. The chondroblasts synthesize cartilage matrix and then undergo endochondral development, ultimately calcifying their extracellular matrix. This is vascularized and osteoprogenitor cells are able to form bone on the calcified cartilage scaffold. Ultimately, the cartilage is replaced with marrow and marrow elements in the same manner as is seen in embryonic bone development. When DBM is implanted in an orthotopic site, endochondral ossification may be initiated, but it is clear that direct induction of osteogenesis also occurs, and in some situations may predominate.

Although allograft has all of the same components as DBM, it is not osteoinductive. Demineralization is an absolute requirement [110] to convey this property. If allograft is implanted in a heterotopic site, it is resorbed [111]. However, if allograft is used orthotopically, it is very effective, more so than would be predicted by osteoconduction alone. This is likely due to the release of osteoinductive factors during osteoclastic resorption.

Most of what we know about osteoinduction has been learned from studies using rat and mouse DBM implanted in mesenchymal tissues of animals with compromised immune systems. Using these models, it is clear that the cascade of events is directed and timed in the same way in each experiment. When DBM is prepared from rats or mice with differing physiologies and ages, some variation exists, but for the most part, the DBM is prepared in a laboratory setting and is very reproducible in its size, shape, and composition. Human DBM is a very different story. Variability in the physiology of the donors is considerable. Donor age is negatively correlated with osteoinduction ability but donor sex does not appear to be a factor [112]. Other issues confound the problem as well. The length of time a donor has been dead can impact on the osteoinductive properties of the DBM, as can the method of procurement [113]. Each bone bank has its own method for processing [2]. Even though there are certain general processing steps, there is no agreed upon mandatory protocol. DBM is not only demineralized; it is washed, extracted with organic solvents, dried, cut, pulverized, sized and sterilized by methods that are subtly unique to each bone bank. Thus, osteoinduction ability may vary as an intrinsic property of the donor bone and also as a consequence of its preparation [114].

Finally, there is no agreed upon assay of osteoinduction activity. It is financially prohibitive for not-for-profit bone banks to test each batch of DBM for osteoinductivity in vivo. While in vitro assays are under development, to date no in vitro assay has been shown in a peer-reviewed publication to be directly correlated with in vivo osteo-induction, although indirect correlations have been noted [115,116]. Thus, the sense of clinicians that DBM is frequently not more osteogenic than allograft is real.

Despite these drawbacks, DBM is an excellent material to use as a bone graft substitute because it is osteoconductive and at the very least, it is osteogenic. DBM is provided to the clinician as a dried powder. Even when it is reconstituted in sterile saline, it has a tendency to float away from the defect site. To improve its handling characteristics, surgeons frequently pre-mix DBM with autologous blood, allowing it to clot slightly before implantation. Commercial preparations have focused on sterility and shelf life, in addition to handling characteristics. Currently, DBM has been formulated with glycerol, calcium sulfate, hyaluronic acid, or a reverse phase polymer, and other possibilities are on the commercial horizon. Each of the carriers confers properties on the composite that differ from DBM alone. Some cause swelling of the particles and some provide a material with a putty-like consistency. By modifying the physical form of the DBM prior to mixing, the final product can be further manipulated to meet a clinical need. While these modifications may add to the attractiveness of DBM in terms of use, it must be remembered that they also may reduce or even destroy completely, the osteoinductive properties of the DBM. Even if the osteoinductive ability of the DBM is not impacted negatively, the carrier may make the composite effectively non-osteoinductive by physically preventing attachment of the appropriate responding cell populations to the DBM.

DBM is itself an excellent carrier. It has been used effectively as a carrier for BMP, thereby enabling clinicians to make use of its excellent osteoconductive properties while ensuring that the implant is osteoinductive [117]. Active DBM can also be made more osteoinductive by addition of osteogenic materials such as proteins derived from porcine fetal enamel [118].

Polymers

Polymers are used in a variety of surgical applications. Non-resorbable polymers include ultra-high molecular weight polyethylene, used as a bearing surface in total joint arthroplasty, and polymethyl methacrylate, used as acrylic cement for implant fixation and filling of defects. These materials are not intended to be replaced with bone, although they may interface with bone tissue.

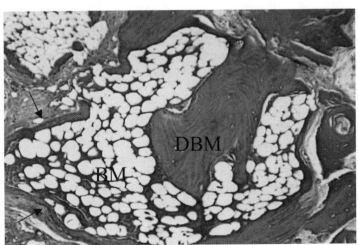

FIG. 3—Photomicrograph of a retrieved implant that contained active DBM after 56 days of implantation in nude mouse calf muscle. Note the new bone formed (arrows), as well as bone marrow (BM) and DBM particles (DBM). Sections were stained with haematoxylin and eosin; original magnification x20.

Biodegradable polymers have several different applications. Early uses included suture materials (polydioxanone, polyglycolide) [119,120] and internal fixation devices, which resorbed thereby theoretically avoiding the need for implant removal [121]. More recently, the use of bioresorbable polymers has expanded to include scaffolds for tissue engineering in various geometric forms including porous membranes, porous blocks and microspheres. These have been developed as carrier materials for cells and growth factors, as well as other proteins [122–128], allowing local introduction of osteogenic substances to the area of the bone defect while providing a framework for ingrowth of new host tissue. One compound has been engineered to allow injection into a bone defect and in-situ polymerization rather than insertion of a preformed block [129].

Most of the bioresorbable polymers in use in tissue engineering at present belong to the polyhydroxy acid family. This group of alpha hydroxy acids includes poly(L-lactide) and poly(D,L-lactide) (PLA), polyglycolide (PGA), and copolymers based on PLA and PGA. Other polymers that have been studied include polypropylene fumarate (PPF), polycaprolactone, tyrosine-derived polymers, and polyanhydrides. When used as a bone graft substitute, either alone or as a composite, the polymers are constructed to form osteoconductive surfaces. The intent is for these materials to resorb as new bone forms, ultimately replacing the tissue engineered medical product.

The bioresorbable polymers described above degrade by hydrolysis. Vert et al. [130] has outlined definitions for polymers based on their breakdown and their elimination or retention in the body, either locally or systemically [130]. The polyhydroxy acids degrade into CO_2 and water, which are completely eliminated from the body. One consequence of hydrolytic degradation is the release of acidic products and a corresponding fall in the local tissue pH. As a result of this, local inflammatory reactions have been reported and intraosseous cysts noted in bone in which resorbable polymer implants have been placed [131], leading to questions regarding the biocompatibility of polymer implants. In general, the normal buffering capacity of biological fluids is sufficient to compensate for the release of acid during degradation, and movement of these fluids ensures that by-products of the degradation are diluted and are able to diffuse from the implant site. However, some polymeric materials undergo bulk degradation, causing the acid load to be greater than can be accommodated by dilution or physiological buffering. Other materials, particularly those that are more crystalline, degrade very slowly, causing the acid insult to become chronic. Either of these two situations may affect tissue response. Fluid flow around polymers can also affect their degradation [132], suggesting that the local pH change may serve as a positive feedback mechanism, increasing the rate of degradation. It should be noted that in vivo and in vitro rates of degradation are variable, and depend both on the polymer composition and physical properties and on local environmental factors [133], including host site vascularity and degree of loading of implant.

Acidic loading can be counteracted by incorporation of basic salts or calcium compounds such as hydroxyapatite or tricalcium phosphate into the polymer [134,135]. In addition to buffering properties, the incorporation of such substances into polymers allows the formation of composites that can be specifically designed to have predictable biomechanical properties and resorption rates. Polymer scaffolds may be fabricated by several different methods, including casting, extrusion, molding and solid free form fabrication, and the pore size and porosity are dependent on the method of manufacture of the scaffold [136]. Other factors influencing the chemical, physical, and biomechanical properties of polymers and their composites include the chemical structure, morphology, composition, ratio of components, addition of low molecular weight components or presence of residual monomers and poly-dispersity. In a rat study, it was seen that different calcium salts incorporated into the polymer scaffold had variable effects on local bone formation and inflammation, in addition to allowing porosity of the polymer composite to be controlled [137].

Much has been written on the pore sizes of ceramic bone graft substitutes and the relationship of pore size, porosity and new tissue ingrowth. It should be noted that the pore sizes of polymers engineered for use as scaffolds depends on the method of fabrication of the 3-D construct, but that many fall below the pore sizes of ceramic materials. However, bone growth has been noted in the smaller pores [138], and it is clear that overall porosity is considerably more important than simple pore size.

One of the most exciting and most studied areas of polymer science in relation to bone grafting is the use of polymer composites as carriers for osteogenic substances and cells. Several studies have reported on the kinetics of protein release from degrading polymers and shown that this is a predictable event. Polymers have been used as carriers for rhBMP-2 and it has been shown that bone formation induced by a polymer/BMP-2 implant exceeds that of polymer alone [125]. Interestingly, BMP-2 also stimulates the degradation of polymer carriers (Fig. 4), perhaps because bone formation is enhanced [125,128]. The incorporation of vascular endothelial growth factor (VEGF) and endothelial cells into polymer implants may be useful in improving the vascularity and incorporation of host bone growth [139,140]. By using various factors to modulate the differentiation of marrow stromal cells and mesenchymal stem cells, and by modifying the physical characteristics with calcium salts or by changing the characteristics of the polymer [141,142], degradable polymer bone graft substitutes have almost limitless potential, particularly if the application does not require load bearing.

DISCUSSION

The work described in this paper gives a snapshot view of the class of materials used as bone graft substitutes. These materials include calcium salts and calcium-based ceramics, synthetic polymers and biopolymers, as well as synthetic composites and biohybrid constructs of cells, proteins, and scaffolds. No one material will work optimally in all applications. By developing improved preclinical models, the ability to identify appropriate bone graft substitutes has moved forward considerably during the past decade. These studies have helped to define the parameters that must be met to determine if a bone graft substitute can be used effectively in humans. Depending on the nature of the defect and the health status of the recipient, there may be specific requirements for structural support, degradation rate, and addition of osteogenic components including growth factors and osteoprogenitor cells.

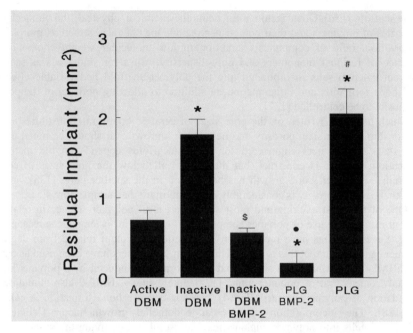

FIG. 4—Effect of BMP-2 on the degradation of bone graft substitutes. BMP-2 (5 μg) was added to DBM previously shown to have no osteoinduction ability or to poly D,L-lactide-co-glycolide (PLG) polymer scaffolds and implanted intramuscularly in nude mice. The graph shows the area of residual DBM and PLG particles in comparison with osteoinductive DBM alone, inactive DBM alone or PLG alone. Each measurement is the mean ± SEM of eight implants harvested from four mice. *P < 0.05 vs. active DBM; #P < 0.05 PLG particles vs. inactive DBM or PLG particles containing rhBMP-2; •P < 0.05 PLG particles containing rhBMP-2 vs. DBM containing rhBMP-2; $P < 0.05 inactive DBM vs. inactive DBM containing rhBMP-2.

In vitro studies can be used to screen specific characteristics of potential bone graft substitutes, but it remains a necessity to test effectiveness in vivo in an animal model. Studies using mice and rats have great utility in determining if a material will be biocompatible and even if a material has clinical value in a bone defect. To this end, the concept of a critical size defect has been of considerable value. Critical size defects are defects in bone that will not heal completely with bone if left untreated. When placed in the cranium or in a long bone, fibrous connective tissue and fibrocartilage fill the defect space, although there may be some bone healing at the margins. The critical size defect can be used to assess the relative effectiveness of a material with respect to rate and quality of healing in comparison with the gold standard autograft, allograft, or another bone graft substitute.

For many applications in orthopedics, however, it is not necessary for a bone graft substitute to be as good as autograft, but it is important that when used to extend autograft, it should not reduce the osteogenicity of autograft to any great extent. Among the most important functions of a bone graft substitute are to stabilize the haematoma that forms at a wound site, and provide a structural support for cell migration and growth factor delivery. Thus, in some circumstances, these materials may enhance the osteogenic activity of autograft and allograft. Until appropriate standards are established and used, unfortunately, the maze of potential bone graft substitutes will continue to confound the orthopedic, neurosurgical, plastic and maxillofacial surgery, and dental communities.

Acknowledgments

The authors thank Drs. Doug Arm and Edwin Shors, Interpore Cross International (Irvine, CA) for sharing their figures with us. We also acknowledge the industry partners of the Center for the Enhancement of the Biology/Biotechnology Interface at the University of Texas Health Science Center at San Antonio for their generous support of our work.

REFERENCES

[1] Younger E. M. and Chapman M. W., "Morbidity at Bone Graft Donor Site," *J Orthop Trauma*, Vol. 3, 1989, pp.192–195.

[2] Schwartz Z., Mellonig J. T., Carnes D. L., Jr., de la Fontaine J., Cochran D. L., Dean D. D., et al., "Ability of Commercial Demineralized Freeze-Dried Bone Allograft to Induce New Bone Formation," *J Periodontol*, Vol. 67, 1996, pp. 918–926.

[3] Bostrom M. P., Saleh K. J., and Einhorn T. A., "Osteoinductive Growth Factors in Preclinical Fracture and Long Bone Defects Models," *Orthop Clin North Am*, Vol. 30, 1999, pp. 647–658.

[4] Muschler G. F., Nitto H., Boehm C. A., and Easley K. A., "Age- and Gender-Related Changes in the Cellularity of Human Bone Marrow and the Prevalence of Osteoblastic Progenitors," *J Orthop Res*, Vol. 19, 2001, pp.117–125.

[5] Huibregtse B. A., Johnstone B., Goldberg V. M., and Caplan A. I., "Effect of Age and Sampling Site on the Chondro-osteogenic Potential of Rabbit Marrow-Derived Mesenchymal Progenitor Cells," *J Orthop Res*, Vol. 18, 2000, pp. 18–24.

[6] Kagel E. M., Majeska R. J., and Einhorn T. A., "Effects of Diabetes and Steroids on Fracture Healing," *Curr Opinion Orthop*, Vol. 6, 1995, pp. 7–13.

[7] Haynesworth S. E., Goshima J., Goldberg V. M., and Caplan A. I., "Characterization of Cells with Osteogenic Potential from Human Marrow," *Bone*, Vol. 13, 1992, pp. 81–88.

[8] Majors A. K., Boehm C. A., Nitto H., Midura R. J., and Muschler G. F., "Characterization of Human Bone Marrow Stromal Cells with Respect to Osteoblastic Differentiation," *J Orthop Res*, Vol. 15, 1997, pp. 546–557.

[9] Ohgushi H., Okumura M., Tamai S., Shors E. C., and Caplan A. I., "Marrow Cell Induced Osteogenesis in Porous Hydroxyapatite and Tricalcium Phosphate: a comparative histomorphometric study of ectopic bone formation," *J Biomed Mater Res*, Vol. 24, 1990, pp. 1563–1570.

[10] Goshima J., Goldberg V. M., and Caplan A. I., "Osteogenic Potential of Culture-Expanded Rat Marrow Cells as Assayed in Vivo with Porous Calcium Phosphate Ceramic," *Biomaterials*, Vol. 12, 1991, pp. 253–258.

[11] Ohgushi H., Goldberg V. M., and Caplan A. I., "Repair of Bone Defects with Marrow Cells and Porous Ceramic. Experiments in Rats," *Acta Orthopedica Scandinavica*, Vol. 60, 1989, pp. 334–339.

[12] Hanada K., Dennis J. E., and Caplan A. I., "Stimulatory Effects of Basic Fibroblast Growth Factor and Bone Morphogenetic Protein-2 on Osteogenic Differentiation of Rat Bone Marrow-derived Mesenchymal Stem Cells," *J Bone Mineral Res*, Vol. 12, 1997, pp. 1606–1614.

[13] Cassiede P., Dennis J. E., Ma F., and Caplan A. I., "Osteochondrogenic Potential of Marrow Mesenchymal Progenitor Cells Exposed to TGF-beta 1 or PDGF-BB as Assayed in Vivo and in Vitro," *J Bone Mineral Res*, Vol. 11, 1996, pp. 1264–1273.

[14] Lennon D. P., Edmison J. M., and Caplan A. I., "Cultivation of Rat Marrow-Derived Mesenchymal Stem Cells in Reduced Oxygen Tension: effects on in vitro and in vivo osteochondrogenesis," *J Cell Physiol*, Vol. 187, 2001, pp. 345–355.

[15] Schwartz Z., Braun G., Kohavi D., Books B. P., Amir D., Sela J., and Boyan B. D., "Effects of Hydroxyapatite Implants on Primary Mineralization During Rat Tibial Healing: Biochemical and morphometric analyses," *J Biomed Materials Res*, Vol. 27, 1993, pp. 1029–1038.

[16] Schwartz Z., Swain L. D., Marshall T. S., Sela J., Gross U., Amir D., Mueller-Mai C., and Boyan B. D., "Modulation of Matrix Vesicle Enzyme Activity and Phosphatidylserine Content by Ceramic Implant Materials During Endosteal Bone Healing," *Calcified Tissue Int*, Vol. 51, 1992, pp. 429–437.

[17] Dennis J. E. and Caplan A. I., "Porous Ceramic Vehicles for Rat-marrow-derived (Rattus norvegicus) Osteogenic Cell Delivery: effects of pre-treatment with fibronectin or laminin," *J Oral Implantol*, Vol. 19, 1993, pp.106–115

[18] Arnaud E., De Pollak C., Meunier A., Sedel L., Damien C., and Petite H., "Osteogenesis with Coral is Increased by BMP and BMC in a Rat Cranioplasty," *Biomaterials*, Vol. 20, 1999, pp. 1909–1918.

[19] Hulbert S. F., Bokros J. C., Hench L. L., Wilson J., and Heimke G., "Ceramics in Clinical Investigations: Past, present and future," *High Tech Ceramics*, Elsevier, Amsterdam, 1987, pp. 189–213.

[20] Oonishi H., Hench L. L., Wilson J., Sugihara F., Tsuji E., Kushitani S., and Iwaki, H., "Comparative Bone Growth Behavior in Granules of Bioceramic Materials of Various Sizes," *J Biomed Mater Res*, Vol. 44, 1999, pp. 31–43.

[21] Frayssinet P., Rouquet N., Fages J., Durand M., Vidalain P. O., and Bonel G., "The Influence of Sintering Temperature on the Proliferation of Fibroblastic Cells in Contact with HA-bioceramics," *J Biomed Mater Res*, Vol. 35, 1997, pp. 337–347.

[22] Frank R. M., Klewansky P., Hemmerle J., and Tenenbaum H., "Ultrastructural Demonstration of the Importance of Crystal Size of Bioceramic Powders Implanted into Human Periodontal Lesions," *J Clin Periodontol*, Vol. 18, 1991, pp. 669–680.

[23] Zreiqat H., Evans P., and Howlett C. R., "Effect of Surface Chemical Modification of Bioceramic on Phenotype of Human Bone-derived Cells," *J Biomed Mater Res*, Vol. 44, 1999, pp. 389–396.

[24] Ray R., Degge G., Gloyd P., and Mooney G., "Bone Regeneration," *J Bone Joint Surg Am*, Vol. 34, 1952, pp. 638–647.

[25] Roy D. and Linnehan S., "Hydroxyapatite Formed from Coral Skeletal Carbonate by Hydrothermal Exchange," *Nature*, Vol. 247, 1974, pp. 220–222.

[26] Cornell C. N., Lane J. M., Chapman M., Merkow R., Seligson D., Henry S., and Gustilo R., and Vincent K., "Multicenter Trial of Collagraft as Bone Graft Substitute," *J Orthop Trauma*, Vol. 5, 1991, pp. 1–8.

[27] Chapman M. W., Bucholz R., and Cornell C., "Treatment of Acute Fractures with a Collagen-calcium Phosphate Graft Material. A Randomized Clinical Trial," *J Bone Joint Surg Am*, Vol. 79, 1997, pp. 495–502.

[28] Porter B. D., Oldham J. B., He S. L., Zobitz M. E., Payne R. G., An K. N., et al., "Mechanical Properties of a Biodegradable Bone Regeneration Scaffold," *J Biomechan Eng*, Vol. 122, 2000, pp. 286–288.

[29] Thomson R. C., Yaszemski M. J., Powers J. M., and Mikos A. G., "Hydroxyapatite Fiber Reinforced Poly (alpha-hydroxy ester) Foams for Bone Regeneration," *Biomaterials*, Vol. 19, 1998, pp. 1935–1943.

[30] Kuhne J. H., Bartl R., Frisch B., Hammer C., Jansson V., and Zimmer M., "Bone Formation in Coralline Hydroxyapatite. Effects of Pore Size Studied in Rabbits," *Acta Orthopedica Scandinavica*, Vol. 65, 1994, pp. 246–252.

[31] Eggli P. S., Muller W., and Schenk R. K., "Porous Hydroxyapatite and Tricalcium Phosphate Cylinders with Two Different Pore Size Ranges Implanted in the Cancellous Bone of Rabbits. A Comparative Histomorphometric and Histologic Study of Bony Ingrowth and Implant Substitution," *Clin Orthop Rel Res*, Vol. 232, 1988, pp. 127–138.

[32] Nakahara H., Goldberg V. M., and Caplan A. I., "Culture-expanded Periosteal-derived Cells Exhibit Osteochondrogenic Potential in Porous Calcium Phosphate Ceramics In Vivo," *Clin Orthop Rel Res*, Vol. 276, 1992, pp. 291–298.

[33] Yamamoto T., Onga T., Marui T., and Mizuno K., "Use of Hydroxyapatite to Fill Cavities after Excision of Benign Bone Tumours. Clinical Results," *J Bone Joint Surg Br*, Vol. 82, 2000, pp. 1117–1120.

[34] Ripamonti U., "Osteoinduction in Porous Hydroxyapatite Implanted in Heterotopic Sites of Different Animal Models," *Biomaterials*, Vol. 17, 1996, pp. 31–35.

[35] Gosain A. K., Song L., Amarante M. T., Nagy P. G., Wilson C. R., Toth J.M., and Ricci J. L., "A 1-year Study of Osteoinduction in Hydroxyapatite-derived Biomaterials in an Adult Sheep Model: part 1," *Plastic Reconstruc Surg*, Vol. 109, 2000, pp. 619–630.

[36] Bucholz R. W., Carlton A., Holmes R., "Interporous Hydroxyapatite as a Bone Graft Substitute in Tibial Plateau Fractures," *Clin Orthop Rel Res*, Vol. 240, 1989, pp. 53–62.

[37] Irwin R. B., Bernhard M., and Biddinger A., "Coralline Hydroxyapatite as Bone Substitute in Orthopedic Oncology," *Am J Orthop*, Vol. 30, 2001, pp. 544–550.

[38] Sakano H., Koshino T., Takeuchi R., Sakai N., and Saito T., "Treatment of the Unstable Distal Radius Fracture with External Fixation and a Hydroxyapatite Spacer," *J Hand Surg*, Vol. 26, 2001, pp. 923–930.

[39] Demers C., Hamdy C. R., Corsi K., Chellat F., Tabrizian M., and Yahia L., "Natural Coral Exoskeleton as a Bone Graft Substitute: a review," *Biomed Mater Eng*, Vol. 12, 2002, pp. 15–35.

[40] White E. and Shors E. C., "Biomaterial Aspects of Interpore-200 Porous Hydroxyapatite," *Dental Clin North Am*, Vol. 30, 1986, pp. 49–67.

[41] Shors E. C., "Coralline Bone Graft Substitutes," *Orthop Clin North Am*, Vol. 30, 1999, pp. 599–613.

[42] Boden S. D., Martin, G. J., Jr., Morone, M., Ugbo, J. L., Titus, L., and Hutton, W. C., "The Use of Coralline Hydroxyapatite with Bone Marrow, Autogenous Bone Graft, or Osteoinductive Bone Protein Extract for Posterolateral Lumbar Spine Fusion," *Spine*, Vol. 24, 1999, pp. 320–327.

[43] Georgiadis N. S., Terzidou C.D., and Dimitriadis A. S., "Coralline Hydroxyapatite Sphere in Orbit Restoration," *Eur J Ophthalmol*, Vol. 9, 1999, pp. 302–308.

[44] Irwin R. B., Bernhard M., and Biddinger A., "Coralline Hydroxyapatite as Bone Substitute in Orthopedic Oncology," *Am J Orthop*, Vol. 30, 2001, pp. 544–550.

[45] Wolfe S. W., Pike L., Slade J. F., 3rd, Katz L. D., "Augmentation of Distal Radius Fracture Fixation with Coralline Hydroxyapatite Bone Graft Substitute," *J Hand Surg*, Vol. 24, 1999, pp. 816–827.

[46] Schwartz Z., Weesner T., van Dijk S., Cochran D. L., Mellonig J. T., Lohmann C. H., et al., "Ability of Deproteinized Cancellous Bovine Bone to Induce New Bone Formation," *J Periodontol*, Vol. 71, 2000, pp. 1258–1269

[47] Albee F. and Morrison H., "Studies in Bone Growth," *Ann Surg*, Vol. 71, 1920, pp. 32–38.

[48] Lange T. A, Zerwekh J. E, Peek R. D, Mooney V, and Harrison B. H., "Granular Tricalcium Phosphate in Large Cancellous Defects," *Ann Clin Lab Sci*, Vol. 16, 1986, pp. 467–472.

[49] Nicholas R. W. and Lange T. A., "Granular Tricalcium Phosphate Grafting of Cavitary Lesions in Human Bone," *Clin Orthop Rel Res*, Vol. 306, 1994, pp. 197–203.

[50] Le Huec J. C., Lesprit E., Delavigne C., Clement D., Chauveaux D., and Le Rebeller A., "Tri-calcium Phosphate Ceramics and Allografts as Bone Substitutes for Spinal Fusion in Idiopathic Scoliosis: comparative clinical results at four years," *Acta Orthopedica Belgica*, Vol. 63, 1997, pp. 202–211.

[51] Termine J. D., Peckhauskas R. A., and Posner A. S., "Calcium Phosphate Formation in vitro: II, Effects of Environment on Amorphous-crystalline Tranformation," *Arch Biophysiol*, Vol. 140, 1970, pp. 318–325.

[52] Wiltfang J., Merten H. A., Schlegel K. A., Schultze-Mosgau S., Kloss F. R., Rupprecht S., et al., "Degradation Characteristics of Alpha and Beta Tri-Calcium-Phosphate (TCP) in Mini-pigs," *J Biomed Mater Res*, Vol. 63, 2002, pp. 115–121.

[53] Fujibayashi S., Jitsuhiko S., Tanaka C., Matsushita M., and Nakamura T., "Lumbar Posterolateral Fusion with Biphasic Calcium Phosphate Ceramic," *J Spinal Disord*, Vol. 14, 2001, pp. 214–221.

[54] Brown W. and Chow L., Dental Restorative Cement Pastes. US Patent No. 4518430, 1985.

[55] Constantz B. R., Ison I. C., Fulmer M. T., Poser R. D., Smith S. T., Van Wagoner M., et al., "Skeletal Repair by In situ Formation of the Mineral Phase of Bone," *Science*, Vol. 267, 1995, pp. 1796–1799.

[56] Larsson S. and Bauer T. W., "Use of Injectable Calcium Phosphate Cement for Fracture Fixation: a review," *Clin Orthop Rel Res*, Vol. 395, 2002, pp. 23–32.

[57] Lobenhoffer P., Gerich T., Witte F., and Tscherne H., "Use of an Injectable Calcium Phosphate Bone Cement in the Treatment of Tibial Plateau Fractures: a prospective study of twenty-six cases with twenty-month mean follow-up," *J Orthop Trauma*, Vol. 16, 2002, pp. 143–149.

[58] Flautre B., Delecourt C., Blary M. C., Van Kanduyt P., Lemaitre J., and Hardouin P., "Volume Effect of Biological Properties of a Calcium Phosphate Hydraulic Cement: experimental study in sheep," *Bone,* Vol. 25, Suppl. 2, 1999, pp. 35S–39S.

[59] Kopylov P., Runnqvist K., Jonsson K., and Aspenberg P., "Norian SRS Versus External Fixation in Redisplaced Distal Radial Fractures: a randomised study in 40 patients," *Acta Orthopedica Scandinavica*, Vol. 70, 1999, pp.1–5.

[60] Thordarson D. B., Hedman T. P., Yetkinler D. N., Eskander E., Lawrence, T. N., and Poser, R. D., "Superior Compressive Strength of a Calcaneal Fracture Construct Augmented with Remodelable Cancellous Bone Cement," *J Bone Joint Surg Am,* Vol. 81, 1999, pp. 239–246.

[61] Keating J. F. and Hajducka C., "The Use of Norian SRS and Minimal Internal Fixation in the Management of Tibial Fractures," *Proc Ann Meeting Orthop Trauma Asso*, 1999.

[62] El-Ghannam A., Ducheyne P., and Shapiro I. M., "Formation of Surface Reaction Products on Bioactive Glass and Their Effects on the Expression of the Oosteoblastic Phenotype and the Deposition of Mineralized Extracellular Matrix," *Biomaterials*, Vol. 18, 1997, pp. 295–303.

[63] Silver I. A., Deas J., and Erecinska M., "Interactions of Bioactive Glasses with Osteoblasts in Vitro: Effects of 45S5 Bioglass, and 58S and 77S bioactive glasses on metabolism, intracellular ion concentrations and cell viability," *Biomaterials*, Vol. 22, 2001, pp. 175–185.

[64] Ducheyne P. and Cuckler J. M., "Bioactive Ceramic Prosthetic Coatings," *Clin Orthop Rel Res*, Vol. 276, 1992, pp. 102–114.

[65] El-Ghannam A., Ducheyne P., and Shapiro I. M., "Effect of Serum Proteins on Osteoblast Adhesion to Surface-modified Bioactive Glass and Hydroxyapatite," *J Orthop Res,* Vol. 17, 1999, pp. 340–345.

[66] Lu H. H., Pollack S. R., and Ducheyne P., "45S5 Bioactive Glass Surface Charge Variations and the Formation of a Surface Calcium Phosphate Layer in a Solution Containing Fibronectin," *J Biomed Mater Res*, Vol. 54, 2001, pp. 454–461.

[67] Garcia A. J., Ducheyne P., and Boettiger D., "Effect of Surface Reaction Stage on Fibronectin-mediated Adhesion of Osteoblast-like Cells to Bioactive Glass," *J Biomed Mater Res*, Vol. 40, 1998, pp. 48–56.

[68] Xynos I. D., Edgar A. J., Buttery L. D., Hench L. L., and Polak J. M., "Gene-Expression Profiling of Human Osteoblasts Following Treatment with the Ionic Products of Bioglass 45S5 Dissolution," *J Biomed Mater Res*, Vol. 55, 2001, pp. 151–157.

[69] Xynos I. D., Edgar A. J., Buttery L. D., Hench L. L., and Polak J. M., "Ionic Products of Bioactive Glass Dissolution Increase Proliferation of Human Osteoblasts and Induce Insulin-like Growth Factor II mRNA Expression and Protein Synthesis," *Biochemical & Biophysical Research Communications*, Vol. 276, 2000, pp. 461–465.

[70] Kaufmann E. A., Ducheyne P., and Shapiro I. M., "Evaluation of Osteoblast Response to Porous Bioactive Glass (45S5) Substrates by RT-PCR Analysis," *Tissue Engineering*, Vol. 6, 2000, pp. 19–28.

[71] Price N., Bendall S. P., Frondoza C., Jinnah R. H., and Hungerford D. S., "Human Osteoblast-like Cells (MG63) Proliferate on a Bioactive Glass Surface," *J Biomed Mater Res,* Vol. 37, 1997, pp. 394–400.

[72] Loty C., Sautier J. M., Tan M. T., Oboeuf M., Jallot E., Boulekbache H., Greenspan, D., and Forest, N., "Bioactive Glass Stimulates in Vitro Osteoblast Differentiation and Creates a Favorable Template for Bone Tissue Formation," *J Biomed Mater Res*, Vol. 16, 2001, pp. 231–239.

[73] Iwashita Y., Yamamuro T., Kasai R., Kitsugi T., Nakamura T., Okumura H., and Kokubo T., "Osteoconduction of Bioceramics in Normal and Osteopenic Rats: comparison between bioactive and bioinert ceramics, *J Appl Biomater*, Vol. 3, 1992, pp. 259–268.

[74] Yuan H., de Bruijn J. D., Zhang X., van Blitterswijk C. A., and de Groot K., "Bone Induction by Porous Glass Ceramic Made from Bioglass (45S5)," *J Biomed Mater Res*, Vol. 58, 2001, pp. 270–276.

[75] Hamadouche M., Meunier A., Greenspan D. C., Blanchat C., Zhong J. P., La Torre G. P., and Sedel L., "Long-term in vivo bioactivity and degradability of bulk sol-gel bioactive glasses," *J Biomed Mater Res*, Vol. 54, 2001, pp. 560–566.

[76] Wheeler D. L., Eschbach E. J., Hoellrich R. G., Montfort M. J., and Chamberland L., "Assessment of Resorbable Bioactive Material for Grafting of Critical-size Cancellous Defects," *J Orthop Res*, Vol. 18, 2000, pp. 140–148.

[77] Santos E. M., Radin S., and Ducheyne P., "Sol-gel Derived Carrier for the Controlled Release of Proteins," *Biomaterials*, Vol. 20, 1999, pp. 1695–1700.

[78] Nicoll S. B., Radin S., Santos E. M., Tuan R. S., and Ducheyne P., "In Vitro Release Kinetics of Biologically Active Transforming Growth Factor-beta 1 from a Novel Porous Glass Carrier," *Biomaterials*, Vol. 18, 1997, pp. 853–859.

[79] Santos E. M., Radin S., Shenker B. J., Shapiro I. M., and Ducheyne P., "Si-Ca-P xerogels and Bone Morphogenetic Protein Act Synergistically on Rat Stromal Marrow Cell Differentiation in Vitro," *J Biomed Mater Res,* Vol. 41, 1998, pp. 87–94.

[80] Bellantone M., Coleman N. J., and Hench L. L., "Bacteriostatic Action of a Novel Four-component Bioactive Glass," *J Biomed Mater Res*, Vol. 51, 2000, pp. 484–490.

[81] Schepers E., De Clercq, M., and Ducheyne, P., "Histological and Histomorphometrical Analysis of Bioactive Glass and Fibre Reinforced Bioactive Glass Dental Root Implants," *J Oral Rehab*, Vol. 15, 1988, pp. 473–487.

[82] Schepers E., de Clercq M., Ducheyne P., and Kempeneers R., "Bioactive Glass Particulate Material as a Filler for Bone Lesions," *J Oral Rehab*, Vol. 18, 1991, pp. 439–452.

[83] Heikkila J. T., Aho H. J., Yli-Urpo A., Happonen R. P., and Aho A. J., "Bone Formation in Rabbit Cancellous Bone Defects Filled with Bioactive Glass Granules," *Acta Orthopedica Scandinavica*, Vol. 66, 1995, pp. 463–467.

[84] Lovelace T. B., Mellonig J. T., Meffert R. M., Jones A. A., Nummikoski P. V., and Cochran D. L., "Clinical Evaluation of Bioactive Glass in the Treatment of Periodontal Osseous Defects in Humans," *J Periodontol*, Vol. 69, 1998, pp. 1027–1035.

[85] Nevins M. L., Camelo M., Nevins M., King C. J., Oringer R. J., Schenk R. K., and Fiorellini J. P., "Human Histologic Evaluation of Bioactive Ceramic in the Treatment of Periodontal Osseous Defects," *Int J Periodon Restor Dentist*, Vol. 20, 2000, pp. 458–467.

[86] Schepers E. J., Ducheyne P., Barbier L., and Schepers S., "Bioactive Glass Particles of Narrow Size Range: a new material for the repair of bone defects," *Implant Dentistry*, Vol. 2, 1993, pp. 151–156.

[87] Kinnunen I., Aitasalo K., Pollonen M., and Varpula M., "Reconstruction of Orbital Floor Fractures Using Bioactive Glass," *J Craniomaxillofacial Surg,* Vol. 28, 2000, pp. 229–234.

[88] Bendall S. P., Gaies M., Frondoza C., Jinnah, R. H., and Hungerford, D. S., "Effect of Particulate Bioactive Glass on Human Synoviocyte Cultures," *J Biomed Mater Res*, Vol. 41, 1998, pp. 392–397.

[89] Tay B. K., Patel V. V., and Bradford D. S., "Calcium Sulfate- and Calcium Phosphate-based Bone Substitutes. Mimicry of the Mineral Phase of Bone," *Orthop Clin North Am*, Vol. 30, 1999, pp. 615–623.

[90] Peltier L. F., "The Use of Plaster of Paris to Fill Large Defects in Bone," *Am J Surg,* Vol. 97, 1959, pp. 311–315.

[91] Peltier L. F. and Jones R. H., "Treatment of Unicameral Bone Cysts by Curettage and Packing with Plaster-of-Paris Pellets," *J Bone Joint Surg Am,* Vol. 60, 1978, pp. 820–822.

[92] Coetzee A. S., "Regeneration of Bone in the Presence of Calcium Sulfate," *Arch Otolaryngol*, Vol. 106, 1980, pp. 405–409.

[93] Kelly C. M., Wilkins R. M., Gitelis S., Hartjen C., Watson J. T., and Kim P. T., "The Use of a Surgical Grade Calcium Sulfate as a Bone Graft Substitute: results of a multicenter trial," *Clin Orthop Rel Res*, Vol. 382, 2001, pp. 42–50.

[94] Turner T. M., Urban R. M., Gitelis S., Infanger S., Berzins A., Hall D. J., et al., "Efficacy of Calcium Sulfate, a Synthetic Bone Graft, Material, in Healing a Large Canine Medullary Defect," *Trans Orthop Res Soc,* Vol. 24, 1999, p. 522.

[95] Hadjipavlou A. G., Simmons J. W., Tzermiadianos M. N., Katonis P. G., and Simmons D. J., "Plaster of Paris as Bone Substitute in Spinal Surgery," *Eur Spine J*, Vol. 10, Suppl. 2, 2001, pp. S189–196.

[96] Hadjipavlou A. G., Simmons J. W., Yang J., Nicodemus C. L., Esch O., and Simmons D. J., "Plaster of Paris as an Osteoconductive Material for Interbody Vertebral Fusion in Mature Sheep," *Spine*, Vol. 25, 2000, pp.10–15.

[97] Turner T. M., Urban R. M., Andersson G. B. J., Lawrence A. M., Igloria R. V., Haggard W. O., et al., "Spinal Fusion Using Synthetic Bone Graft Calcium Sulfate Compared to Autogenous Bone in a Canine Model," *Trans Soc Biomater*, Vol. 24, 1999, p. 90.

[98] Elkins A. D. and Jones L. P., "The Effects of Plaster of Paris and Autogenous Cancellous Bone on the Healing of Cortical Defects in the Femurs of Dogs," *Vet Surg*, Vol. 17, pp. 71–76.

[99] Gitelis S., Piasecki P., Turner T., Haggard W., Charters J., and Urban R., "Use of a Calcium Sulfate-based Bone Graft Substitute for Benign Bone Lesions," *Orthopedics*, Vol. 24, 2001, pp.162–166.

[100] Alexander D. I., Manson N. A., and Mitchell M. J., "Efficacy of Calcium Sulfate Plus Decompression Bone in Lumbar and Lumbosacral Spinal Fusion: preliminary results in 40 patients," *Can J Surg*, Vol. 44, 2001, pp. 262–266.

[101] Wilkins R. M., Kelly C. M., and Giusti D. E., "Bioassayed Demineralized Bone Matrix and Calcium Sulfate: use in bone-grafting procedures," *Annales Chirurgiae et Gynaecologiae*, Vol. 88, 1999, pp. 180–185.

[102] Damien C. J., Parsons J. R., Benedict J. J., and Weisman D. S., "Investigation of a Hydroxyapatite and Calcium Sulfate Composite Supplemented with an Osteoinductive Factor," *J Biomed Mat Res*, Vol. 24, 1990, pp. 639–654.

[103] Robinson D., Alk D., Sandbank J., Farber R., and Halperin N., "Inflammatory Reactions Associated with a Calcium Sulfate Bone Substitute," *Ann Transplantation*, Vol. 4, 1999, pp. 91–97.

[104] Urist M. R. and Strates B. S., "Bone Formation in Implants of Partially and Wholly Demineralized Bone Matrix. Including Observations on Acetone-fixed Intra and Extracellular Proteins," *Clin Orthop Rel Res*, Vol. 71, 1970, pp. 271–278.

[105] Urist M. R. and Dawson E., "Intertransverse Process Fusion with the Aid of Chemosterilized Autolyzed Antigen-extracted Allogeneic (AAA) Bone," *Clin Orthop Rel Res*, Vol. 154, 1981, pp. 97–113.

[106] Sampath T. K. and Reddi A. H., "Distribution of Bone Inductive Proteins in Mineralized and Demineralized Extracellular Matrix," *Biochemical Biophysical Res Comm*, Vol. 119, 1984, pp. 949–954.

[107] Rosenthal R. K., Folkman J., and Glowacki J., "Demineralized Bone Implants for Nonunion Fractures, Bone Cysts, and Fibrous Lesions," *Clin Orthop Rel Res*, Vol. 364, 1999, pp. 61–69.

[108] Upton J. and Glowacki J., "Hand Reconstruction with Allograft Demineralized Bone: twenty-six implants in twelve patients," *J Hand Surg*, Vol. 17, 1992, pp. 704–713.

[109] Yamashita K. and Takagi T., "Calcification Preceding New Bone Formation Induced by Demineralized Bone Matrix Gelatin," *Arch Histol Cytol*, Vol. 55, 1992, pp. 31–43.

[110] Lohmann C. H., Andreacchio D., Koster G., Carnes D. L., Jr., Cochran, D. L., Dean D. D., et al., "Tissue Response and Osteoinduction of Human Bone Grafts in Vivo," *Arch Orthop Trauma Surg*, Vol. 121, 2001, pp. 583–590.

[111] Glowacki J. and Cox K. A., "Osteoclastic Features of Cells that Resorb Bone Implants in Rats," *Calcified Tissue Int*, Vol. 39, 1986, pp. 97–103.

[112] Schwartz Z., Somers A., Mellonig J. T., Carnes D. L., Jr., Dean D. D., Cochran D. L., et al., "Ability of Commercial Demineralized Freeze-dried Bone Allograft to Induce New Bone Formation is Dependent on Donor Age But Not Gender," *J Periodontol*, Vol. 69, 1998, pp. 470–478.

[113] Yazdi M., Bernick S., Paule W. J., and Nimni M. E., "Postmortem Degradation of Demineralized Bone Matrix Osteoinductive Potential. Effect of Time and Storage Temperature," *Clin Orthop Rel Res*, Vol. 262, 1991, pp. 281–285.

[114] Russell J. L. and Block J. E., "Clinical Utility of Demineralized Bone Matrix for Osseous Defects, Arthrodesis, and Reconstruction: impact of processing techniques and study methodology," *Orthopedics*, Vol. 22, 1999, pp. 524–531.

[115] Adkisson H. D., Strauss-Schoenberger J., Gillis, M., Wilkins R., Jackson M., and Hruska K. A., "Rapid Quantitative Bioassay of Osteoinduction," *J Orthop Res*, Vol. 18, 2000, pp. 503–511.

[116] Zhang M., Powers R. M., Jr., and Wolfinbarger L., Jr., "A Quantitative Assessment of Osteoinductivity of Human Demineralized Bone Matrix," *J Periodontol*, Vol. 68, 1997, pp.1076–1084.

[117] Schwartz Z., Somers A., Mellonig J. T, Carnes D. L., Jr., Wozney J. M., Dean D. D., et al., "Addition of Human Recombinant Bone Morphogenetic Protein-2 to Inactive Commercial Human Demineralized Freeze-dried Bone Allograft Makes an Effective Composite Bone Inductive Implant Material," *J Periodontol*, Vol. 69, 1998, pp.1337–1345.

[118] Boyan B. D., Weesner T. C., Lohmann C. H., Andreacchio D., Carnes, D. L., Dean D. D., et al., "Porcine Fetal Enamel Matrix Derivative Enhances Bone Formation Induced by Demineralized Freeze Dried Bone Allograft in Vivo," *J Periodontol*, Vol. 71, 2000, pp. 1278–1286.

[119] Ray, J. A., Doddi, N., Regula, D., Williams, J. A., and Melveger, A., "Polydioxanone (PDS), a Novel Monofilament Synthetic Absorbable Suture," *Surg, Gynaecol, Obstet*, Vol. 153, 1981, pp. 497–507.

[120] Hermann J. B., Kelly R. J., and Higgins G. A., "Polyglycolic Acid Sutures," *Arch Surg*, Vol. 100, 1970, pp. 486–490.

[121] Bucholz R. W., Henry S., and Henley M. B., "Fixation with Bioabsorbable Screws for the Treatment of Fractures of the Ankle," *J Bone Joint Surg Am,* Vol. 76, 1994, pp. 319–324.

[122] Athanasiou K. A., Singhal A. R., Agrawal C. M., and Boyan B. D., "In vitro Degradation and Release Characteristics of Biodegradable Implants Containing Trypsin Inhibitor," *Clin Orthop Rel Res*, Vol. 315, 1995, pp. 272–281.

[123] Lu L., Stamatas G. N., and Mikos A. G., "Controlled Release of Transforming Growth Factor Beta 1 From Biodegradable Polymer Microparticles," *J Biomed Mater Res*, Vol. 50, 2000, pp. 440–451.

[124] Oldham J. B., Lu L., Zhu X., Porter B. D., Hefferan T. E., Larson D. R., et al., "Biological Activity of rhBMP-2 Released from PLGA Microspheres," *J Biomechanical Eng*, Vol. 122, 2000, pp. 289–292.

[125] Heckman J. D., Ehler W., Brooks B. P., Aufdemorte T. B., Lohmann C. H., Morgan T., et al., "Bone Morphogenetic Protein but Not Transforming Growth Factor-beta Enhances Bone Formation in Canine Diaphyseal Nonunions Implanted with a Biodegradable Composite Polymer," *J Bone Joint Surg Am*, Vol. 81, 1999, pp. 1717–1729.

[126] Agrawal C. M., Best J., Heckman J. D., and Boyan B. D., "Protein Release Kinetics of a Biodegradable Implant for Fracture Non-unions," *Biomaterials*, Vol. 16, 1995, pp. 1255–1260.

[127] Whang K., Tsai D. C., Nam E. K., Aitken M., Sprague S. M., Patel P. K., et al., "Ectopic Bone Formation via rhBMP-2 Delivery from Porous Bioabsorbable Polymer Scaffolds," *J Biomed Mater Res*, Vol. 42, 1998, pp. 491–499.

[128] Boyan B. D., Lohmann C. H., Somers A., Niederauer G. G., Wozney J. M., Dean D. D., et al., "Potential of Porous Poly-D,L-lactide-co-glycolide Particles as a Carrier for Recombinant Human Bone Morphogenetic Protein-2 During Osteoinduction in Vivo," *J Biomed Mater Res*, Vol. 46, 1999, pp. 51–59.

[129] He S., Yaszemski M. J., Yasko A. W., Engel P. S., and Mikos A. G., "Injectable Biodegradable Polymer Composites Based on Poly (propylene fumarate) Crosslinked with Poly (ethylene glycol)-dimethacrylate," *Biomaterials*, Vol. 21, 2000, pp. 2389–2394.

[130] Vert M., Li, M. S., Spenlehauer G., and Guerin P., "Bioresorbability and Biocompatibility of Aliphatic Polyesters," *J Mater Sci*, Vol. 3, 1992, pp. 432–446.

[131] Bostman O. M. and Pihlajamaki H. K., "Adverse Tissue Reaction to Bioresorbable Fixation Devices," *Clin Orthop Rel Res*, Vol. 371, 2000, p. 216.

[132] Agrawal C. M., McKinney J. S., Lanctot D., and Athanasiou K. A., "Effects of Fluid Flow on the in Vitro Degradation Kinetics of Biodegradable Scaffolds for Tissue Engineering," *Biomaterials*, Vol. 21, 2000, pp. 2443–2452.

[133] Lu L., Peter S. J., Lyman M. D., Lai H. L., Leite S. M., Tamada J. A., et al., "In Vitro and in Vivo Degradation of Porous Poly (DL-lactic-co-glycolic acid) Foams," *Biomaterials*, Vol. 21, 2000, pp. 1837–1845.

[134] Thomson R. C., Yaszemski M. J., Powears J. M., and Mikos A. G., "Hydroxyapatite Fiber Reinforced Poly (alpha-hydroxy ester) Foams for Bone Regeneration," *Biomaterials*, Vol. 19, 1998, pp. 1935–1943.

[135] Agrawal C. M. and Athanasiou K. A., "Technique to Control pH in Vicinity of Biodegrading PLA-PGA Implants," *J Biomed Mater Res*, Vol. 38, 1997, pp. 105–114.

[136] Hutmacher D. W., "Scaffolds in Tissue Engineering Bone and Cartilage," *Biomaterials*, Vol. 21, 2000, pp. 2529–2543.

[137] Lewandrowski K-U., Gresser, J. D., Wise, D. L., and Trantolo, D. J., "Bioresorbable Bone Graft Substitutes of Different Osteoconductivities: a

histologic evaluation of osteointegration of poly(propylene glycol-co-fumaric acid)-based cement implants in rats," *Biomaterials*, Vol. 21, 2000, pp. 757–764.

[138] Whang K., Healy K. E., Elenz D. R., Nam E. K., Tsai D. C., Thomas C. H., et al., "Engineering Bone Regeneration with Bioabsorbable Scaffolds with Novel Microarchitecture," *Tissue Engineering*, Vol. 5, 1999, pp. 35–51.

[139] Suggs L. J. and Mikos A. G., "Development of Poly(propylene fumarate-co-ethylene glycol) as an Injectable Carrier for Endothelial Cells," *Cell Transplant*, Vol. 8, 1999, pp. 345–350.

[140] Murphy W. L., Peters M. C., Kohn D. H., and Mooney D. J., "Sustained Release of Vascular Endothelial Growth Factor from Mineralized Poly(lactide-co-glycolide) Scaffolds for Tissue Engineering," *Biomaterials*, Vol. 21, 2000, pp. 2521–2527.

[141] Lu L., Yaszemski M. J., and Mikos A. G., "TGF-beta1 Release from Biodegradable Polymer Microparticles: its effects on marrow stromal osteoblast function," *J Bone Joint Surg Am,* Vol. 83, Suppl. 1(Pt 2), 2001, pp. S82–91.

[142] Peter S. J., Lu L., Kim D. J., and Mikos A. G., "Marrow Stromal Osteoblast Function on a Poly(propylene fumarate)/beta-tricalcium Phosphate Biodegradable Orthopedic Composite," *Biomaterials*, Vol. 21, 2000, pp. 1207–1213.

Calcium Sulfate-Based Bone Void Substitutes

by Warren O. Haggard, [1] *Ph.D., Kelly C. Richelsoph,* [1] *M.S., and Jack E. Parr,* [1] *Ph.D.*

INTRODUCTION

THE USE OF CALCIUM SULFATE as a bone graft implant has been reported in the clinical literature for more than a century. The history of calcium sulfate usage for both dental and orthopedic applications can be found in reviews by many authors including Bahn, Damien, Hulbert, Mackey, Peltier, and Smith [2,5,10,14,19,23]. A review of the recent development of multiple calcium sulfate bone graft products, their clinical performance, regulatory status, and standard activity will be surveyed and presented.

DEVELOPMENT

The chemical form of calcium sulfate as a bone graft implant or a bone void filler can be found in two primary formulations:

$CaSO_4 \bullet 2\,H_2O$ Calcium Sulfate Dihydrate

$CaSO_4 \bullet \frac{1}{2}\,H_2O$ Calcium Sulfate Hemihydrate

Currently, calcium sulfate-based bone void filler products can be found in two applications that are directly related to the chemical formulations of the calcium sulfate. One type is a bone void filler in a solid shaped morphology, such as a cylindrical pellet. The pellet is composed of calcium sulfate dihydrate. A photograph of this product application is shown in Fig. 1. The second type of clinical product is a bone void filler where calcium sulfate hemihydrate is provided in a powder form, which is intended to be mixed with a diluent of water, saline, or other aqueous liquid and liquid composites to form a paste or putty. The paste or putty can have other additives to improve osteoconductivity, osteoinductivity, and handling or setting characteristics. Upon mixing with the diluent, the calcium sulfate hemihydrate powder will begin conversion into a calcium sulfate dihydrate, producing a paste or putty with a solid structure or partially solid structure. A photograph of this type of product can be found in Fig. 2.

---

[1] Wright Medical Technology, Inc., 5677 Airline Road, Arlington, TN 38002-9501.

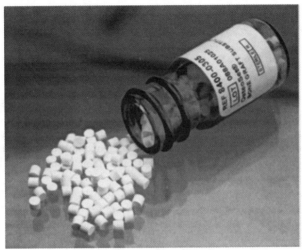

FIG. 1—Calcium sulfate dihydrate pellet.

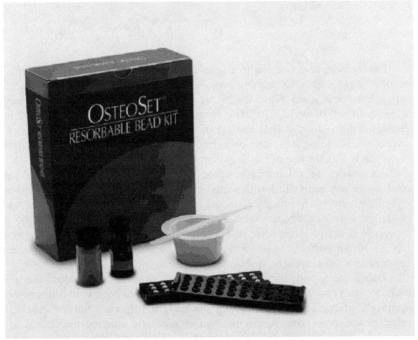

FIG. 2—Calcium sulfate paste/putty product.

Another application of calcium sulfate is as an excipient in an allograft tissue device that has paste or putty characteristics. These products are currently regulated by the Federal Food and Drug Administration (FDA) as allogenic tissue devices. These products may contain human demineralized bone and cancellous bone particles.

Calcium sulfate can be found in a native state as gypsum. Chemically, gypsum is primarily calcium sulfate dihydrate. In its pure form, gypsum is a white crystalline material with a density of 2.31–2.33 g/cc and a Mohs hardness of 1.5–2.0. Gypsum is found in nature in a variety of shapes, forms, and colors, with the most commercially important forms being rock gypsum, alabaster, selenite, satin spar, and gypsite. The most useful property of gypsum is its ability to lose water at elevated temperatures (conversion from a dihydrate to a hemihydrate) and then re-combine with water at low temperatures to re-form the dihydrate [21].

The process of converting from a dihydrate to a hemihydrate is called calcination, where the crushed dihydrate is heated with or without pressure to a temperature exceeding 100°C. The hemihydrate created from the calcination reaction will have different crystalline morphologies and characteristics, depending upon the rate of heating, use of pressure, and incorporation of other chemical additives.

$$CaSO_4 \bullet 2H_2O \xrightarrow[\text{Proprietary Processing}]{\text{Heat}} CaSO_4 \bullet 1/2H_2O$$

| Dihydrate | | Hemihydrate |

Hemihydrate, also referred to as plaster of Paris or stucco, will react with water at ambient temperatures to re-form gypsum. When used as a bone void filler, calcium sulfate acts as a space filler, which restores morphological contour and prevents the ingrowth of soft tissue [2,5,20]. This biomaterial provides an osteoconductive matrix for the ingrowth of blood vessels and osteogenic cells. An important advantage of calcium sulfate is the resorption rate of carefully selected and processed material, which corresponds with the rate of new bone formation [11,25].

Historically, the calcination reaction used to produce calcium sulfate has varied, resulting in calcium sulfate with varied crystalline structures. The use of these varied crystalline materials has resulted in sporadically successful outcomes [3,14]. An example of the hemihydrate crystal structure (surgical-grade) used in a series of clinically successful calcium sulfate bone void filler products with optimized handling is shown in Fig. 3. In comparison, an alternative hemihydrate crystal structure (non-surgical), not optimized for clinical usage, is shown in Fig. 4.

Contaminants and non-uniform crystalline structure can alter the dissolution characteristics and biological response to calcium sulfate bone void fillers and may have negatively affected bone growth and histological response. Special care in material selection and processing of calcium sulfate materials must be maintained to produce consistent bone restoration. The dissolution of calcium sulfate in aqueous solution generates the ions described in the following diagram [17]:

$$CaSO_4 \bullet 2\ H_2O \xrightarrow{\text{aqueous solution}} Ca^{2+},\ SO_4^{2-},\ CaSO_4$$

Calcium sulfate dihydrate

The ions and undissociated calcium sulfate are metabolized or excreted [6].

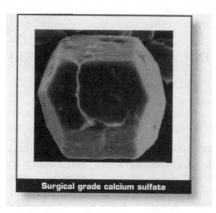

FIG. 3—Controlled crystalline structure found in surgical grade calcium sulfate hemihydrate.

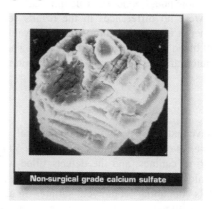

FIG. 4—Irregular crystalline structure found in non-surgical grade calcium sulfate hemihydrate.

The mechanical properties of calcium sulfate material and human bone are given in Table 1. These values are for reference only since bone graft substitutes based on calcium sulfate are not indicated for load bearing applications. Calcium sulfate implants are designed to bioresorb and be replaced by new bone, which will provide mechanical strength for the graft site. Calcium sulfate dihydrate is also naturally radiopaque, which allows X-ray observation of the implant location and its replacement by bone.

TABLE 1—Mechanical properties.

Typical Mechanical Properties	Wet Calcium Sulfate [8]	Dry Calcium Sulfate [8]	Cancellous Bone [12,13]	Cortical Bone [22]
Compressive Strength (psi)	1,500	3,340	800	23,500
Tensile Strength (psi)	300	600	1,000	22,000

PRECLINICAL AND CLINICAL PERFORMANCE

Preclinical

Spinal Applications

The use of calcium sulfate to promote fusions in the spine has been explored in several animal models. Cunningham et al. used a sheep animal model to evaluate the fusion rate at L2-3 and L4-5 of four treatments: decortication alone, autograft, autograft/calcium sulfate pellets in a 1:1 blend, and calcium sulfate pellets alone [4]. The autograft/calcium sulfate pellets combination demonstrated radiographic and bio-mechanical equivalency to autograft alone at two and four months post-op.

Nicodemus et al. used a sheep model to determine the fusion rate of titanium cages filled with either autogenous bone or calcium sulfate [18]. Biomechanically and histologically there were no differences in the results seen with autogenous bone or calcium sulfate. Turner et al. used a canine model to evaluate the use of calcium sulfate alone and in a 50:50 blend with autogenous bone [24]. There were no differences in the fusion rates when autograft was compared to the calcium sulfate/autograft blend. See Fig. 5.

Non-spinal Applications

Turner et al. have extensive experience in animal studies with calcium sulfate materials [25]. In a series of animal studies, large (13 × 50 mm) cylindrical defects were created in the humeri of canines, and the defects filled with calcium sulfate dihydrate pellets, autograft, calcium sulfate pellets containing demineralized bone matrix, or calcium sulfate pellets containing tobramycin sulfate. In all of these studies, the defects healed and were filled with new bone in a manner comparable to autograft. (See Fig. 6.)

In another study, Turner et al. evaluated a putty containing calcium sulfate, demineralized bone matrix, and cancellous bone chips to heal defects created in the canine humerus. When compared to an unfilled control, the putty was shown to heal the defects, with new bone formation present at the DBM margins [26].

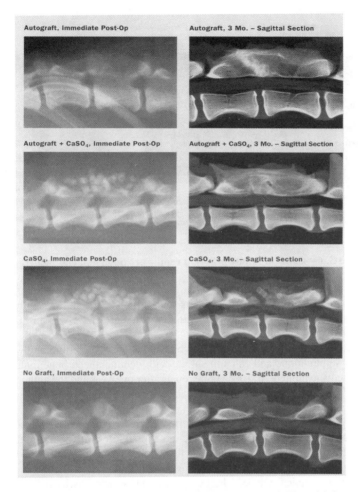

FIG. 5—Calcium sulfate pellet and autograft blend (50:50 ratio) in canine spinal fusion model.

Clinical

Numerous published papers attest to the successful usage of calcium sulfate in clinical applications. Alexander et al. [1], in a randomized prospective clinical trial, compared the results of calcium sulfate dihydrate pellets with local autograft to iliac crest autograft in lumbar and lumbosacral spinal fusion. The authors found that calcium sulfate was an effective extender to local bone, providing bone formation equivalent to autologous iliac crest bone in the majority of patients.

Kelly et al. reported on a study of 109 patients in a non-randomized prospective study where calcium sulfate (alone and mixed with DBM, bone marrow aspirate, and autograft)

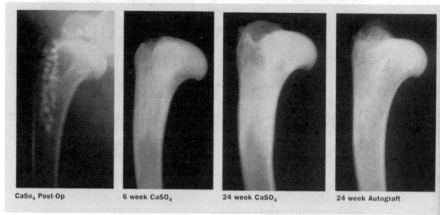

CaSo₄ Post-Op   6 week CaSO₄   24 week CaSO₄   24 week Autograft

FIG. 6—Calcium sulfate pellets in canine proximal humeral model.

was used in bone defects caused by trauma, periprosthetic bone loss, tumor, or fusion [11]. In this study, resorption of the pellets and filling of the defects with bone was demonstrated, leading the author to conclude that calcium sulfate was an effective and convenient bone graft substitute.

Gitelis et al. [9] reported on 23 patients who had benign bone lesions and were treated with calcium sulfate alone and calcium sulfate with demineralized bone matrix. In this study, 21 patients exhibited 76–100% bone repair after one year and the author concluded that calcium sulfate is a reasonable alternative to autogenous bone graft for benign legions.

In another study on the use of calcium sulfate to treat benign bone lesions, Mirzayan et al. [16] reported on 13 patients where calcium sulfate dihydrate pellets had been used to fill a variety of defects. In this study, all defects healed in an average of 13.4 weeks and the authors concluded that the material was an acceptable alternative to autograft.

In all of these clinical studies, the use of calcium sulfate has been found to be an effective bone graft substitute, either alone, or as extender to autograft.

Multiple clinical products are available in both the dihydrate and hemihydrate form of calcium sulfate. A list of some of these clinical products with their regulatory status can be found in Table 2. Representative clinical cases with these products are shown in Figs. 7 and 8.

STANDARD ACTIVITY

A draft standard on calcium sulfate as an implant material is being currently reviewed by the Ceramic Subcommittee of ASTM Division 04. The contents of the current draft standard are the trace element compositions, overall composition and purity and suggested evaluation methods for calcium sulfate implant materials and finished components.

TABLE 2—Calcium sulfate based bone void filler products.

Chemical Formulation	Product Shape/Morphology	Additives	Trade Name	Company	Regulatory Approval
$CaSO_4 \bullet 2H_2O$	Cylindrical Pellet	None	OSTEOSET®	Wright Medical Technology	510(k)
$CaSO_4 \bullet 2H_2O$	"Jack" Shaped	None	JAX™	Smith & Nephew	510(k)
$CaSO_4 \bullet 2H_2O$	Cylindrical Pellet	None	STIMULAN®	BioComposites	510(k)
$CaSO_4 \bullet 2H_2O$	Cylindrical Pellet	None	CALCEON™ 6	Synthes	510(k)
$CaSO_4 \bullet 2H_2O$	Cylindrical Pellet	None	PROFUSION™	Biogeneration	510(k)
$CaSO_4 \bullet 1/2 H_2O$	Kit with powder and diluent, transforms to a hardened shape	None	Resorbable Bead Kit	Wright Medical Technology	510 (k)
$CaSO_4 \bullet 1/2 H_2O$	Kit with powder and diluent, transforms to a hardened shape	None	BONE PLAST™	Interpore Cross	510(k)
$CaSO_4 \bullet 1/2 H_2O$	Kit with powder and diluent, transforms to a hardened shape	None	MIIG™ 115	Wright Medical Technology	510(k)

TABLE 3— Allogenic tissue products with calcium sulfate.

Chemical Formulation	Product Shape/Morphology	Major Component	Trade Name	Company	Regulatory Approval
$CaSO_4 \bullet 1/2 H_2O$	Kit with powder and diluent, transforms into a putty	Demineralized Bone Matrix	ALLOMATRIX® Injectable Putty	Wright Medical Technology	Classified as an allogenic tissue device by FDA in 2002
$CaSO_4 \bullet 1/2 H_2O$	Kit with powder and diluent, transforms into a putty	Demineralized Bone Matrix, Cancellous Bone	ALLOMATRIX® Injectable Putty-C, DR and Custom	Wright Medical Technology	Classified as an allogenic tissue device by FDA in 2002

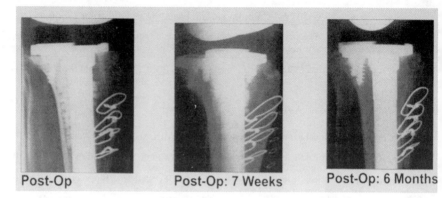

FIG. 7— Proximal tibia revision knee surgery with calcium sulfate pellets.

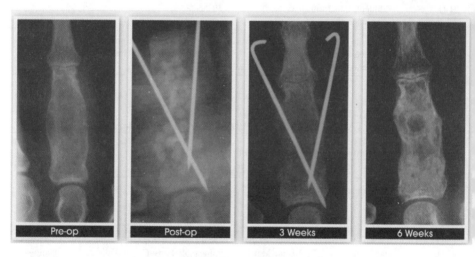

FIG. 8—Aneurysmal bone cyst of the middle phalanx surgery with calcium sulfate pellets and ALLOMATRIX® Injectable Putty.

DISCUSSION

Calcium sulfate has been found to be effective as a bone graft material, carrier, or extender of other bone graft materials. With continued research and development, the clinical uses for calcium sulfate-based products can be expanded and enhanced. The unique characteristic of calcium sulfate resorption in conjunction with bone formation continues to be investigated preclinically and clinically, and defined with standards development.

REFERENCES

[1]   Alexander D. I., Manson N. A., and Mitchell M. J., "Efficacy of Calcium Sulfate Plus Decompression Bone in Lumbar and Lumbosacral Spinal Fusion: Preliminary Results in 40 patients," *Can J Surg*, Vol. 44, 2001, pp. 262–266.

[2]   Bahn S., "Plaster: A bone substitute," *Oral Surg, Oral Med Oral Pathol*, Vol. 21, 1966, pp. 672–681.

[3]   Coetzee A. S., "Regeneration of Bone in the Presence of Calcium Sulfate," *Arch Otolaryngol*, Vol. 106, 1980, pp. 405–409.

[4]   Cunningham B., Oda I., Sefter J. C., Buckley R., Geobel M., Haggerty C. J., Fedder I. L. and McAfee P. C., "An Investigational Study of Calcium Sulfate for Posterolateral Spinal Arthrodesis—An In-Vivo Animal Model," NASS Abstracts, 13th Annual Meeting, San Francisco, 28–31 October, 1998, pp. 216–217.

[5]   Damien C. and Parsons J. R., "Bone Graft and Bone Graft Substitutes: A review of current technology and applications," *J Appl Biomater*, Vol. 2, 1991, pp. 187–208.

[6]   DeWet I. S. and Jansen C., "The Use of Plaster of Paris to Fill Large Defects in Bone," *South African J Surg*, Vol. 11, 1973, pp. 1–8.

[7]   Dreesmann H., "Ueber knochenplombierung," *Beitr Klin Chir*, Vol. 9, 1892, pp. 804–810.

[8]   Earnshaw R. and Smith D. C., "The Tensile and Compressive Strength of Plaster and Stone," *Aus Dental J*, Vol. 11, 1966, pp. 415–422.

[9]   Gitelis S., Piaseki P., Turner T., Haggard W., Charters J., and Urban R., "Use of a Calcium Sulfate-Based Bone Graft Substitute for Benign Bone Lesions," *Orthopedics*, Vol. 24, 2001, pp. 162–166.

[10] Hulbert S. F., "History of Bioceramics," *Ceramics Int*, Vol. 8, 1982, pp. 131–140.

[11] Kelly C. M., Wilkins, R. M., Gitelis, S., Hartjen, C., Watson, J. T., and Kim, P. T., "The Use of a Surgical Grade Calcium Sulfate as a Bone Graft Substitute," *Clin Orthop Rel Res*, Vol. 382, 2001, pp. 42–50.

[12] Lee R. W., Volz R. G., and Sheridan D. C., "The Role of Fixation and Bone Quality on the Mechanical Stability of Tibial Knee Components," *Clin Orthop Rel Res*, Vol. 273, 1991, pp. 177–183.

[13] Linde F., Hvid I., and Pongsoipeetch B., "Energy Absorptive Properties of Human Trabecular Bone Specimens During Axial Compression," *J Orthop Res*, Vol. 7, 1989, pp. 432–439.

[14] Mackey D., Varlet A., and Debeaumont D., "Antibiotic Loaded Plaster of Paris Pellets: An in vitro study of a possible method of local antibiotic therapy in bone infection," *Clin Orthop Rel Res*, Vol. 167, 1982, pp. 263–268.

[15] McGee P., "Calcium Sulfate Demonstrates Efficacy for Spinal Fusion in Sheep," *Orthopedics Today*, Vol. 19, 1999.

[16] Mirzayan R., Panossian V., Avedian R., Forrester D. M., and Menendez L. R., "The Use of Calcium Sulfate in the Treatment of Benign Bone Lesions," *J Bone Joint Surg Am,* Vol. 83, 2001, pp. 355–358.

[17] Nakayama F. and Rasnick B., "Calcium Electrode Method for Measuring Dissociation and Solubility of Calcium Sulfate Dihydrate," *Ann Chem*, Vol. 39, 1967, pp. 1022–1023.

[18] Nicodemus C., Simmons J., Hadjipavlou A., Yang J., and Simmons D., "Lumbar Spine Stabilization With Osteoconductive and Osteoinductive Graft Materials in Mature Sheep," Abstract, *Presented at the North American Spine Society Meeting*, 1997, p. 20.

[19] Peltier L. F., "The Use of Plaster of Paris to Fill Defects in Bone," *Clin Orthop Rel Res*, Vol. 21, 1961, pp. 1–31.

[20] Peltier L. F. and Speer D. P., "Calcium Sulfate," *Bone Grafts and Bone Substitutes*, W. B. Saunders, Philadelphia, PA, 1992, pp. 243–251.

[21] Randolph, D. A., "Gypsum," *Encyclopedia of Industrial Chemical Analysis*, Vol. 14, 1971, John Wiley & Sons, pp. 87–102.

[22] Reilly D. and Burstein A. H., "The Mechanical Properties of Cortical Bone," *J Bone Joint Surg Am*, Vol. 56, 1974, pp. 1001–1022.

[23] Smith D., "Implantation of Plaster of Paris of Recontouring and Regeneration of Alveoli, " *Dental Students' Magazine*, November 1966, pp. 121–166.

[24] Turner T. M., Urban R. M., Andersson G. B. J., Lawrence A. M., Igloria, R.V., Haggard W.O., et al., "Spinal Fusion Using Synthetic Bone Graft Calcium Sulfate Compared to Autogenous Bone in a Canine Model," *Tran Soc Biomaterials*, Vol. 22, 1999, p. 90.

[25] Turner T. M., Urban R. M., Gitelis S., Kuo K. N., and Andersson G. B. J., "Radiographic and Histologic Assessment of Calcium Sulfate in Experimental Animal Models and Clinical Use as a Resorbable Bone-Graft Substitute, a Bone-Graft Expander, and a Method for Local Antibiotic Delivery: One institution's experience," *J Bone Joint Surg Am*, Vol. 83, 2001, pp. 355–358.

[26] Turner T. M., Urban R. M., Hall D. J., Infanger S., Lawrence-Smith A. M., Gitelis S., et al., "Injectable Calcium Sulfate-Based Putty for the Delivery of DBM and Cancellous Bone Chips, *Tran Soc Biomaterials,* Vol. 25, 2002, p. 221.

The Development of Coralline Porous Ceramic Graft Substitutes

by Edwin C. Shors,[1] Ph.D.

INTRODUCTION

BONE, UNLIKE MOST TISSUES, HAS a unique ability to regenerate, reforming completely without a scar. Surgeons have learned over the centuries to capitalize on this natural and invaluable attribute for the repair of large defects or to generate bone where it does not normally form. Autograft is the undisputed "gold standard" today for generating or regenerating bone. Over 250,000 autograft procedures are performed annually for orthopedic and neurosurgical treatments in the United States alone. However, autografting is not without disadvantages. Clinical studies show that it causes increased donor site morbidity to the patient, such as pain, blood loss, and scarring [1]. In addition, harvesting bone adds additional operating room time to the procedure. Further, the volume or quantity of autograft may be limited. Therefore, other bone grafting materials have been developed.

The conventional wisdom attributes three biological processes to the efficacy of autografting: osteogenesis, growth factors, and osteoconduction. These processes constitute the Triad of Tissue Regeneration. Osteogenesis is the process by which bone grows directly from living cells. For a bone graft, these are cells from the donor site, which are transplanted to the host site. The transplanted cells are also supplemented with and eventually replaced by host cells that migrate into the bone graft site. This migration and proliferation of bone cells is stimulated by the local release of growth factors, chemotactic factors and mitogens. It may also be complemented by morphogens which trigger the osteoinduction or conversion of pluripotential cells to form bone. A third process is osteoconduction. It is the process whereby bone cells grow into and along the surface of a biocompatible structure. The living, "conductive" cells migrate from the host bone or from the donor cells in the autograft. Osteoconduction has three requirements that must always be achieved. First, the implant must be placed in direct apposition to host bone, generally within 1–2 mm. Secondly, the host bone must be viable. Conditions that decrease viability are vascular impairment, infection, radiation and metabolic bone diseases. Therefore, viability is supported by the ingrowth of neovascular tissues, which nourish the regenerated bone. Thirdly, the construct must be stable, without significant macromotion. The dependence of osteoconduction on

---

[1] Research and New Technology, Interpore Cross International, 181 Technology Drive, Irvine, CA 92618.

proximity to surrounding cells, viability of these cells and stability of the tissues and implant in relationship to each other is the Triad of Osteoconduction [2] (Fig.1).

Bone grafting materials and techniques in use today have adopted the Triad of Bone Regeneration in varying degrees. The ideal bone graft may require all three processes. However, evidence accumulated over the past two decades indicates that there are clinical cases, which can be successfully treated strictly with osteoconductive implants, as long as all three components of the Triad of Osteoconduction are achieved. One such implant is derived from coral. However, the implant is not coral. Instead, it is processed from coral and, therefore, called coralline. The purpose of this chapter is to summarize the development, material properties, experimental and clinical experience with coralline porous ceramics used as implants for bone regeneration.

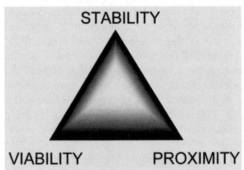

STABILITY

VIABILITY   **PROXIMITY**

FIG. 1—Triad of Osteoconduction. The three essential processes for osteoconduction are proximity of the implant to surrounding bone, viability of the osteogenic cells that grow into the porosity, and stability of the interface between the implant and the surrounding bone.

ORIGIN OF CORALLINE PROCESS

The concept of converting coral to useful bone grafting materials was developed at Pennsylvania State University more than two decades ago [3]. It was a case of serendipity, fortuitous collaborations and insight into both biology and materials sciences. It was not the creation of a single, omniscient inventor, who recognized the similarity of coral to cancellous bone. Instead, it shows the more typical creative process, which often germinates when divergent expertise from a team converges. In this case, a professor of materials sciences at Pennsylvania State University was developing instrumentation for materials characterization using scanning electron microscopes (SEM). A friend and colleague in Marine Geology proposed looking under the SEM at marine invertebrates because some of them have predictable interconnected porosity. A medical student working in the laboratory recognized the similarity of some corals to porous ceramics and metals, which were being developed for bone ingrowth. The three inventors fabricated negative replicates of the structures in metal, ceramics and polymers, using a variation of the "lost wax" technology. They also made positive replicates of coral by a direct conversion of its calcium carbonate to calcium phosphate [4]. This has now become the basis for a family of osteoconductive materials, trade named Pro Osteon™ (Interpore Cross, Irvine, CA).

MANUFACTURING PROCESS

The stony corals, phylogenetically called scleractinia, are a large family with hundreds of genera [5]. A limited number of these genera have significant porosity. An even more limited number have interconnected porosity. Two genera have been identified as having porosity in the range that is optimal for bone conduction. They grow in abundance and in large, boulder-like forms that are amenable for manufacturing into blocks or granules. One of the genera is *Goniopora* and the other is *Porites* (Fig. 2). *Goniopora* coral has pores of approximately 500 microns and a porosity of approximately 65%. *Porites* has pore diameters of approximately 200 microns and a porosity of approximately 50%.

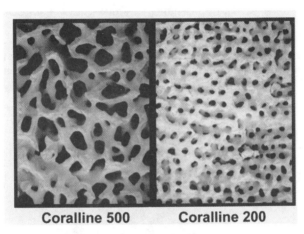

Coralline 500   Coralline 200

FIG. 2—Microstructures. Scanning electron micrographs of coralline porous implants made with 500 micron pores (left) and with 200 micron pores (right). Note the interconnected porosity and the relative densities of the two materials, accounting for the higher strength of coralline 200 implants.

The calcium carbonate skeleton of specific marine corals is converted to hydroxyapatite, the mineral component of bone, using temperature, water and a phosphate donor (Fig. 3). This hydrothermal exchange reaction is a solid-state and topotactic reaction (i.e., progressive conversion on the calcium carbonate surface). Therefore, it preserves the inherent interconnected porosity of the original coral structure. The carbonate is directly replaced with phosphate. A modification of the original process was recently introduced. It is manufactured using a partial conversion of the coral such that all of the internal porous surfaces are transformed to calcium phosphate, leaving the core of the trabecular struts as calcium carbonate (Trade name Pro Osteon 500R or Pro Osteon 200R). The thickness of this calcium phosphate layer is several microns (Fig. 4). However, it is adequately thick to retard the rapid resorption of calcium carbonate by osteoclasts. The thickness of this calcium phosphate layer can therefore directly control the resorption rate of the implant. The rationale for a resorbable form is three-fold. It eases the post-operative diagnosis of bone formation using conventional radiographic, CT and densitometry techniques [6–8]. It increases the available space for bone formation. Lastly, it decreases the rare potential for long term complications. However, it is vitally important that the implant not resorb before it has served its function as an osteo-conductive matrix and provided biomechanical support. For some indications, such as identifying recurrent tumors, the hydroxyapatite form may be preferential.

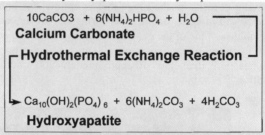

$$10CaCO_3 + 6(NH_4)_2HPO_4 + H_2O$$

Calcium Carbonate

Hydrothermal Exchange Reaction

$$Ca_{10}(OH)_2(PO_4)_6 + 6(NH_4)_2CO_3 + 4H_2CO_3$$

Hydroxyapatite

FIG. 3—Hydrothermal exchange reaction. Calcium carbonate is converted directly to calcium phosphate in the form of hydroxyapatite supplied from a phosphate donor in the presence of heat and water.

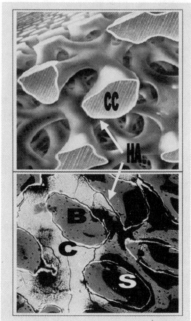

FIG. 4—Resorbable Pro Osteon™. An artist rendition illustrates the interconnected porosity with a thin layer of hydroxyapatite on calcium carbonate. (top). A scanning electron micrograph shows regenerated bone growing into the pores and the calcium carbonate significantly resorbing with bone growing into that space, as well (bottom).

The relatively high temperature and long processing time of the hydrothermal reaction, the caustic environment of phosphate solution and the inherently minimal amount of organics within the calcium carbonate of the original coral assure that there are no antigenic components in the implant. The chemical stability and durability of calcium-based ceramics allows the implant to be terminally sterilized with high dose, gamma sterilization or conventional steam sterilization.

PHYSICAL PROPERTIES

The interconnectivity of the porosity with optimal pore diameters for bone ingrowth in coralline ceramics is the key and unique property that cannot be made by any other known synthetic method. Using a hydrothermal process, two implant materials have been developed: Pro Osteon 200 and Pro Osteon 500 porous hydroxyapatite. They have average pore diameters of 200 and 500 microns and average porosity of 50% and 65%, respectively. The large surface area relative to its volume is critical for bone osteointegration [9]. The physical parameters, including surface area as estimated by histomorphometry and inert gas absorption, are provided in Table 1. This high surface area accounts for the higher than expected resorption rate of coralline hydroxyapatite, compared to sintered materials. It also accounts for the osteoconductive properties, providing a large internal surface for bone formation.

TABLE 1—Physical properties of coralline ceramics.

	Coralline 500 μm (HA and Resorbable)	Coralline 200 μm (HA and Resorbable)
Interconnectivity	Complete	Complete
Pore Diameter, Average	500 μm	200 μm
Pore Diameter, Range	270–880 μm	180–220 μm
Porosity, Average	65%	50%
Porosity, Range	60–70%	45–55%
Density	0.8 gm/cc	1.3 gm/cc
Compressive Strength, Average	6 MPa	10 MPa
Tensile Strength, Average	1 MPa	2 MPa
Surface Area (atomic)	1.5 m^2/gm	2.0 m^2/gm
Surface Area (morphometric)	5.3 mm^2/mm^3	8.0 mm^2/mm^3
Forms	Blocks and Granules	Blocks and Granules

The mechanical properties of the block form of porous hydroxyapatite are important if a bone graft substitute is to be used for mechanical support. The main goal of the surgeon when using coralline porous ceramic is to set up an environment for bone incorporation within the pores of the implant. This includes having the implant in direct apposition to the host bone and to minimize motion at the interface between the bones and implant. Long term, the regenerated bone that grows into and onto the pores of the ceramic must provide the mechanical strength. Nevertheless, in the short term, the implant must not collapse or subside into the host bone. The mechanical properties of coralline implants are similar to cancellous bone: compressive strength for Pro Osteon 200 is approximately 10 MPa, whereas the compressive strength of Pro Osteon 500 is 6 MPa and its modulus is 2.5 GPa [10]. Wittenberg et al. tested the compressive force of various bone graft materials, including coralline porous hydroxyapatite [11]. They found that the more dense material, i.e., Pro Osteon 200 HA, was as strong as anterior or posterior iliac crest corticocancellous bone graft. Even though Pro Osteon 200 has less porosity (approximately 50%), there is adequate available room for regeneration of mature cancellous bone. Clearly, these results should not be overextended. Compressive strength is only one mode of loading. Ceramics have low tensile strength and poor impact properties, as manifested by their brittleness. In contrast, bone, because of its collagen component, is tough. Therefore, it is imperative for long term durability of the construct that bone grows into the porous hydroxyapatite. These ceramic implants are not designed to be permanent mechanical constructs. They are a temporary trellis for bone regeneration.

CHEMICAL PROPERTIES

The conventional method for characterizing the chemistry of a ceramic is to use X-ray powder diffraction (Fig. 5). Coralline porous ceramics can be completely or partially converted to calcium phosphate, by adjusting the degree of conversion (Table 2). The conversion of calcium phosphate is a solid-state reaction, occurring from the surface of the calcium carbonate inward. After complete conversion, more than 95% of the calcium phosphate is in the form of hydroxyapatite. A trace of either tricalcium phosphate or whitlockite may also be present. The conversion is a relatively low temperature process, unlike most ceramic processing. As a consequence, the crystallites are relatively small, approximately 1 micron, and cause significant line broadening of the X-ray pattern. The crystallite size is approximately an order of magnitude smaller than that found in high temperature, sintered ceramics. Although an order of magnitude larger than bone crystals, the relative smaller crystallite size, in part, may cause the relatively faster resorption of coralline implants compared to sintered ceramics. Another contributing factor may be the substitution of some carbonate apatite into the structure. This substitution makes coralline ceramics more similar to bone apatite than conventional, synthetic ceramics. Although the small crystallite size, carbonated apatite structure, and high surface area of the interconnected porosity account for the resorption that does occur with coralline hydroxyapatite, there is a clinician need for an even more resorbable ceramic. This stimulated the development of a composite coralline implant, now called Pro Osteon™ 500R and Pro Osteon™ 200R. The "R" indicates it is highly resorbable.

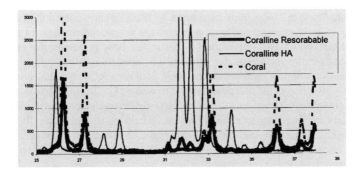

FIG. 5—X-ray Diffraction of Coralline Implants. XRD patterns are for coral composed of calcium carbonate in the form of aragonite (dashed line), coralline implant completely converted to hydroxyapatite (thin line) and resorbable coralline implant consisting of aragonite and a minority component of hydroxyapatite (thick line).

TABLE 2—Chemical properties of coralline ceramics.

	Coralline HA (200 µm and 500 µm)	Coralline Resorbable (200 µm and 500 µm)
Osteoconductive	Yes	Yes
Interconnectivity	Yes	Yes
Calcium Phosphate Content	100%	15%
Calcium Phosphate Layer on Interface Surface	No layer, completely converted to HA	2–10 microns
Resorption Rate	Months to years	Weeks to Months

The resorbable form has a layer of hydroxyapatite on all the internal surfaces of the implant. This layer has a chemical composition identical to the completely converted material. Under this layer, the original calcium carbonate is unconverted, remaining as aragonite. This is seen in the X-ray diffraction pattern. The composition of the entire implant is approximately 15% calcium phosphate; however, the layer of calcium phosphate is only about 2–10 microns.

ANIMAL STUDIES

Osteoconduction

Coralline ceramics are completely biocompatible. They are without antigens. Because they are made of the same materials as the mineral content of bone, they are not seen by the body as being foreign. Consequently, this property facilitates bone conduction and bone bonding by osteoblasts and osteocytes. Moreover, it has a microstructure that is strikingly similar to that of cancellous bone and composed of the same chemistry as that of the mineral content of bone. When placed next to bone, the osteoconductive process promotes bone regeneration within and throughout the porosity. This is the definition of osteoconduction. That is, the bone preferentially grows on and intimately bonds to the surface of the implant. Studies using a variety of biomaterials, including metals, ceramics, and polymers, have consistently shown that pore diameters must be 100–500 microns for osteoconduction to occur [4]. Therefore, two pore sizes of coralline implants were developed. Osteoclasts resorb bone in part by dissolving the mineral content by secreting an acidic solution. These cells, then, have the capacity to resorb the calcium salts of the coralline implants. Osteoclasts lacunae can be seen, apparently dissolving the surface. They resorb the hydroxyapatite, but at a slow rate. They can resorb the calcium carbonate at a faster rate.

Trauma Models

Osteoconduction and resorption of coralline hydroxyapatite was shown by repairing clinically relevant defects in the metaphysis and the diaphysis of dogs [12,13]. Histometry using a scanning electron microscope with a backscatter electron detector (SEM-BSE) was validated and then used to quantify bone regeneration within the porosity [14]. SEM-BSE histometry can determine the volume fraction of implant, bone, and soft tissue and it can determine the surface area of the implant covered by bone. Histometry was used to calculate the volume fraction of implant, bone and soft tissue at intervals of 1, 2, 3, 4, and 12 months. The volume fraction of bone was approximately 10% at one month for both groups. In metaphyseal sites, the volume fraction averaged 17% at one year. However, the volume fraction of bone for the same type of material when placed in cortical defects increased to 55% at one year. Further, no statistical resorption occurred when coralline implants were used to reconstruct metaphyseal defects, yet 25% of the implant resorbed when used to reconstruct cortical defects. The osteoconductive property of the coralline implants was proven because more than 50–55% of the surface area was covered by bone [13]. These results demonstrate an appropriate biological response to Pro Osteon in accordance with Wolff's Law. The biomechanics of the reconstructed radius was completely restored. Further, histometry showed that the strength of the reconstruction was exponentially related to the volume fraction of bone.

Spinal Fusion Models

Coralline porous hydroxyapatite has been evaluated for anterior interbody spine fusion. Dawson was the first to implant blocks into intervertebral space of the lumbar spine in beagle dogs [15]. He found that bone grew throughout the porosity. He reported incomplete resorption of the implant at one year, which may be a benefit in this application. He further concluded that the implant's lack of antigenic potential and uniform pore size makes it a potentially ideal bone graft substitute. Porous hydroxyapatite has been experimentally tested for cervical fusion [16]. Zdeblick et al. reported the histologic, radiographic and biomechanical outcomes after using porous hydroxyapatite (500) blocks for cervical fusion in goats at 12 weeks [16]. The hydroxyapatite group was compared to sham, autograft, and allograft. Each of the groups was analyzed to determine the effects from anterior plating, as well. The results indicated that using a rigid plate was vital for bone incorporation regardless of the implant material. However, the biomechanical stiffness of the spine after grafting with porous hydroxyapatite was lower than after autografting. This study and other studies have shown the importance of achieving limited motion at the interface between the porous hydroxyapatite and the surrounding host bone [17]. Recently, the use of coralline material in a rigid interbody fusion cage allowed for complete bone formation without the addition of autograft [18].

Porous hydroxyapatite has been used on the posterior spine, as well. Holmes et al. used porous hydroxyapatite (IP200 HA) blocks as large "match sticks" to perform posterior mass fusion on dogs [19]. After decorticating the facets and lamina, the blocks were layered between the transverse processes and against the facets, similar to constructing a brick wall. They compared the histological performance at 3, 6, 12, and 24 months using this osteoconductive porous ceramic to autograft derived from the spinous process. It is very important to recognize that no fixation or immobilization was used for either grafting material. The failure for bone regeneration and fusion in either model (implant or autograft) must be largely attributed to the lack of rigid fixation used in this model.

For all clinical application, but especially posterior lateral fusion, it is vital to recall the Triad of Osteoconduction. Osteoconduction can only be achieved if all three components (i.e., proximity, viability, and stability) are successfully met. Therefore, it is incumbent on the surgeon to use osteoconductive materials only when appropriate. If the condition cannot be met, then it should not be used or the appropriate condition must be made available. This typically requires the addition of either bone cells and/or growth factors. The bone cells can be obtained from autograft, bone marrow or other stem cells. The growth factors can be autologous, allogenic, xenogenic or recombinant. Coralline implants have been shown to respond favorably to combinational therapy.

Contrary to conventional thinking, bone can form within coralline hydroxyapatite even without direct apposition to surrounding bone or the addition of either cells or growth factors. It has been seen in dogs, baboons, monkeys, and even humans [20–22]. It is rarely seen in small animals. The explanation for this phenomenon remains elusive, but it is theorized that it may be due to the unique protein binding properties of hydroxyapatite. The bone is limited in quantity and late forming; therefore it is more an academic curiosity than a clinical therapy.

Osteoconduction and Osteogenesis

Bone Graft and Bone Marrow

Posterior lumbar fusion represents an environment that is extremely challenging for a purely osteoconductive material. The amount of surrounding bone is limited generally to only the decorticated inferior surface of the fusion mass. It is aggravated by the long span of fusion mass required to bridge from one transverse process level to the next transverse process. Lastly, it is further compromised by the relative instability even with posterior instrumentation to rely solely on osteoconduction. The rabbit model for posterior lumbar fusion without instrumentation has been widely used to test various implants materials, including coralline implants. Used alone without autograft, coralline implants were unsuccessful. However, when mixed 1:1 with autograft, fusion rates were equivalent to autograft alone. The addition of bone marrow cells, rather than bone autograft, has had contradictory results [23]. In small animals and in vitro using both syngeneic bone marrow and human marrow in nude rats, bone marrow has been shown to form abundant bone within coralline implants [24,25]. Therefore, the potential for the clinical use of bone marrow is high.

Recently, a sheep model for posterior lateral spine fusion using pedicle screw fixation was reported using coralline implants [26,27]. The model was a two level lumbar fusion from L3 to L5 with 30 cc of graft material. The model was validated by comparing the biomechanical stiffness at 5 months of an autograft group with a sham control group. Two experimental groups were then tested: porous hydroxyapatite granules alone and porous hydroxyapatite mixed 1:1 with autograft harvested from local bone. Coralline porous hydroxyapatite granules alone improved the stiffness over sham controls and they were not significantly different from autograft alone. However, mixing the synthetic bone graft substitute with autograft improved the stiffness further. These results show the efficacy of recruiting hosts cells into the construct. Perhaps, more importantly, when the resorbable coralline granules were mixed with local bone, the fusion was superior to autograft and significant resorption of the implant occurred.

Osteoconduction and Growth Factors

Growth factors are proteins with one of three functions. They can be chemotactic, recruiting cells into the implants; they can be mitogenic, causing the proliferation of existing cells: or they can be morphogenic, initiating the conversion of stem cells to mature, tissue specific cells. Using contemporary technology, they can be derived using one of three methods. Growth factors can be purified and concentrated from the patient, for example from the buffy coat (i.e., platelets and white cells) in peripheral blood. They can also be purified and concentrated from the bone of the same species or another species. They can be produced using recombinant molecular engineering for direct inoculation or indirectly from cells using gene therapy. Coralline implants have been evaluated and shown to have increased bone formation using each of these technologies.

Coralline implants have been shown to be effective for an instrumented, spinal fusion sheep model when combined with bone marrow and platelet derived growth factors. Chemotactic and mitogenic factors, such as TGF-beta, PDGF, FGF, IGF, and FGF were able to increase the levels of endogenous BMP resulting in increased biomechanical stiffness of the construct. "Autologous growth factors" from human blood were shown also to be effective for increasing both the bone formation and soft tissue formation in bone chambers installed in nude rats [28].

Coralline hydroxyapatite has been used very effectively with allograft. The most effective allograft has been demineralized bone matrix, which has particles sufficiently small to percolate into the interconnected porosity [29,30].

Xenogenic, purified growth factors combined with coralline implants are also a potentially viable therapy. A soup of growth factors, including bone morphogenic proteins was purified from cow bone and shown to be active in a variety of clinically relevant models when inoculated and freeze dried onto the internal surface of the coralline implants [31–33]. In the rabbit posterior lateral model, the fusion rates were superior to autograft [34]. The regenerated bone typically grows uniformly throughout the implant rather than from the surrounding bone as seen when autograft is used.

Mitogenic growth factors, including basic FGF, PDGF, and TGF-beta, have been shown to increase the osteogenic response in the porosity of coralline ceramics [35–37]. Bone proteins have been made using recombinant techniques and inoculated into the pores of coralline implants [38]. The bone forms directly on the internal surface of the implant. Apparently, the added bone increases the resorption rate of the implant. The efficacy of recombinant proteins with coralline implants is now well accepted in a variety of animal models.

CLINICAL STUDIES

Coralline implants have been proven to be biocompatible, osteoconductive, and resorbable in a variety of experimental animal models. These attributes have also been shown in human clinical trials in a variety of applications, including plastic, oral, periodontal and orthopedic surgery [39–45]. Controlled clinical studies began in 1982 to substantiate the safety and efficacy of the coralline hydroxyapatite (Pro Osteon 500 hydroxyapatite) for the repair of long bone defects under an investigational device exemption and subsequent pre-market approval [46]. These clinical studies clearly indicate its safety and efficacy as a bone graft substitute for the repair of long bone fractures. The clinical trials consisted of 167 patients with 174 defects enrolled at nine clinical centers. The study patients had defects caused by fractures, cysts/tumors, and delayed unions and non-unions. The locations included diaphyseal and metaphyseal bones. Clinical effectiveness was evaluated for degree of pain, weight bearing, functional impairment and radiographically (Fig. 6). The median time to clinical and radiographic healing was approximately 4.5 months, which was not significantly different from a concurrent control population receiving autograft. Histological and histometric evaluation of biopsy specimens was also performed on 25 patients reconstructed with coralline hydroxyapatite at a mean post-operative time of 14 months [47]. This provided a unique opportunity to evaluate the healed implant/bone composite in humans. The volume fraction of new bone in the implant averaged 34%, with the remainder of the volume being occupied by the Pro Osteon implant (31%) and soft tissue (35%). The osteointegration index was 55%. These biopsies provide conclusive evidence of the effectiveness of the Pro Osteon 500 as a scaffold material for bony ingrowth with direct contact of bone tissue to the implant surface. Biopsy specimens were also analyzed to determine the rate of implant degradation (Fig. 7). Linear regression of the volume fraction of implant versus time indicates that the rate of resorption is between 5–10% per year. These results indicate that coralline in the slowly resorbing hydroxyapatite form is suitable for use as a bone graft substitute in the reconstruction of long bone defects. More recent studies have indicated that the resorbable form is also appropriate for long bone defects (Fig. 8).

These results have been substantiated in a variety of other clinical studies. Coralline hydroxyapatite was shown to be clinically and biologically effective for the treatment of 21 consecutive fractures of the distal radius [48].   Patients were treated with external fixation and K-wires and subjected to a battery of tests for wrist function. Coralline

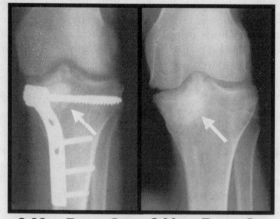

FIG. 6— Radiographs of a patient treated with coralline hydroxyapatite (arrows) for a tibial plateau fracture. The implant is readily visible at 2 months (left). After more than two years and hardware removal, the implant remains visible although there is a distinct blurring of the interface surface. Therefore, bone has ingrown the implant and some residual implant remains (right).

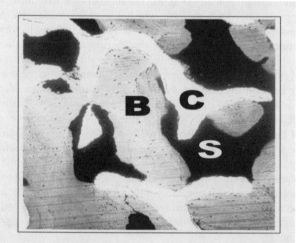

FIG. 7— Scanning electron micrographs of biopsy taken from a patient treated with coralline hydroxyapatite after 14 months. The regenerated bone (B) forms directly on the surface of the ceramic implant (C). Soft tissue (S) supports the ingrown bone. There is no evidence of implant resorption.

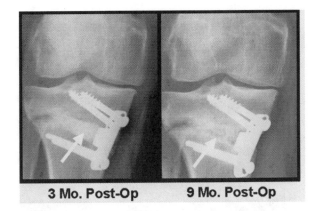

3 Mo. Post-Op   9 Mo. Post-Op

FIG. 8— **Radiographs of patient treated with resorbable coralline implant for tibial osteotomy (arrows). The implant is readily visible at 3 months after surgery (left). After only 9 months of implantation, the implant is virtually all resorbed and replaced with regenerated bone (right). (Courtesy of Jean Potvin, MD, Montmagny, QC, Canada.)**

hydroxyapatite was effective at achieving articular surface reduction and a result consistent with bone grafting. A retrospective study in patients was conducted to treated small bones of the foot and ankle. The authors concluded that the material was safe for use in small defects with low loads [49–52].

Coralline implants were also found to be effective for the treatment of tumors. Coralline porous hydroxyapatite 500 was used to treat 71 consecutive patients and followed for 2.4 years [53]. The patients returned to pre-operative function in 7.6 weeks with minimal complications. One major advantage of the coralline hydroxyapatite is its relatively slow resorption increasing the identification of recurrent tumors.

Anterior cervical interbody fusions require significant compressive strength. Therefore, coralline hydroxyapatite implants with 200 microns pores, which has a lower porosity and a higher strength, was evaluated in patients [54]. A clinical study treated 26 patients with single and multi-level from C3 to T1 in combination with a rigid locking plate [55]. With a minimum follow-up of 2 years, there was reduced pain in 75% of the patients, no significant complications and no visible resorption of the hydroxyapatite implant.

Posterolateral lumbar spinal fusion requires the combination of osteoconductive materials like coralline implants with other therapies, including autograft [54]. Preliminary studies indicated that platelet derived growth factors with resorbable coralline ceramics can enhance the fusion rates of autograft mixed with coralline implants [56]. The process also concentrated the fibrinogen in the buffy coat of the patient's own blood to form a fibrin gel. The gelling provides a biomechanical role by maintaining the grafting materials in position, as well as initiating the release of the chemotactic and mitogenic growth factors. Early clinical results are consistent with the large animal models. Clinical biopsies show bone regeneration and significant implant resorption when grafting with the resorbable form of coralline implants (Fig. 9).

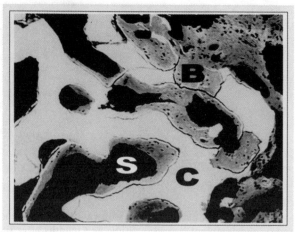

FIG. 9—Scanning electron micrograph of patient treated with resorbable coralline implant and autograft for posterior lumbar spinal fusion. The regenerated bone (B) forms directly on surface of the ceramic implant (C). In addition, the calcium carbonate has significantly resorbed. Bone and soft tissue (S) has also grown into this vacated space.

CONCLUSIONS

Coralline porous ceramics have been part of the surgeon's armamentarium for almost two decades. However, for the first 10 years, they were used clinically solely for oral, periodontal, and plastic surgery, due to regulatory issues. For almost a decade now, they have been widely available for orthopedic applications. Over the past 20 years, scientists and clinicians have learned a great deal about the appropriate clinical applications for osteoconductive materials. There is little controversy that matrices have an essential role to play for treating bone defects or to aid in the generation of bone where it does not normally grow. However, the surgical team must always apply the three essential requirements for osteoconduction: proximity, viability, and stability. Coralline hydroxyapatite implants resorb but slowly through the action of osteoclasts. For some indications, it is desirable to have the implants resorb after they have conducted bone. Resorbable coralline implants have osteoconductive properties and they resorb after bone incorporation, typically in 6–18 months. There are numerous clinical applications for coralline implants in block and granular form as osteoconductive matrices used alone. If the Triad of Osteoconduction cannot be met, then combinational therapy must be used. Coralline implants have been shown experimentally and clinically to be the primary candidates for the use with growth factors and cellular therapies. Although the field of tissue engineering has come to understand the specific limitations of osteoconduction, the most surprising awareness has been the inability of growth factors and cellular therapies to function without a matrix. Therefore, coralline implants will remain contemporary when used alone or in combination with other treatment modalities available to the surgeon.

REFERENCES

[1]   Chapman M. W., "Bone Grafting," *Operative Orthop*, M. W. Chapman and M. Madison, Eds., J. B. Lippincott Company, Philadelphia, 1993, pp. 139–149.

[2]   Shors E. C., "Coralline Bone Graft Substitutes," *Orthop Clin North Am*, Vol. 30, 1999, pp. 599–613.

[3]   White E. W., "Biomaterials Innovation: It's a Long Road to the Operating Room," *Mater Res Innovat*, Vol. 1, 1997, pp. 57–63.

[4]   White E. and Shors E. C., "Biomaterial Aspects of Interpore-200 Porous Hydroxyapatite," *Dental Clin North Am*, Vol. 30, 1986, pp. 49–67.

[5]   Vernon J. E. N., *Coral of Australia and the Indio-Pacific*, University of Hawaii Press, Honolulu, 1986.

[6]   Preidler K. W., Lemperle S. M., Holmes R. E., Calhoun C. J., Shors E. C., Brossmann J., et al. "Coralline Hydroxyapatite Bone Graft Substitutes. Evaluation of Bone Density with Dual Energy X-ray Absorptiometry," *Invest Radiol*, Vol. 31, 1996, pp. 716–723.

[7]   Sires B. S., Holds J. B., and Archer C. R., "Variability of Mineral Density in Coralline Hydroxyapatite Spheres: Study by Quantitative Computed Tomography," *Ophth Plastic Reconstruct Surg*, Vol. 9, 1993, pp. 250–253.

[8]   Sires B. S., Holds J. B., and Archer C. R., "Post-implantation Density Changes in Coralline Hydroxyapatite Orbital Implants," *Ophth Plastic Reconstruct Surg*, Vol. 14, 1998, pp. 318–322.

[9]   Shors E. C., White E. W., and Edwards R. M., "A Method for Quantitative Characterization of Porous Biomaterials Using Automated Image Analysis," *Quantitative Characterization and Performance of Porous Implants for Hard Tissue Applications, ASTM STP 953*, J. E. Lemons, Ed., ASTM International, West Conshohocken, 1987, pp. 347–358.

[10] Haddock S. M., Debes J. C., Nauman E. A., Fong K. E., Arramon Y. P., and Keaveny T. M., "Structure-function Relationships for Coralline Hydroxyapatite Bone Substitute," *J Biomed Mater Res*, Vol. 47, 1999, pp. 71–78.

[11] Wittenberg R. H., Moeller J., Shea M., White A. A., and Hayes W. C., "Compressive Strength of Autogenous and Allogenous Bone Grafts for Thoracolumbar and Cervical Spine Fusion," *Spine*, Vol. 15, 1990, pp. 1073–1078.

[12] Martin R. B., Chapman M. W., Sharkey N.A., Zissimos S. L., Bay B., and Shors E. C., "Bone Ingrowth and Mechanical Properties of Coralline Hydroxyapatite 1 Year After Implantation," *Biomaterials*, Vol. 14, 1993, pp. 341–348.

[13] Bay B. K., Martin R. B., Sharkey N. A., and Chapman M. W., "Repair of Large Cortical Defects with Block Coralline Hydroxyapatite," *Bone*, Vol. 14, 1993, pp. 225–230.

[14] Holmes R. E., Hagler H. K., and Coletta C. A., "Thick-Section Histometry of Porous Hydroxyapatite Implants Using Backscattered Electron Imaging," *J Biomed Mater Res*, Vol. 21, 1987, pp. 731–739.

[15] Dawson E., "The Fate of Bone Substitution with Porous Hydroxyapatite Implant in the Dog Spine," *Transact Orthop Res Soc*, Vol. 27, 1981, p. 206.

[16] Zdeblick T. A., Cooke M. E., Kunz D. N., Wilson D., and McCabe R. P., "Anterior Cervical Discectomy and Fusion Using a Porous Hydroxyapatite Bone Graft Substitute," *Spine 15*, Vol. 19, 1994, pp. 2348–2357.

[17] Emery S. E., Fuller D. A., and Stevenson S., "Ceramic Anterior Spinal Fusion. Biologic and Biomechanical Comparison in a Canine Model," *Spine,* Vol. 21, 1996, pp. 2713–2719.

[18] Mooney V., Massie J. B., Lind B. I., Rah J. H., Negri S., and Holmes R. E., "Comparison of Hydroxyapatite Granules to Autogenous Bone Graft in Fusion Cages in a Goat Model," *Surg Neurol*, Vol. 49, 1998, pp. 628–633.

[19] Holmes R. E., Bucholz R. W., and Mooney V., "Synthetic Hydroxyapatite as a Bone Graft Substitute," *Clin Orthop Rel Res*, Vol. 188, 1984, pp. 252–262.

[20] Ripamonti U., "Osteoinduction in Porous Hydroxyapatite Implanted in Heterotopic Sites of Different Animal Models," *Biomaterials*, Vol. 17, 1996, pp. 31–35.

[21] Pollick S., Shors E. C., Holmes R. E., and Kraut R. A., "Bone Formation and Implant Degradation of Coralline Porous Ceramics Placed in Bone and Ectopic Sites," *J Oral Maxillofacial Surg,* Vol. 53, 1995, pp. 915–922.

[22] Nunery W. R., Heinz G. W., Bonnin J. M., Marin R. T., and Cepela M. A., "Exposure Rate of Hydroxyapaite Spheres in the Anophthalmic Socket: Histopathologic Correlation and Comparison with Silicone Sphere Implants," *Ophth Plastic Reconstruct Surg*, Vol. 9, 1993, pp. 96–104.

[23] Bozic K. J., Glazer P. A., Zurakowski D., Simon B. J., Lipson S. J., and Hayes W. C., "In Vivo Evaluation of Coralline Hydroxyapatite and Direct Current Electrical Stimulation in Lumbar Spinal Fusion," *Spine 15*, Vol. 24, 1999, pp. 2127–2133.

[24] Sempuku T., Ohgushi H., Okumura M., and Tamai S., "Osteogenic Potential of Allogeneic Rat Marrow Cells in Porous Hydroxyapatite Ceramics: A Histological Study," *J Orthop Res*, Vol. 14, 1996, pp. 907–913.

[25] Norman M. E., Elgendy H. M., Shors E. C., El-Amin S. F., and Laurencin C. T., "An In-vitro Evaluation of Coralline Porous Hydroxyapatite as a Scaffold for Osteoblast Growth," *Clin Mater,* Vol. 17, 1994, pp. 85–91.

[26] Baramki H. G., Steffen T., Lander P., Chang M., and Marchesi D., "The Efficacy of Interconnected Porous Hydroxyapatite in Achieving Posterolateral Lumbar Fusion in Sheep," *Spine*, Vol. 25, 2000, pp. 1053–1060.

[27] Steffen T., Marchesi D., and Aebi M., "Posterolateral and Anterior Interbody Spinal Fusion Models in the Sheep," *Clin Orthop Rel Res,* Vol. 371, 2000, pp. 28–37.

[28] Siebrecht M. A., De Rooij P. P., Arm D. M., Olsson M. L., and Aspenberg P., "Platelet Concentrate Increases Bone Ingrowth into Porous Hydroxyapatite," *Orthopedics,* Vol. 25, 2002, pp. 169–172.

[29] Damien C. J., Parsons J. R., Prewett A. B., Huismans F., Shors E. C., and Holmes R. E., "Effect of Demineralized Bone Matrix on Bone Growth Within a Porous HA Material: a Histologic and Histometric Study," *J Biomater Appl*, Vol. 9, 1995, pp. 275–288.

[30] El Deeb M., Hosny M., and Sharawy M., "Osteogenesis in Composite Grafts of Allogenic Demineralized Bone Powder and Porous Hydroxylapatite," *J Oral Maxillofacial Surg*, Vol. 47, 1989, pp. 50–56.

[31] Ashby E. R., Rudkin G. H., Ishida K., and Miller T. A., "Evaluation of a Novel Osteogenic Factor, Bone Cell Stimulating Substance, in a Rabbit Cranial Defect Model," *Plastic Reconstruct Surg*, Vol. 98, 1996, pp. 420–426.

[32] Gao T., Lindholm T. S., Martinen A., Urist M. R., "Composites of Bone Morphogenetic Protein (BMP) and Type IV Collagen, Coral-derived Coral Hydroxyapatite, and Tricalcium Phosphate Ceramics," *Int Orthop*, Vol. 20, 1996, pp. 321–325.

[33] Sires B. S., Holds J. B., Kincaid M. C., and Reddi A. H., "Osteogenin-enhanced Bone-Specific Differentiation in Hydroxyapatite Orbital Implants," *Ophth Plastic Reconstruct Surg*, Vol. 13, 1997, pp. 244–251.

[34] Boden S. D., Martin G. J., Jr., Morone M., Ugbo J. L., Titus L., and Hutton W. C., "The Use of Coralline Hydroxyapatite with Bone Marrow, Autogenous Bone Graft, or Osteoinductive Bone Protein Extract for Posterolateral Lumbar Spine Fusion," *Spine 15*, Vol. 24, 1999, pp. 320–327.

[35] Wang J. S. and Aspenberg P., "Basic Fibroblast Growth Factor Promotes Bone Ingrowth in Porous Hydroxyapatite," *Clin Orthop Rel Res*, Vol. 333, 1996, pp. 252–260.

[36] Aspenberg P., Jeppsson C., Wang J. S., and Bostrom M., "Transforming Growth Factor Beta and Bone Morphogenetic Protein 2 for Bone Ingrowth: A Comparison Using Bone Chambers in Rats," *Bone*, Vol. 19, 1996, pp. 499–503.

[37] Arm D. M., Tencer A. F., Bain S. D., and Celino D., "Effect of Controlled Release of Platelet-derived Growth Factor from a Porous Hydroxyapatite Implant on Bone Ingrowth," *Biomaterials*, Vol. 17, 1996, pp. 703–709.

[38] Han B., Perelman N., Tang B., Hall F., Shors E. C., and Nimni M., "Collagen-Targeted BMP3 Fusion Proteins Arrayed on Collagen Matrices or Porous Ceramics Impregnated with Type I Collagen Enhance Osteogenesis in a Rat Cranial Defect Model," *J Orthop Res*, (in press), 2002.

[39] Choi S. H., Levy M. L., and McComb J. G., "A Method of Cranioplasty Using Coralline Hydroxyapatite," *Ped Neurosurg*, Vol. 29, 1998, pp. 324–327.

[40] El Deeb M. E., Tompach P. C., and Morstad A. T., "Porous Hydroxylapatite Granules and Blocks as Alveolar Ridge Augmentation Materials," *J Oral Maxillofacial Surg*, Vol. 46, 1988, pp. 955–970.

[41] Ayers R. A., Simske S. J., Nunes C. R., and Wolford L. M., "Long-term Bone Ingrowth and Residual Microhardness of Porous Block Hydroxyapatite Implants in Humans," *J Oral Maxillofacial Surg*, Vol. 56, 1998, pp. 1297–1301.

[42] Cottrell D. A. and Wolford L. M., "Long-term Evaluation of the Use of Coralline Hydroxyapatite in Orthognathic Surgery," *J Oral Maxillofacial Surg*, Vol. 56, 1998, pp. 935–941.

[43] Oreamuno S., Lekovic V., Kenney E. B., Carranza F. A., Takei H. H. and Prokic B., "Comparative Clinical Study of Porous Hydroxyapatite and Decalcified Freeze-Dried Bone in Human Periodontal Defects," *J Periodontol*, Vol. 61, 1990, pp. 399–404.

[44] Rosen H. M. and McFarland M. M., "The Biologic Behavior of Hydroxyapatite Implanted into the Maxillofacial Skeleton," *Plastic Reconstruct Surg*, Vol. 85, 1990, pp. 718–723.

[45] Bucholz R. W., Carlton A., and Holmes R., "Interporous Hydroxyapatite as a Bone Graft Substitute in Tibial Plateau Fractures," *Clin Orthop Rel Res,* Vol. 240, 1989, pp. 53–62.

[46] Shors E. C., "Bone Graft Substitutes: Clinical Studies Using Coralline Hydroxyapatite," *Biomater Surg*, G. H. I. M. Walenkamp, Ed., Georg Thieme Verlag, Stuttgart Germany, 1998, pp. 83–89.

[47] Shors E. C. and Holmes R. E., "Bone Formation in Porous Hydroxyapatite Obtained from Human Biopsies," *Bioceramics,* Vol. 6, P. Ducheyne and D. Christiansen, Eds., Butterworth-Heinemann Ltd., 1993, pp. 375–379.

[48] Wolfe S. W., Pike L., Slade J. F., III, and Katz L. D., "Augmentation of Distal Radius Fracture Fixation with Coralline Hydroxyapatite Bone Graft Substitute," *J Hand Surg Am,* Vol. 24, 1999, pp. 816–827.

[49] Mahan K. T. and Carey M. J. "Hydroxyapatite as a Bone Substitute," *J Am Podiatr Med Assoc*, Vol. 89, 1999, pp. 392–397.

[50] Nesheiwat F., Brown W. M., and Healey K. M., "Post-traumatic First Metatarsal Reconstruction Using Coralline Hydroxyapatite," *J Am Podiatr Med Assoc*, Vol. 88, 1998, pp. 130–134.

[51] Rahimi F., Maurer B. T., and Enzweiler M. G., "Coralline Hydroxyapatite: A Bone Graft Alternative in Foot and Ankle Surgery," *J Foot Ankle Surg*, Vol. 36, 1997, pp. 192–203.

[52] Elsinger E. C. and Leal L., "Coralline Hydroxyapatite Bone Graft Substitutes," *J Foot Ankle Surg*, Vol. 35, 1996, pp. 396–399.

[53] Irwin R. B., Bernhard M., and Biddinger A., "Coralline Hydroxyapatite as Bone Substitute in Orthopedic Oncology," *Am J Orthop*, Vol. 30, 2001, pp. 544–550.

[54] Thalgott J. S., Kabins B. B., Timlin M., Fritts C. K., and Giuffre J. M., "Treated Coral for Bone Replacement in Spinal Surgery," *Manual of Internal Fixation of the Spine,* J. S. Thalgott and M. Aebi, Eds., Lippincott-Raven Publishers, Philadelphia, 1996, pp. 285–295.

[55] Thalgott J. S., Fritts K., Giuffre J. M., and Timlin M., "Anterior Interbody Fusion of the Cervical Spine with Coralline Hydroxyapatite," *Spine*, Vol. 24, 1999, pp. 1295–1299.

[56] Lowery G. L., Kulkarni S., and Pennisi A. E., "Use of Autologous Growth Factors in Lumbar Spinal Fusion," *Bone,* Vol. 5, 1999, pp. 47S–50S.

Clinical Issues in the Development of Bone Graft Substitutes in Orthopedic Trauma Care

by Robert W. Bucholz,[1] M.D.

INTRODUCTION

MORE THAN 500,000 SURGICAL PROCEDURES using bone grafts or bone graft substitutes are performed annually in the United States. Fractures and traumatic bone defects constitute a large proportion of these procedures, second only to spinal arthrodeses. This expanding market for grafts has stimulated the development over the last 20 years of a host of different bone graft substitutes composed of calcium phosphate or calcium sulfate biomaterials. No fewer than 30 bone graft substitutes and allograft products are currently in various stages of clinical development. The purpose of this chapter is to discuss the critical clinical issues in the development of bone graft substitutes in orthopedic trauma care.

GOALS OF CLINICAL TRIALS

As with any new orthopedic device, pilot and pivotal clinical trials are designed to test safety and efficacy. Most bone graft substitutes pose little or no risk for either local or systemic toxicity. Despite the fact that small particles of crystalline hydroxyapatite can incite an inflammatory reaction, no clinical or histologic data have shown such a reaction to the block, granular, or cement formulations of substitutes that have been implanted in humans. Similarly, the prevalence of surgical infection does not seem to be increased by the use of bone graft substitutes. Although antibodies to collagen carriers of various substitutes have been documented, no adverse local or systemic effects have been noted [1]. Extrusion of graft substitutes, especially cement formulations inserted percutaneously, can occur through a peri-articular fracture into an adjacent joint or into surrounding soft tissues. The long-term effect of such ectopic graft substitute is not known. Overall, however, safety issues are of lesser concern than efficacy in most clinical trials.

In the simplest of terms, efficacy is judged by the ability of a graft substitute to enhance or accelerate bone regeneration in a fracture or traumatic defect. Most bone graft substitutes are only osteoconductive with no inductive properties unless supplemented with autologous marrow, demineralized allograft or recombinant growth

[1]Department of Orthopaedic Surgery, University of Texas Southwestern Medical School, 5323 Harry Hines Boulevard, Dallas, TX 75390-8883.

factors. As regenerated bone predictably fills in fractures and traumatic bone defects, the efficacy of any given substitute must be measured by the rapidity and volume of new bone formation.

ASSESSMENT OF EFFICACY

Because there is no widely applicable non-invasive method of quantitating bone formation or healing, all clinical trials have relied on indirect measures of efficacy. The following are the most commonly used.

Comparison of Healing Time to Autograft

Fracture patterns, which predictably are known to heal slowly, will often require autogenous bone grafting in addition to internal fixation. Comminuted fractures of the diaphyses of the radius and ulna are such injuries. Although there is no consensus on which fractures routinely require bone grafting, a well designed protocol to compare the efficacy of autograft and bone graft substitute is a reasonable model to test efficacy. Precisely defined inclusion and exclusion criteria are critical to ensure that only fractures with a high nonunion rate without the use of supplemental graft are included.

Most studies have merely tried to show comparability of the healing times of autograft and substitute. In the pivotal study using Collagraft® (Zimmer, Warsaw, IN) substitute, various complex fractures of the humerus, radius, ulna, femur, and tibia were included, and only simple fracture patterns excluded [1]. A major criticism of this study was the unfocused, overly broad inclusion criteria necessitating stratification of data for analysis.

Another problem with using healing times for measuring efficacy is the discrepancy between clinical and radiographic healing. Clinical healing with full functional use of the limb often precedes radiographic healing. If clinical healing is used as an endpoint, it must be explicitly defined.

Comparison of Nonunion Rate

Nonunion of a long bone fracture is difficult to define. Qualitatively a nonunion implies that a fracture has not healed within an expected period of time and will not heal unless some intervention (e.g., internal fixation or grafting) is undertaken. A quantitative definition is more elusive. Most investigators consider a nonunion to be present if a fracture has failed to heal within 6–9 months of injury and there has been no radiographic progression of healing over three months. Nonunions, even in bones at risk such as tibia, occur in less than 10% of fractures.

Because nonunions are uncommon, this criterion for efficacy (nonunion rate) is rarely used in clinical trials because a prohibitively large study population would have to be accrued.

Comparison of Malunion Rate

In certain peri-articular and metaphyseal fractures, autograft may be used to assist in maintenance of a reduction. For example, elevated osteochondral fragments of a depressed tibial plateau fracture or of a distal radius fracture can be supported by filling the underlying metaphyseal defect with a bone graft. In such settings, the graft serves primarily as a spacer and contributes little to healing of any major cortical fractures. The first FDA-approved substitute in the American market, Pro-Osteon™ (Interpore Cross International, Irvine, CA) is used principally as a filler of traumatic metaphyseal defects [2]. More recently, Alpha-BSM® (Depuy, Warsaw, IN) and NORIAN SRS® (Synthes, Paoli, PA) have been investigated as bone graft substitutes for similar defects. In such applications, efficacy is measured by comparison of the post-operative and follow-up radiographs to detect any fracture subsidence of the articular surface (Figs. 1–3).

Comparison of Need for Subsequent Surgeries

At various stages of fracture healing, additional surgeries may be deemed necessary for achieving union. For example, open tibial shaft fractures stabilized with non-reamed intramedullary nails often are treated with staged secondary procedures, such as nail dynamization, bone grafting or exchange nailing. The early application of a bone graft substitute or growth factor may sufficiently enhance early bone formation to obviate the need for secondary surgery. This measure of efficacy was used in a pivotal study of rhBMP-2 (Genetics Institute, Cambridge, MA) applied at the time of wound closure in open tibial fractures [3]. The avoidance of secondary procedures would offer substantial clinical and economic benefits.

PROBLEMS WITH TESTING EFFICACY

The treatment effect of bone graft substitutes is best tested through randomized controlled trials. Problems with the design, conduct, and analysis of bone graft trials are universally encountered. The following are common investigational problems in all such studies.

Difficulty in Measuring In Vivo Bone Formation

All non-invasive methods to measure bone formation within or about bone grafts and bone graft substitutes are flawed to some degree. Plain radiographs are most commonly used. Even with plain radiographic views, the evaluation of callus size and location and fracture union are subjective. Although blinded radiographic assessment enhances accuracy and lessens potential bias, interobserver and intraobserver reliability are often poor. The definition of fracture union (usually defined as bridging callus on two or more cortices or obliteration of all fracture lines) is frequently imprecise. Other imaging studies, such as computerized tomographic scans are of limited usefulness due to the scatter effect of metallic implants and the cost and radiation exposure of the studies.

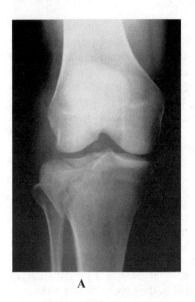

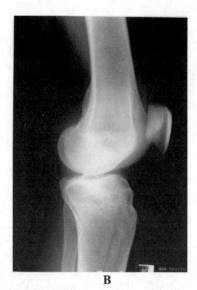

A   B

FIG. 1A/1B—Anteroposterior and lateral radiograph of a split depression fracture of the lateral tibial plateau with greater than 10 mm of articular depression.

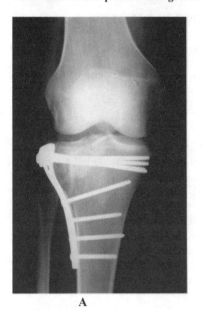

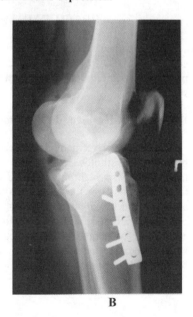

A   B

FIG. 2A/2B—Anteroposterior and lateral radiographs following open reduction and internal fixation of fracture. Following elevation of the articular surface, the metaphyseal defect was filled with Alpha-BSM® cement.

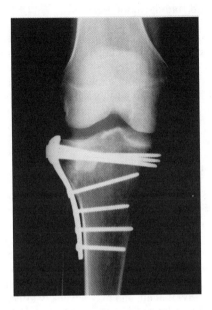

FIG. 3—Anteroposterior radiograph at six months after injury showing fracture union and maintenance of the articular reduction.

Investigational techniques to measure bone/callus strength and stiffness, such as resonance frequency and ultrasound, are not widely available. Thus, a convenient, reproducible, and accurate method to measure bone regeneration into bone graft substitutes is as yet unavailable.

Choice of Controls

The treatment effect of bone graft substitutes is most often compared to that of autogenous graft. Comparison to autograft alone may, however, be insufficient if the inclusion and exclusion criteria are controversial. Most fractures heal without graft and the addition of autograft or bone graft substitute will have little impact on the radiographic or clinical result. Thus, if a fracture that has a high probability of healing with standard care is used in a study, the treatment effect of bone graft substitute must be compared to both autograft and no graft. Many studies on fracture healing such as the original Collagraft® trial, suffer from the lack of any concurrent control group without any graft material. Similar problems arise in the testing of substitutes on fracture nonunions. The pivotal trial of OP-1 or rhBMP-7 (Stryker Corp., Mahwah, NJ) involved the treatment of tibial nonunions with reamed intramedullary nails and either autograft or OP-1 [4]. Because the union rate with reamed intramedullary nailing of such nonunions may be as high as 80–90%, the comparison of the effect of adjunctive autograft versus OP-1 is more difficult and necessitates a larger study population.

Disparate Functional and Radiographic Results

The ultimate goal of fracture care is improved patient outcome. It is widely appreciated in the orthopedic trauma community that functional results of treatment do not necessarily parallel radiographic results. A healed fracture with excellent callus formation may be associated with a poor clinical outcome. For example, an open tibial shaft fracture may heal but associated soft tissue problems such as muscle contractures, neural defects, vascular compromise, or compartment syndromes may leave the patient functionally impaired. Thus, functional outcome measures must be used cautiously in any study of graft efficacy.

Large Enrollment of Patients

If a graft substitute is being compared to autograft, a large patient accrual is necessary to ensure an adequately powered study. Using standard statistical methodologies, most studies should enroll a minimum of 150 patients to show comparability. Enrollment of such a large number of patients requires a multicenter study. Trauma patients are often poorly compliant and lost to follow-up. Additionally, the volume of trauma patients is seasonal and unpredictable, frequently delaying the completion of studies.

Follow-up is also problematic in that some substitutes such as the highly crystalline hydroxyapatite resorb slowly, if at all, and may adversely affect bone remodeling. Long-term follow-up to determine the prevalence of refracture is thus desirable, but rarely achievable.

Subjective Assessment of Secondary Intervention

The use of the number of secondary interventions to achieve union as a measure of efficacy is fraught with several problems. The clinical decision for additional surgery deemed necessary to achieve fracture union may be based on poorly defined criteria. A consensus on such guidelines is lacking for most fractures. Additionally, the decision may be biased if the surgeon is not blinded to the original treatment with autograft or bone graft substitute. A major critique of the pivotal rhBMP-2 trial using secondary intervention as an efficacy measure was the potential for surgeon's bias [3]. Thus, the need for secondary intervention, although an important clinical issue, is perceived as an imprecise variable.

Limited Biopsy Specimens

Routine histomorphometric measurement of regenerated bone in graft substitutes is not feasible. Biopsy specimens of substitutes at fractures or bone defects generally are available only at the time of elective hardware removal or reconstructive surgery for a nonunion. Elective hardware removal rarely is scheduled before 1–2 years after fracture and grafting at a time when the callus or regenerated bone has remodeled. Such late biopsies are thus of limited value. Similarly, biopsy tissue at the time of reconstructive surgery for a nonunion does not provide an accurate qualitative or quantitative assessment of bone growth.

Biopsy specimens are primarily useful in evaluating the amount of retained implant (e.g., calcium phosphate) using standardized histomorphometric techniques. In one of the few published series of human biopsies, Shors and Holmes measured the new bone, implant, and soft tissue volume fractions [5]. All specimens were obtained well past the critical first three months after implantation and, therefore, could not be used to measure efficacy.

FACTORS INFLUENCING CHOICE OF CLINICAL TRIALS

Multiple factors must be taken into consideration in the choice of a clinical trial. The fabrication technique, chemical composition, pore dimensions, crystallinity, biomechanical properties, resorptive rates, and setting properties of substitutes vary widely, and all must be considered in selecting a preferred trial protocol for a given substitute [1,6–8].

Inductive Properties of Graft Substitutes

Most bone graft substitutes are osteoconductive, acting as scaffolds for bone regeneration. Their usefulness in nonunions and diaphyseal fractures is thus limited. Most trials to date have focused on simple metaphyseal and peri-articular defects where the substitute acts primarily as a spacer [2,6]. The additions of bone marrow aspirate, demineralized bone matrix, or growth factors enhance the osteoinductive potential of bone graft substitutes. The volume, preparation, and binding properties of these osteoinductive adjuncts to the substitute determine the magnitude of the osteoinductive stimulus. Nevertheless, the size of defects treatable by synthetic substitutes is limited by their poor osteoinductive properties. For example, Collagraft®, whose osteoinductive properties are enhanced with autogenous bone marrow, is approved for only relatively small defects of less than 30 cc in volume.

Structural Properties of Graft Substitutes

Calcium phosphate and calcium sulfate substitutes, whether porous or dense in structure and crystalline or amorphous in composition, are brittle and weak, especially in bending and shear [9]. Thus, they serve as poor substitutes for cortical bone. Their ideal applications are traumatic non-load defects and defects whose bending, shear, and torsional stresses have been neutralized by internal fixation implants. Anterior spinal applications similarly necessitate the use of protective cages or other instrumentation to prevent fragmentation of the substitute from excessive loading. Although the NORIAN SRS® cement substitute was originally conceived as a fracture fixation implant, its brittle mechanical properties restricts its utility in this regard.

Injectability

Bone graft substitutes may be fabricated as blocks, granules, or paste. Only this latter formulation is suitable for percutaneous injectable delivery. Injectable applications have focused primarily on the self-setting hydroxyapatite and amorphous calcium phosphates such as NORIAN SRS®, BONE SOURCE™ (Stryker, Corp., Mahwah, NJ), and Alpha-

BSM®. These materials harden over 10–30 min. depending on the solute used. During the mixing process, various pharmaceuticals such as antibiotics and growth factors can be added. Injection of such a composite into a fracture hematoma conceivably might accelerate callus formation.

Several major concerns about injectable delivery systems have surfaced. First, the percutaneous insertion of the substitute, whether performed blindly or under fluoroscopic control, does not permit any preparation of the recipient site. Organized fracture hematoma, scar tissue, or superimposed soft tissue may prevent the accurate placement of the substitutes adjacent to viable bone. Various systems have been developed to irrigate the graft site free of hematoma and soft tissue but they remain unproven. Second, percutaneous injection of a viscous substitute risks inadvertent extravasation of the substitute into the surrounding soft tissues. Adjacent neurovascular structures may be at risk. Injection into a peri-articular defect may lead to intra-articular extravasation through a subchondral fracture. Such intra-articular extravasation was noted in several patients during the pivotal trial in distal radius fractures of NORIAN SRS®. The adverse effect, if any, of such ectopic substitutes is unknown.

Properties as Carriers

Antibiotics, growth factors, and other pharmaceuticals bond to different substitutes to a variable degree [10]. Most proteins are not appreciably denatured when added to these materials, even the self-curing calcium phosphate and sulfate cements. With gradual resorption of the substitute, sustained release of the drug is feasible. Clinical trials designed to test the efficacy of bone graft substitutes as carriers will be complex and costly.

CONCLUSIONS

The testing of efficacy of bone graft substitutes in orthopedic trauma trials is a difficult task. Few, if any, study designs have been free of bias and controversy. None to date have met the CONSORT standards for randomized controlled trials [11].

Clinical trials in orthopedic trauma care are especially costly, often to a prohibitive extent. Trials with strict inclusion criteria necessitate the recruitment of multiple Level I or II trauma centers serving primarily indigent populations. The high cost limits the feasibility of long-term follow-up trials and extended indications trials. Generalization of trial results is often flawed since fractures in different anatomic locations behave differently. The efficacy of a substitute in a tibial plateau fracture may not extrapolate into efficacy in a forearm fracture.

Despite the inherent challenges of orthopedic trauma trials of bone graft substitutes, it is anticipated that the large potential market for such substitutes will continue to drive clinical research.

REFERENCES

[1] Chapman M., Bucholz R., and Cornell C., "Treatment of Acute Fractures with a Collagen Calcium Phosphate Graft Material: A randomized clinical trial," *J Bone Joint Surg Am*, Vol. 79, 1997, pp. 495–502.

[2] Bucholz R., Carlton A., and Holmes R., "Interporous Hydroxyapatite as a Bone Graft Substitute in Tibial Plateau Fractures," *Clin Orthop Rel Res*, Vol. 240, 1989, pp. 53–62.

[3] Govender S., Csimmia C., Genant H., and Valentin-Opram A., "Recombitant Human Bone Morphogenetic Protein-2 for Open Tibial Fractures: A prospective, controlled, randomized study of 450 patients," *J Bone Joint Surg,* Vol. 84, 2002, pp. 2123–2134.

[4] Friedlander G., Cole J., Cook S., Cierny G., Muschler G., Zych G., Calhoun J., LaForte A., and Yin S., "Osteogenic Protein – 1 (Bone Morphogenetic Protein-7) in the Treatment of Tibial Nonunions: A prospective, randomized clinical trial comparing rhOP-1 with fresh bone autograft," *J Bone Joint Surg Am*, Vol. 83, 2001, pp. 83–90.

[5] Shors E. and Holmes R., "Bone Formation in Porous Hydroxyapatite Obtained from Human Biopsies," *Bioceramics*, Vol. 6, 1993, pp. 375–379.

[6] Wolfe J., Pike L., Slade J., and Katz L., "Augmentation of Distal Radius Fracture Fixation with Coralline Hydroxyapatite Bone Graft Substitute," *J Hand Surg Am*, Vol. 24, 1999, pp. 816–827.

[7] Blaha D., "Calcium Sulfate Bone-Void Filler," *Orthopaedics*, Vol. 21, 1998, pp. 1017–1019.

[8] Kelly C., Wilkins R., Gitelis J., et al., "The Use of a Surgical Grade Calcium Sulfate as a Bone Graft Substitute: Results of a multicenter trial," *Clin Orthop Rel Res*, Vol. 382, 2000, pp. 42–50.

[9] Martin R., Chapman M., Holmes R., et al., "Effects of Bone Ingrowth on the Strength and Non-Invasive Assessment of a Coralline Hydroxyapatite Material," *Biomaterials*, Vol. 10, 1989, pp. 481–488.

[10] McKee M., Schemitsch E., Wild L., and Waddell J., "Osteoset-Tobramycin Pellets in Infected Nonunions," *Presented at the 15ᵗʰ Annual Meeting of the Orthopaedic Trauma Association*, Charlotte, North Carolina, 1999.

[11] Begg C., Cho M., Eastwood S., Horton R., Moher D., Oikin R., et al., "Improving the Quality of Reporting Randomized Controlled Trials," *J Am Med Assoc*, Vol. 274, 1996, pp. 637–639.

Issues Involving Standards Development for Synthetic Material Bone Graft Substitutes

17

by Marc Long, [1] Ph.D., Robert Talac, [2] M.D., Ph.D., and
Michael J. Yaszemski,[2] M.D., Ph.D.

INTRODUCTION

MODERN ORTHOPEDIC SURGERY HAS become complex and technically sophisticated. Orthopedic surgeons and basic scientists have translated recent advances in chemistry, molecular biology, physiology, and biomaterials science into novel management options for their patients. In particular, the development of new synthetic bone graft substitutes (BGS) represents a rapidly evolving area. These synthetic biomaterials may be used alone, as scaffold, or as carrier for bioactive agents (proteins, antibiotics, blood derived or bone marrow derived agents, and cells). To date, most BGS materials available on the market have been classified as Bone Void Fillers (BVF) "intended to be gently packed into bone voids or gaps that are not intrinsic to the stability of the bony structure" [12]. These graft alternatives are subjected to varying degrees of regulatory scrutiny, and thus their true safety and effectiveness in patients may not be known prior to their clinical use [22]. Continuous innovation and the development of new implants raise important issues for technology testing, clinical performance, risk assessment and regulation. It is therefore not surprising that the development of standards for these implants represents an issue that increasingly confronts the professionals from industrial and health care sectors.

SAFETY AND BIOCOMPATIBILITY

The first issue in standards development for synthetic bone graft substitutes is most appropriately an assessment of their safety. A wide spectrum of tests exists that may be used to determine the biological response to a particular material. The unique nature of each individual synthetic bone graft substitute demands that the tests be selected on a case-by-case basis. This selection process should give consideration to the common goal of convincing the public, the surgeons, and the regulatory agencies that the group of tests

---

[1] Smith &Nephew, Inc., 1450 Brooks Road, Memphis, TN 38116.
[2] Department of Orthopedic Surgery and Bioengineering, Mayo Clinic, Medical Sciences Bldg. 3-75, 200 First St., SW, Rochester, MN 55905.

chosen demonstrate that the particular BGS under consideration is safe. Detailed guidelines on the selection of individual tests to consider for a particular biological interaction have been developed (i.e., ASTM standard F 748, ISO 10993 or OECD guidelines) [1–3,10]. These guidelines have been developed in cooperation with the U.S. Food and Drug Administration (FDA), the International Standards Organization (ISO), and other voluntary standardization organizations. However, these guidelines have been insufficient in addressing all safety and biocompatibility issues related to new materials. Additionally, the US Pharmacopeia (USP), National Formulary (NF), Food Chemical Codex (FCC), European Pharmacopeia and British Standards Institute databases have all been used to establish the safety and biocompatibility of some current BGS materials. These additional standards [11] have generally been used to verify the chemical composition of BGS and the minor constituents typically used during processing. These documents also include standard procedures and their methodology. However, most of those tests provide information only on the response of host tissue to the material. Test methods for assessment of the material's response to the host (intended or unintended biodegradation) are often available, but have not yet been standardized.

ASTM standards for particular bone graft substitutes used in musculoskeletal applications have historically been developed after the introduction of these materials into clinical practice. Standards that cover bioceramics such as hydroxyapatite and β-tricalciumphosphate show this sequence [1,2]. A standard on calcium sulfate materials is currently being finalized [3]. It should be noted that specific standards are typically developed from a consensus of several parties and usually become available after the material is already on the market. For instance, the calcium sulfate ASTM standard, when completed, will have become available about seven years after the introduction of the modern form of this material, and 40 years after Peltier's reintroduction of this material to clinical practice in the late 1950s [27]. Furthermore, this standard is not exacting, but rather is a guide, as several test methods are dependent on the physical form and chemical composition of the particular calcium sulfate BGS product. It would be extremely difficult to define standards for all BGS materials being developed, as new materials in a variety of forms and shapes are constantly developed and introduced into the market. However, a guidance document that suggests safety and biocompatibility evaluation methods for these devices would move researchers, industry, and clinicians toward consensus on this issue.

Due to the increasing use of calcium-based materials as bone void fillers, the FDA has recently issued a guidance document entitled "Resorbable Calcium Salt Bone Void Filler Device; Draft Guidance for Industry and FDA" [12]. This document is to be used as a guide for the clearance of new bioceramics based on calcium salt materials. The safety and biocompatibility issues include infection, adverse tissue reaction, allergy to the material, disease transmission, incomplete bone growth, and the strength of the newly formed bone. This is the type of guidance document that could serve as a baseline for the development of standard guides for other BGS materials.

A special ASTM committee has started defining new standards to address specific issues associated with bone graft substitutes and tissue engineered products. This Tissue-Engineered Medical Products (TEMPs) committee is focusing on establishing standards directly applicable to tissue-engineered materials that include the new generation of BGS materials. First attempts at new standards include guides for terminology and definitions related to tissue engineering, and for characterization and testing of substrate materials and biomaterial scaffolds used in tissue-engineered medical products [5,6]. Due to the rapid changes that occur as tissue engineering evolves, the aforementioned documents may only be developed at this time as standards guidelines and not as standards per se. As all BGS materials serve the purpose of providing temporary mechanical support and facilitating bone regeneration through osteogenesis, osteoinduction, or osteoconduction, a set of guidelines may indeed be established that covers the common aspects associated with the nature of bone healing. Specific standards for certain classes of materials or particular implant-host interactions may later be defined.

It is obvious that these new standards require the collaboration of engineers, scientists, and medical professionals from a variety of fields. A strong collaboration with the different regulatory bodies is also critical. The TEMPs committee has undertaken a multidisciplinary approach to the development of these standards. This committee is leading the way in terms of standards development for these new biomaterials and will have a strong influence on the international scene of standardization.

EFFICACY AND PERFORMANCE

Once a synthetic bone graft substitute has been proven safe, it then must be evaluated for measures of efficacy. The assessment of efficacy varies according to the particular clinical application under consideration. The nature of potential clinical applications is diverse, including many types of trabecular voids, defects in areas of tendinous or ligamentous attachment, voids arising from periarticular defects, and voids associated with pseudarthroses. Each of these types of defects presents a unique bony environment with specific structural, mechanical, and biological requirements. Thus, validation of a particular bone graft substitute in one anatomic site does not necessarily predict its performance in another location [22]. Efficacy and performance standards as they relate to the properties of newly formed bone are lagging behind safety and biocompatibility standards. In general, any BGS should show sufficient ability to provide mechanical support to the particular anatomic area and facilitate bone regeneration.

Mechanical testing as it applies to conventional structural orthopedic materials (e.g., metal alloys and structural ceramics) is generally not directly applicable to synthetic BGS materials. The physical characteristics of many of the new BGS materials and products are not amenable to the fabrication of standard test samples representative of the actual product. Testing of the actual product (granules, porous blocks, in situ setting cements) is essential to determine the true structural behavior of the BGS product, the latter rarely being supplied as bars or plates amenable to the usual mechanical tests applied to musculoskeletal devices. In addition, the variety of BGS forms and shapes makes it difficult to directly compare different materials and products. Compression testing appears to be an appropriate choice for the mechanical testing of BGS materials being offered in block forms. Likewise, confined compression testing would be appropriate for those BGS materials that are processed into granule, pellet or tablet forms. Finally, compression testing of in situ polymerizable devices after they have hardened would be appropriate for those BGS materials offered in settable cement or slurry forms. It then seems that a standard compression protocol may be able to cover the range of shapes and forms of synthetic BGS materials such that strength standards could be established for different clinical applications. It should however be noted that all cleared BGS products currently on the market in their fabricated form are intended to be used in non-load bearing applications — therefore the label "bone void filler."

The mechanical properties of BGS materials are important, but additional properties, such as their handling strength, are also critical to their validation for use. There is a test from the pharmaceutical industry that may be appropriate to verify the handling strength of calcium sulfate BGS materials. The USP "Tablet Friability" test [14] has been shown to be an appropriate test for quality inspection and assurance of packaging stability for calcium sulfate granules [13]. This test is commonly used for pharmaceutical tablets. Briefly, this test consists of "tumbling" a specific mass of material for a determined amount of time using a calibrated rotating drum (friabilitor machine). The change in mass after friability testing is measured and the granules are inspected for any breakage. The material passes the test if not a single granule is cracked or broken and if the mass loss is less than 1%. This test could be easily adapted to a block form or any type of solid form. Ultimately, the efficacy of these BVF shows in the mechanical properties of the new bone formed in defects where these materials are implanted. This issue is discussed in the next section on performance.

Polymerizable materials, such as cements and resins, represent a separate class of bone graft substitutes. The final properties of these cements are highly dependent on the setting conditions (e.g., time and mixing method) specific to each BGS material. Standards for settable orthopedic materials (PMMA acrylic bone cement) have already been developed [7]. Such standards could be used as a platform for the development of a standard for settable BGS cements. Standards from other industries have been suggested and applied to bioceramic BGS cements (e.g., plaster of Paris) [8,9].

The efficacy and performance of synthetic BGS materials as they relate to the characteristics of the new bone formed have generally been shown using pre-clinical studies based on animal models representative of clinical conditions. A variety of animal models have been used [18–20,23,24,29–32]. Animals that are most commonly used include rabbits, dogs, rats, and sheep. The nature and location of the defects used for implantation in these models most commonly include distal and proximal femur, proximal tibia, ulna, and lumbar spine [15,17].

The main issues associated with a new synthetic BGS material relate to incomplete bone regeneration and the mechanical properties of the newly formed bone at the reconstruction site. The FDA guidance document for calcium salt BVF materials states that animal testing may be necessary "to evaluate bone formation, device resorption and the biomechanical properties of the newly formed bone over the time required for complete resorption of the device material." The evaluation techniques typically associated with an animal study are radiographic, histological, and biomechanical analyses [12].

Although radiographic analyses are routinely used, these evaluations do not always correlate with the actual biologic and mechanical properties of the newly formed bone. There is a need for improved imaging techniques for evaluation of synthetic bone graft substitutes. Furthermore, the resolution associated with radiographic techniques has not been sufficient to detect small differences in healing responses between test groups. New techniques, such as computerized tomography (CT), are becoming increasingly popular. However, this technique is subjective and there is need for an imaging test method that correlates with bone properties. The amount of bone growth and the nature of the newly formed bone are best characterized using histology techniques. Quantitative bone histomorphometry has become a standard component of BGS material evaluations.

Biomechanical testing of the new bone formed in the anatomic location of the BGS is critical to assessing the efficacy of a BGS material. Conventional mechanical testing includes bending, compression, tensile, and torsional methods [16]. Newer minimally destructive techniques are gaining acceptance. One of these new techniques is nanoindentation, in which a diamond indenter advances slowly into a bone specimen using controlled load and displacement [28]. Elastic modulus and hardness can be determined at any location within the defect. This allows for the measurement of local bone properties at the micron and sub-micron level. This technique has been used to characterize individual lamellae within osteons, anisotropy in small bone specimens, and bone-implant interfaces. The variety of biomechanical testing methods applied to specific animal models and bone defects would be difficult to standardize in a single document, but a guidance document on the requisites for biomechanical testing and the outcome of such testing would be beneficial. It is interesting to note that although BVF materials are not associated with any strength or load-bearing claims, biomechanical testing is almost always required by regulatory bodies for clearance of BGS products. Although biomechanical testing has generally been used in most studies in correlation with histology, radiographs, or imaging techniques, the current BVFs cannot be categorized as load-bearing materials.

The testing regimen for porous biodegradable BGS materials must address two additional issues. These include assessment and quantification of porosity and interconnectivity of pores within the BGS. Currently available testing methods provide only estimates of porosity. There is no test available to quantify interconnectivity. Porosity and interconnectivity are essential prerequisites for bone growth throughout the scaffold. Thus, there is a need for development and standardization of such methods.

Synthetic BGS are increasingly being used as scaffolds or carriers for biologically active agents such as proteins, antibiotics, or cells. The addition of these biologic molecules to the tissue-engineering scaffold or controlled drug delivery system increases the bioactivity of these BGS materials such that they become osteoinductive osteogenic BGS products. Although bioactive BGS materials are not the topic of this chapter, the acceptance of standards for the synthetic BGS materials are likely to provide a sound basis for the inevitable subsequent standards that will involve the bioactive agent. It should also be noted that potential interactions may exist between the components and that a guide is desired to define the type of testing and requirements needed for this emerging class of combined products. The increasing importance of these combined products is clearly illustrated by the recent establishment of a combined product division at the USFDA that will be in charge of examining this class of products. Again, a general guidance document for these combined products needs to be developed to address critical issues such as safety, biocompatibility, interaction between the synthetic scaffold and the biological agent, elution rates of the biologic agent into the surrounding tissues, and maximum local concentrations of the biological agent.

Most BGS materials are now designed to resorb within a timeframe desirable for new bone growth. Non-resorbable scaffolds are less desirable, as their continued presence will affect the long-term ability of the newly formed bone to remodel. Scaffolds that dissolve too quickly do not provide appropriate support for new bone growth. Therefore, one of the key performance parameters is the rate of degradation of the synthetic materials. Animal models and in vitro tests are both used to evaluate the degradation of BGS materials [19]. A parallel situation exists in the wear testing of joint prostheses, in which in vitro wear simulator testing has now become widely accepted as an indicator of in vivo total joint replacement component performance. In vitro BGS degradation testing includes dissolution in various solutions and resorption in tissue culture [25,26]. However, no specific standard has been defined for synthetic bone graft substitute materials. Standards established for other materials have been applied, occasionally with material specific modifications, to bioceramic and biopolymeric materials [4]. In vitro dissolution may suffice to demonstrate equivalence to a predicate device currently in clinical use. An in vitro dissolution protocol modified from ASTM F 1636 for PLLA resin was used to demonstrate the equivalence in dissolution between two different calcium sulfate products [13]. However, in vitro testing also has its limitations. For example, when calcium sulfate shaped granules are mixed with a carboxymethylcellulose (CMC) hydrogel, in vitro dissolution testing does not suffice because it is not representative of the in vivo biologic conditions, and differs significantly from the testing of any available predicate devices. In this particular situation, an in vivo pre-clinical study was required to demonstrate that the CMC-hydrogel did not affect the bone healing process supported by the calcium sulfate porous scaffold [29]. Thus, one major issue facing standards recommendations for synthetic BVF devices is the development of a standard for in vitro dissolution for resorbable biomaterials. Animal studies are currently required to assess new materials since no in vitro standard is available. An appropriate standard would allow for the clinical acceptance and possibly regulatory clearance of synthetic materials without the need of animal testing. It should be noted that in vitro testing may include the use of non-biological fluids, such as Ringer's solution or phosphate buffered saline, as well as the use of biological fluids. The mechanisms of dissolution or resorption in vivo may differ among the different types of materials. As an example, calcium phosphate bioceramics require either the use of acids to simulate osteoclastic resorption in vivo, or the use of osteoclasts or macrophage cell cultures. Calcium sulfate materials, on the other hand, are more prone to dissolve than to resorb. Thus, in vitro dissolution of these materials would not necessarily require the use of cell cultures but could be evaluated using simple fluids like Ringer's solution.

In vitro tests provide essential baseline information on both tissue and cellular responses to the biomaterial under consideration. In order to further understand the biological behavior of a synthetic BGS and assess its actual performance in a physiological environment, animal studies have become the accepted mode of pre-clinical evaluation. Several animal models have been used to demonstrate the safety and efficacy of synthetic BGS materials [18–20,23,24,29–32]. These studies generally compare the new material or product to a product currently used clinically, or to biological standards such as allogeneous or autogeneous bone. There are several issues related to the use of animal models. These include the appropriateness of the chosen animal species as representative of the response in humans, and the selected defect and reconstruction method. Additional considerations include the selection of positive and negative controls, the success criteria selected to declare efficacy, and the extrapolation of the data from animal studies to human disease [21]. As the efficacy assessment of a particular BGS material depends on the particular clinical application, it is clear that experimental success depends on the use of clinically relevant models [33].

APPLICATION TO CLINICAL PRACTICE

It is evident that more standards are needed to support a broader and safer clinical use of BGS materials. As a start, consensus on the definitions of several terms as they relate to medical devices needs to occur. Definitions of commonly used terms applied to bone graft substitutes, such as osteoinductivity and osteoconductivity, and standards that then use these definitions would enhance communication among colleagues in the many disciplines that must contribute to the successful clinical application of these materials.

One of the primary uses of BGS standards would be to suggest minimum requisites for clinical efficacy and performance. Dissolution guidance for in vitro evaluation and animal model guidance for in vivo evaluation would be a reasonable starting point for the uniform evaluation of new BGS products. These guidelines will also allow comparisons between the various BGS materials. One of the most critical current needs is a definition of bone healing and a method to quantify it as it relates to the use of BGS materials. Radiographic evaluations are still the standard for observing bone healing clinically. However, radiographic evaluations are limited in their ability to determine the mechanical characteristics of the newly formed bone. The clinical outcome criteria will need to include both imaging data and patient reported functional data.

Every BGS material is required to be validated for shelf life through aging stability studies. These studies are material and device specific, and aging protocols have to be established individually. A general guidance document is desirable, in the same spirit as a guidance document for animal models, to define the minimum requisites for aging stability studies. BGS products have been developed in cement or resin forms [20,24]. The performance of these products is highly dependent on their characteristics after setting. Therefore, the setting time (or polymerization time) is a critical parameter that needs attention. Specific standards are not available for BGS and standards for other applications are being used as alternatives. For instance, the setting times for calcium sulfate cements are tested in accordance with ASTM C 59 and C 472 for plaster of Paris. These are standards from the masonry industry. The example of standards developed for bone cement setting times [7] may be followed for synthetic BGS materials. The above issues, suggestions, and challenges related to new BGS standards development may best be illustrated by giving an example of the tests applied to a new calcium sulfate bone void filler (JAX® Advanced Bone Void Filler, Smith & Nephew, Inc.). This product consists of calcium sulfate granules with a carboxymethylcellulose hydrogel as a handling agent. Table 1 summarizes the tests and requirements used for clearance and commercialization of this device and their associated standards in those instances for which standards were available. The number of tests that were considered important to show the safety and efficacy of this device that yet had no existing standards, illustrates the importance of continuing current efforts toward standards or guidance documents for tissue-engineered medical products.

TABLE 1—Tests used for clearance and commercialization of calcium sulfate granules and CMC-hydrogel and the associated standards when available (N/A = not available).

Requirement/Test	Standard
Calcium Sulfate Granules:	
Calcium Sulfate Purity (Chemical Analysis)	USP XXIV
Processing Aids Purity (Chemical Analysis)	NF19
Calcium Sulfate Structure (X-ray Diffraction)	N/A
Density (Pycnometry)	N/A
Porosity (Mass to Volume Ratio Measurements)	N/A
Interlocking (Timed flow of granules through a funnel)	N/A
In vitro Degradation (Dissolution)	ASTM F 1635-95, modified
Mechanical Testing (Friability)	USP XXIV
Safety (Clinical history, LD50 values)	N/A
Biocompatibility	ASTM F 648, F 763, F 981
	ISO 10993-1
Pyrogenicity	USP XXIV
Sterility (gamma radiation)	ANSI/AAMI/ISO 11137, EN 552
CMC-Hydrogel (handling agent):	
Constituents Purity-Water,Glycerin(Chemical Analysis)	USP XXIV
Constituents Purity – CMC (Chemical Analysis)	N/A
Consistency (Viscometry, Consistometry)	N/A
Interlocking (Timed flow of device through a funnel)	N/A
In vitro Degradation (Dissolution)	N/A (modified ASTM F1635-95)
Safety (Clinical history, LD50 values, Animal study I)	N/A
Biocompatibility	ISO 10993-1
Pyrogenicity	USP XXIV
Sterility (aseptic fill followed by EtO)	ISO 13408-1, USP XXIV
	ANSI/AAMI/ISO 11135
Syringe	ISO 7886-1, USP XXIV
Microbial Testing (Bioburden)	N/A
Effect on Bone Healing (Animal Study II)	N/A

CONCLUSIONS

Current standards for BGS have shown that their limitations have in many ways curbed the development and commercialization of synthetic BGS materials and products. New standards are needed to address specific issues related to this new generation of biomaterials. Standard guides for characterization and testing of substrate materials and biomaterial scaffolds are being developed through the ASTM, ISO, and other voluntary standards groups. Standards guidance for in vitro dissolution/resorption, mechanical testing after implantation, animal models and evaluation protocols, and cement setting times represent good starting points for BGS testing protocols. These standards for BGS materials will require collaboration between several fields of expertise, such as bioengineering, biology, pharmaceutical science, orthopedic surgery, and regulatory agencies.

REFERENCES

[1] "Standard Specification for Composition for Ceramic Hydroxylapatite for Surgical Implants," ASTM F 1185, *Annual Book of ASTM Standards*, Vol. 13.01, ASTM International, West Conshohocken, PA, 1993.

[2] "Beta Tricalcium Phosphate for Surgical Implantation," ASTM F 1088, *Annual Book of ASTM Standards*, ASTM International, West Conshohocken, PA, 2000.

[3] "Standard Specification for High Purity Calcium Sulfate Hemihydrate or Dihydrate for Surgical Implants," ASTM Draft 09, submitted to ASTM F04.13.15 Subcommittee, 2002.

[4] "Test Method for In Vitro Degradation Testing of Poly (L-lactic acid) Resin and Fabricated Form for Surgical Implants," ASTM F 1635, *Annual Book of ASTM Standards*, Vol. 13.01, ASTM International, West Conshohocken, PA, 2000.

[5] "Standard Guide for Characterization and Testing of Substrate Materials for Tissue-Engineered Medical Products," ASTM F 2027-00e1, *Annual Book of ASTM Standards*, Vol. 13.01, ASTM International, West Conshohocken, PA, 2002.

[6] "Standard Guide for Characterization and Testing of Biomaterial Scaffolds Used in Tissue-Engineered Medical Products," ASTM F 2150-02$^{\varepsilon}$, *Annual Book of ASTM Standards*, Vol. 13.01, ASTM International, West Conshohocken, PA, 2002.

[7] "Standard Specification for Acrylic Bone Cement," ASTM F 451, *Annual Book of ASTM Standards*, Vol. 13.01, ASTM International, West Conshohocken, PA, 1999.

[8] "Standard Specification for Gypsum Casting Plaster and Gypsum Molding Plaster," ASTM C 59, *Annual Book of ASTM Standards*, Vol. 04.01, ASTM International, West Conshohocken, PA, 2000.

[9] "Physical Testing of Gypsum, Gypsum Plasters and Gypsum Concrete," ASTM C 472, *Annual Book of ASTM Standards*, Vol. 04.01, ASTM International, West Conshohocken, PA, 1999.

[10] "Biological Evaluation of Medical Devices," ISO 10993-1, International Organization for Standardization, Genève, Switzerland.

[11] "Official Monograph for Calcium Sulfate," National Formulary (NF), Vol. 19, 2000, p. 2425.

[12] "Class II Special Controls Guidance Document: Resorbable Calcium Salt Bone Void Filler Device; Draft Guidance for Industry and FDA," U. S. Food and Drug Administration—Center for Devices and Radiological Health, Draft released for comment on February 7, 2002.

[13] "JAX™ Granules Bone Void Filler," 510(k) Summary, K010557, U.S. Food and Drug Administration, May 25, 2001.

[14] "Tablet Friability," United States Pharmacopeia (USP) XXIV, USP<1216>, Rockville, MD, 2000, p. 2148.

[15] An Y. H. and Friedman R. J., "Animal Selections in Orthopedic Research," *Animal Models in Orthopedic Research*, Chapt. 3, Y. H. An and R. J. Friedman, Eds., CRC Press, Boca Raton, FL, 1999, pp. 15–38.

[16] An Y. H. and Draughn R. A., "Mechanical Properties and Testing Methods of Bone," *Animal Models in Orthopedic Research*, Chapter 12, Y. H. An and R. J. Friedman, Eds., CRC Press, Boca Raton, FL, 1999, pp. 219–240.

[17] An Y. H. and Friedman R. J., "Animal Models of Bone Defect Repair," *Animal Models in Orthopedic Research*, Chapt. 13, Y. H. An and R. J. Friedman, Eds., CRC Press, Boca Raton, FL, 1999, pp. 241–260.

[18] Bucholz R. W., "Nonallograft Osteoconductive Bone Graft Substitutes," *Clin Orthop Rel Res*, Vol. 395, 2002, pp. 44–52.

[19] Erbe E., Clineff T., Lavagnino M., Dejardin L., and Arnoczky S., "Comparison of Vitoss and ProOsteon 500R in a Canine Model at One Year," *47th Annual Meeting of the Orthopedic Research Society*, San Francisco, CA, Abstract 975, 2001.

[20] Frankenburgh E. P., Goldstein S. A., Bauer T. W., Harris S. A., and Poser R. D., "Biomechanical and Histological Evaluation of a Calcium Phosphate Cement," *J Bone Joint Surg Am*, Vol. 80, 1998, pp. 1112–1124.

[21] Frondoza C., Aberman H., and Jones L. C., "Bringing a Biomaterial-based Product from the Bench to the Clinic," *Biomaterials Forum*, Vol. 24, 2002, p. 10.

[22] Greenwald A. S., Boden S. C., Goldberg V. M., Khan Y., Laurencin C. T., and Rosier R. N., "Bone-graft Substitutes: Facts, Fictions, and Applications, *J Bone Joint Surg Am,* Vol. 83, Suppl. 2, 2001, pp. 98–103.

[23] Holmes R., Bucholz R., and Mooney V., "Porous Hydroxyapatite as a Bone Graft Substitute in Metaphyseal Defects: a histometric study," *J Bone Joint Surg Am*, Vol. 68, 1986, pp. 904–911.

[24] Knaack D., Goad M. E. P., Aiolova M., Rey C., Tofighi A., Chakravarthy P., and Lee D. D., "Resorbable Calcium Phosphate Bone Substitute," *J Applied Biomater*, Vol. 43, 1998, pp. 399–409.

[25] Leeuwenburgh S., Payrolle, Barrère F., de Bruijn J., van Blitterswijk C. A., and de Groot K., "Osteoclastic Resorption of Biomimetic Calcium Phosphate Coatings *in vitro*," *J Biomed Mater Res*, Vol. 56, 2001, pp. 208–215.

[26] LeGeros R. Z. and Daculsi G., "*In vivo* Transformation of Biphasic Calcium Phosphate Ceramics: ultrastructural and physicochemical characterizations," CRC Handbook of Bioactive Ceramics, Volume II, Calcium Phosphate and Hydroxylapatite Ceramics, T. Yamamuro, L. L. Hench, and J. Wilson, Eds., CRC Press, Boca Raton, FL, 1990, pp. 17–28.

[27] Peltier L. F., "The Use of Plaster of Paris to Fill Large Defects in Bone. A Preliminary Report," *Am J Surg*, Vol. 97, 1959, pp. 11–15.

[28] Rho J.-Y. and Pharr G. M., "Nanoindentation Testing of Bone," *Mechanical Testing of Bone and the Bone-implant Interface*, Chapt. 17, Y. H. An and R. A. Draughn, Eds., CRC Press, Boca Raton, FL, 2000.

[29] Smith R. A., et al., "Evaluations of a Calcium Sulfate Bone Void Filler Used with a CMC-based Hydrogel in an Experimental Rabbit Model," *submitted to ORS 2003.*

[30] St. John K. R., Zardiackas L. D., Terry R. C., Teasdall, R. D. Cooke S. E., and Mitias H. M., "Histological and Electron Microscopic Analysis of Tissue Response to Synthetic Composite Bone Graft in the Canine," *J Appl Biomater*, Vol. 6, 1995, pp. 89–97.

[31] Tay B. K. B., Patel V. V., and Bradford D. S., "Calcium Sulfate and Calcium Phosphate Based Bone Substitute: mimicry of the mineral phase of bone," *Bone Grafting and Bone Graft Substitutes*, S. D. Boden and S. Stevenson, Guest Eds., The Orthopedic Clinics of North America, Philadelphia, PA, Vol. 30, 1999, pp. 615–624.

[32] Turner T., Urban, R. Gitelis, S., Infanger S., Berzins A., Hall D. J., et al., "Efficacy of Calcium Sulfate, a Synthetic Bone Graft Material, in Healing a Large Canine Medullary Defect," *45th Annual Meeting of Orthopedic Research Society*, Anaheim, CA, Abstract 522, 1999.

[33] Winet, H., Emmanual J., and Jones L.C., "Implant Pathology," *Biomaterials Forum*, Vol. 24, 2002, p. 3.

Index